Complications of
Shoulder Surgery

Complications of Shoulder Surgery

Edited by

Louis U. Bigliani, M.D.

Chief, The Shoulder Service
Associate Professor of Orthopaedics
New York Orthopaedic Hospital
Columbia-Presbyterian Medical Center
New York, New York

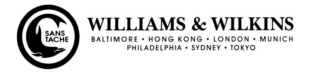

WILLIAMS & WILKINS
BALTIMORE • HONG KONG • LONDON • MUNICH
PHILADELPHIA • SYDNEY • TOKYO

Editor: Timothy H. Grayson
Project Manager: Kathleen Courtney Millet
Copy Editor: Judith F. Minkove
Designer: Wilma E. Rosenberger
Illustration Planner: Ray Lowman
Cover Designer: Dan Pfisterer

Copyright © 1993
Williams & Wilkins
428 East Preston Street
Baltimore, Maryland 21202, USA

Printed in the United States of America

Chapter reprints are available from the Publisher.

Library of Congress Cataloging in Publication Data

Complications of shoulder surgery / edited by Louis U. Bigliani.
    p.   cm.
    Includes bibliographical references and index.
    ISBN 0-683-00751-3
    1. Shoulder—Surgery—Complications.   I. Bigliani, Louis U.
    [DNLM: 1. Postoperative Complications. 2. Shoulder—surgery. WE
810 C737]
RD557.5.C65   1993
617.5′7201—dc20
DNLM/DLC
for Library of Congress   92-49883
                                                  CIP

                93 94 95 96 97
        1 2 3 4 5 6 7 8 9 10

*This book is dedicated
to improving the quality of care
provided to our patients*

Preface

Shoulder surgery has become increasingly popular in the last decade. It has even prompted some to say that the shoulder will be the "joint of the '90s." Anatomically, the shoulder is a complex structure. The intricate soft tissue and bony relationships allow for almost global motion yet maintain stability permitting functional use. The scope of shoulder surgery has recently been enlarged and now encompasses a full spectrum of operative techniques, many of which can be difficult to perform. Unfortunately, complications do occur and require prompt diagnosis and treatment to ensure the well-being of our patients.

The goal of *Complications of Shoulder Surgery* is to share knowledge about specific complications, to foster prevention, and to enhance diagnosis and treatment of these complications. The rewards will be reflected in the improved quality of patient care.

This book would not be possible without the hard work and expertise of the contributing authors. I appreciate the time taken from their busy schedules to help complete this project. Also, I am indebted to my wonderful office staff for their time and devotion to this volume. Finally, I would like to thank the editorial staff of Williams & Wilkins for all of their help and professionalism.

Louis U. Bigliani, M.D.

Contributors

Craig T. Arntz, M.D.
Clinical Assistant Professor
Department of Orthopaedics
University of Washington School of Medicine
Seattle, Washington

Louis U. Bigliani, M.D.
Chief, The Shoulder Service
Associate Professor of Orthopaedics
New York Orthopaedic Hospital
Columbia-Presbyterian Medical Center
New York, New York

James P. Bradley, M.D.
Assistant Clinical Professor
University of Pittsburgh
Department of Orthopaedics
Team Physician, Pittsburgh Steelers
Pittsburgh, Pennsylvania

John J. Brems, M.D.
Cleveland Clinic Foundation
Cleveland, Ohio

James D. Cash, M.D.
Central States Orthopaedic and Sports Medicine
    Center
Tulsa, Oklahoma

Daniel E. Cooper, M.D.
W. B. Carrell Memorial Clinic
Associate Attending
Baylor University Medical Center
Dallas, Texas

Efrain D. Deliz, M.D.
The Shoulder Service
New York Orthopaedic Hospital
Columbia-Presbyterian Medical Center
New York, New York

Xavier A. Duralde, M.D.
Shoulder Fellow
The New York Orthopaedic Hospital
Columbia-Presbyterian Medical Center
New York, New York

Evan L. Flatow, M.D.
The Shoulder Service
The New York Orthopaedic Hospital
Columbia-Presbyterian Medical Center
New York, New York

Carl P. Giordano, M.D.
Senior Resident
Hospital for Joint Diseases, Orthopaedic Institute
New York, New York

Thomas P. Goss, M.D.
Professor of Orthopaedic Surgery
Department of Orthopaedic Surgery
University of Massachusetts Medical Center
Worcester, Massachusetts

Douglas T. Harryman, II, M.D.
Department of Orthopaedics
University of Washington School of Medicine
Seattle, Washington

Richard J. Hawkins, M.D., F.R.C.S.(C)
Steadman Hawkins Clinic
Vail, Colorado

Christopher M. Jobe, M.D.
Assistant Professor, Orthopaedic Surgery
Department of Orthopaedic Surgery
Loma Linda University, School of Medicine
Loma Linda, California

Frederick A. Matsen, III, M.D.
Professor and Chairman
Department of Orthopaedics
University of Washington School of Medicine
Seattle, Washington

Peter D. McCann, M.D.
Attending Surgeon
Insall Scott Kelly Institute for Orthopaedics and
    Sports Medicine
New York, New York

Stephen J. McIlveen, M.D.
Assistant Professor in Orthopaedic Surgery
New York Orthopaedic Hospital
Columbia-Presbyterian Medical Center
New York, New York

Seth R. Miller, M.D.
Greenwich Orthopaedic Associates
Greenwich, Connecticut
Instructor in Orthopaedic Surgery
College of Physicians and Surgeons of Columbia
    University
New York, New York

David S. Morrison, M.D.
Director of Shoulder and Elbow Surgery
Southern California Center for Sports Medicine
Long Beach, California

Robert J. Neviaser, M.D.
Professor and Chairman
Department of Orthopaedic Surgery
The George Washington University
School of Medicine and Health Sciences
Director, Hand and Upper Extremity Surgery
    Service
The George Washington University Medical Center
Washington, DC

Tom R. Norris, M.D.
California-Pacific Medical Center
San Francisco, California

Melvin Post, M.D.
Chicago, Illinois

Charles A. Rockwood, Jr., M.D.
Professor and Chairman Emeritus
Department of Orthopaedics
The University of Texas Health Science Center
San Antonio, Texas

Howard Rosen, M.D.
Chief, Problem Trauma Service
Hospital for Joint Diseases, Orthopaedic Institute
Clinical Professor of Orthopaedic Surgery
Mt. Sinai School of Medicine
New York, New York

Gregory W. Soghikian, M.D.
Tahoe Fracture and Orthopaedic Clinic
South Lake Tahoe, California

James S. Thompson, M.D.
Carolina Hand Surgery Associates
Asheville, North Carolina

James E. Tibone, M.D.
Clinical Associate Professor
University of Southern California
Los Angeles, California
Kerlan-Jobe Orthopaedic Clinic
Inglewood, California

Jon J.P. Warner, M.D.
Assistant Professor
Department of Orthopaedics
University of Pittsburgh
The Sports Medicine Institute
Pittsburgh, Pennsylvania

Russell F. Warren, M.D.
Professor of Orthopaedic Surgery
Cornell Medical College
Director, Sports Medicine/Shoulder Service
The Hospital for Special Surgery
New York, New York

Keith C. Watson, M.D.
Assistant Director
Orthopaedic Residency Program
John Peter Smith Hospital
Fort Worth, Texas

Michael A. Wirth, M.D.
Assistant Professor
Department of Orthopaedics
The University of Texas Health Science Center
San Antonio, Texas

Joseph D. Zuckerman, M.D.
Chief, Shoulder Service
Hospital for Joint Diseases, Orthopaedic Institute
New York, New York

Contents

1
Anatomy of the Shoulder

Christopher M. Jobe

INTRODUCTION

Avoidance of complications is the first principle of surgery: *"Primumnon nocere."* A thorough knowledge of anatomy, especially of those areas where problems are most likely to arise, is essential to help reduce the incidence of complications. Ultimately, the surgeon will learn to recognize the main structures at risk.

The shoulder is the region where the arm moves relative to the axial skeleton. It is a multiarticulated system which, taken as a whole, produces the largest range of motion of any joint in the body. The range of motion of the arm via this multiarticulated system has implications for the joints, muscles, and neurovascular connections. Complications of shoulder surgery must be considered not only for their effect upon individual structures, but upon the complex as a whole.

Three diathrodial joints make up the shoulder: the glenohumeral, the sternoclavicular, and the acromioclavicular joints. The scapulothoracic joint is made up of the fascial planes where motion of the scapula occurs relative to the thoracic wall.

The purpose of this chapter is to review the anatomy of the shoulder, with emphasis on the dangerous relationships of each structure rather than on anatomic variants. The chapter begins with bones and joints and proceeds outward through the muscles that control these articulations, the nerves that control the muscles, the arteries that supply the muscles, and the skin.

BONES AND JOINTS

Sternoclavicular Joint

The articulation of the sternum with the proximal end of the clavicle is the only diathrodial be-tween the upper limb and the axial skeleton. The articular surfaces of this joint are relatively flat, and the joint itself is usually (97% of specimens) divided by a complete disc (Fig. 1.1) (9). The orientation of the joint in the transverse plane is from anterolateral to posteromedial, and in the coronal plane from superomedial to inferolateral.

Several ligaments are associated with this joint. The most important ligaments in terms of stability are the paired sternoclavicular ligaments (2), which are located anterior and posterior, particularly the posterior sternoclavicular ligament (8). In addition, these are supplemented by the interclavicular ligament, which is superior, and by the anterior and posterior costoclavicular ligaments. The anterior of these costoclavicular ligaments resists lateral displacement of the clavicle on the thoracic cage, and the posterior ligament prevents medial displacement of the clavicle. The posterior of these ligaments also resists rotation of the clavicle in a forward direction (6).

This joint serves as the primary static stabilizer that maintains the elevation of the shoulder at rest (2). Motion in the joint occurs on both sides of the disc, with elevation and depression occurring in the joint between the clavicle and disc, and the anteroposterior motion and rotary motions occurring between the disc and the sternum. The motion at this joint contributes to the motion of the scapulothoracic joint with two actions. The first of these is upward elevation. This is a motion in the coronal plane of the joint that is limited to about 35° and tends to occur between 30–90° of arm elevation. The second of these motions is upward rotation, which occurs in the sagittal plane and occurs mainly after 70–80° of arm elevation. Fusion of the sternoclavicular joint may limit arm abduction to about 100°. In addition, the strength of the top of this range is diminished (3).

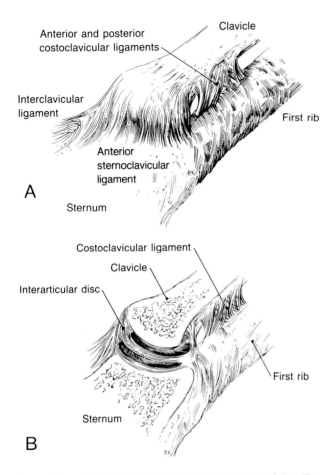

Figure 1.1. **A**, The ligaments of the sternoclavicular articulation. The sternoclavicular ligaments are the most important for suspending the lateral end of the clavicle. The posterior and anterior costoclavicular ligaments constrain medial and lateral displacement of the clavicle on the thorax, respectively. **B**, A cross-section of the sternoclavicular joint showing the complete disc dividing the joint into two sections.

The most perilous anatomic relationship with respect to complications is the presence of the large vessels and trachea immediately posterior to the joint, protected only by the very thin sternohyoid and sternothyroid muscles (Fig. 1.2) (21). It is in relationship to these structures that most of the complications with sternoclavicular surgery have occurred.

Clavicle

The clavicle is an S-shaped bone whose convexity is anterior medially and posterior laterally, the lateral curve being somewhat larger than the medial (Fig. 1.3). The bone functions as a strut for support of the shoulder. It maintains the length tension curves of the muscles, going from the chest wall to the scapula and humerus, and also functions as the site of support for the scapula. Although earlier authors have suggested that patients have few functional problems after claviculectomy (1) and only with overhead activity, other opinions indicate that the loss of the clavicle may have more profound effects, depending upon how much soft tissue suspension remains or is absent.

The clavicle is divided for clinical purposes into thirds. The middle third contains the hard cortical bone and the least soft tissue reinforcement. It is in this section that the rare nonunions of the clavicle occur (20). The ends of the bone are related to the adjacent joints. The endangered adjacent soft tissues are those that cross the first rib: the subclavian vein, the subclavian artery and the inferior trunk of the brachial plexus (17, 20).

Acromioclavicular Joint

The acromioclavicular joint is an articulation of limited range of motion, but of a complex ligament arrangement (Fig. 1.4) (8). It is the sole articulation between the scapula and the clavicle, although occasionally there is a second articulation between the coracoid and the clavicle in the area where we usually find the coracoclavicular ligaments. The joint itself has a meniscus that is perforated in the majority of cases. The joint is stabilized by a surrounding cuff of ligaments, the acromioclavicular ligaments, which are thicker on the superior surface (8). The joint is, in addition, reinforced by two coracoclavicular ligaments, the conoid and the trapezoid (15, 16, 43). The conoid ligament is more vertical and posterior than the trapezoid. These two ligaments are longer and thicker than the acromioclavicular ligaments and play an important role in trauma and surgery of the acromioclavicular joint.

Cadaver acromioclavicular joints have more than 20° of rotation, about the longitudinal axis of the clavicle, although there is little evidence yet to suggest that patients utilize all of this motion in vivo. In the coronal plane there is about 3° of motion, and in the transaxial plane there is about 3° of motion.

In everyday situations, the acromioclavicular ligaments, because they are shorter, make use of the integrity of the acromioclavicular joint to control most of the motion at the joint (10). For larger displacements, other ligaments may play a large role. The inferior displacement of the scapula relative to the clavicle is resisted mainly by the conoid ligament, with some help from the trapezoid and acromioclavicular ligaments (10). Anterior translation of the acromion on the end of the clavicle is prevented mainly by the A–C ligaments (43), whereas posterior translation of the acromion on the clavicle is controlled mainly by the conoid ligament (10). Large axial compressions of the joint are controlled mainly by the trapezoid ligament. Because motion is greatly limited in this joint, complications resulting in stiffness usually have little consequence; however, large acromioclavicular dissociations can be disabling because of the loss of scapular suspension. Important structures in the vicinity to remember are: (a) the acromial branch of the thoracoacromial artery along the anterior portion of the acromioclavicular joint, and (b) the supraspinatus outlet with the subacromial bursa immediately inferior to this joint.

A great deal of stability is afforded to the acromioclavicular joint from muscle fascia of the deltoid and trapezius muscles. If all of these stabilizers along with the coracoclavicular and acromioclavicular ligaments are torn, the scapulothoracic rhythm can be disrupted, and the shoulder can become dependent and painful.

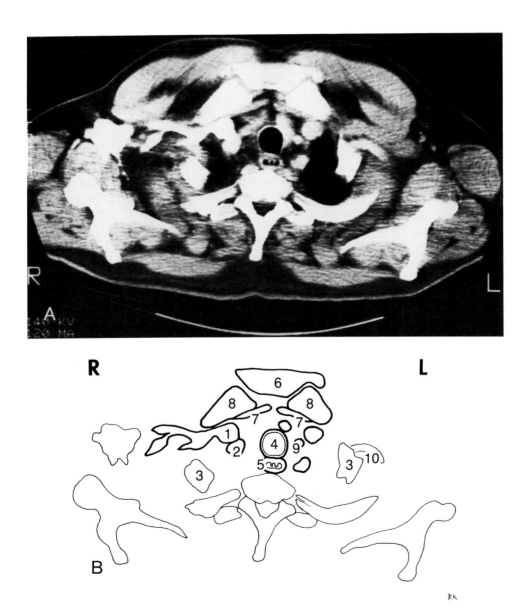

Figure 1.2. **A**, A CT angiogram at the level of the sternoclavicular joints showing the close proximity of the great vessels and trachea to the posterior surface of the sternoclavicular joint. **B**, A labeled diagram of the CT scan: (1) the junction of subclavian and jugular veins; (2) innominate artery; (3) first rib; (4) trachea; (5) esophagus; (6) sternum; (7) sternohyoid muscle origin; (8) clavicle; (9) carotid artery; and (10) axillary artery.

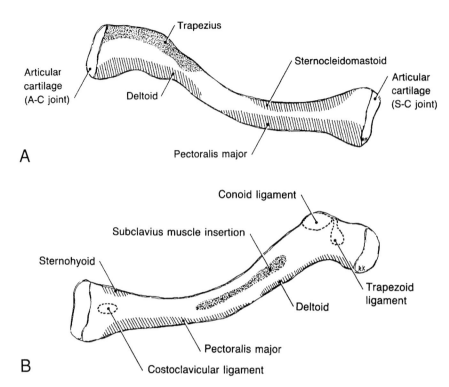

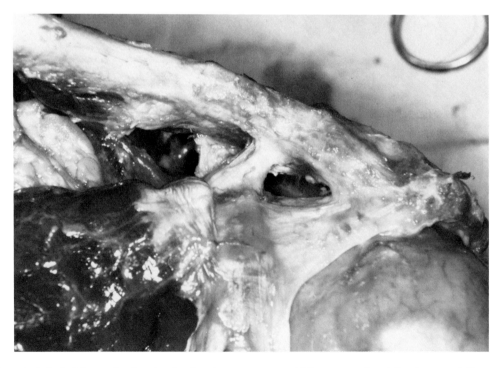

Figure 1.3. **A**, A superior view of the clavicle and its attachments showing the S-shape, the medial end to the right, and the lateral end to the left. **B**, An inferior view of the clavicle showing ligament insertions and muscle origins. The medial end of the clavicle is to the left, the lateral end is to the right, and the anterior surface is inferior in this drawing.

Figure 1.4. Acromioclavicular joint anterior view showing the orientation of the two coracoclavicular ligaments in the center and the cora-coacromial ligament running obliquely upward. The acromioclavicular ligaments blend in with the acromion and clavicle.

Scapula

The scapula is mainly a thin plate of a metaphyseal (5) type of bone that serves as a source for muscle attachment (Fig. 1.5). It has several important bony processes including the glenoid, coracoid, acromion, and spine of the scapula. The glenoid will be discussed with the glenohumeral joint. The remaining three processes serve as sources of muscle attachment and provide the lever arm for the action of these muscles.

Scapular bone is metaphyseal in quality, which means there are abundant and large connections be-

tween the intraosseous blood supply and the blood supply of the surrounding soft tissues, mainly the muscles. Because of this, there can be more interoperative bleeding than with usual subperiosteal dissection. In addition to the vessels, the suprascapular nerve travels adjacent to bone on the deep surfaces of the supraspinatus and infraspinatus muscles, close to the coracoid at its base and close to the glenoid at the spinoglenoid notch. In the latter location, the nerve may be as close as 11 mm to the rim of the glenoid (4). Also, this nerve is accompanied by the suprascapular artery, and there are abundant branches from the circumflex scapular artery that run adja-

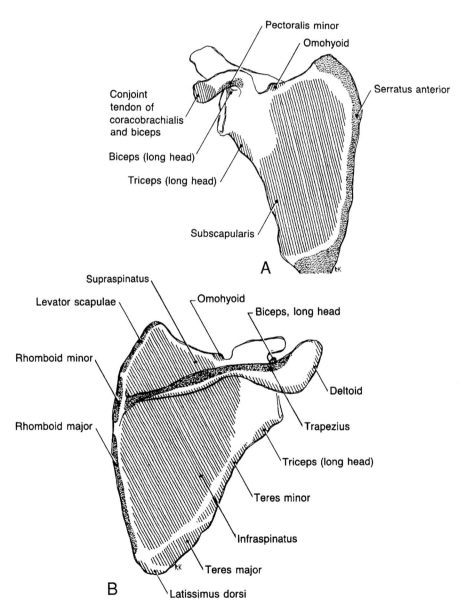

Figure 1.5. **A**, An anterior drawing of the scapula showing the muscle and tendon origins and insertions. **B**, A posterior view of the scapula, showing the muscle origins and insertions and important bony processes.

cent to bone. This bone has a nutrient artery entering in either the supraspinatus or infraspinatus fossa (58).

The acromion serves as an attachment for the deltoid and trapezius and produces the lever arm of the deltoid muscle (16). Anteriorly, the acromion is the point of attachment of the coracoacromial ligament. This is a very interesting ligament in that it connects two parts of the same bone. There are tremendous forces on the acromion process, so that sacrifice of this lever arm or of the mechanical integrity of the acromion may have disastrous effects on the mechanics of the shoulder. In addition, the acromion forms the roof of the subacromial space, or supraspinatus outlet, so that its arrangement in the sagittal plane becomes as important as its anterior and lateral reach in the transaxial plane (3, 27, 28).

Anterior-superiorly on the scapula is the coracoid process, to which are attached the short head of the biceps, the coracobrachialis, and pectoralis minor muscles. It forms the roof of the axillary space, and represents a boundary to safe dissection. A higher order of caution is required in dissection inferior or medial to the coracoid. In addition, the coracoid is the point of attachment of the coracoclavicular and coracoacromial ligaments, mentioned earlier and the coracohumeral ligament, discussed with the glenohumeral joint.

The spine of the scapula has a function similar to that of the acromion, as a point of attachment of muscle—in this case the middle portion of the trapezius and the posterior portion of the deltoid—and it suspends the acromion. The spine of the scapula is sacrificed in some head and neck reconstructions, and this is done safely as long as one maintains the acromion suspending function. Sacrifice of the attachment of the acromion has disastrous consequences for the function of the shoulder.

Glenohumeral Joint

This is probably the most interesting joint of the body and certainly one of the most studied. The socket of this joint is the glenoid process of the scapula. It has an inverted "comma"-shaped surface that averages about 35 mm in its vertical length, and about 25 mm in its greatest horizontal dimension. It has two small bony processes superior and inferior for the attachment of the long heads of the biceps and triceps, respectively. The glenoid articular surface is a little deepened and widened by the presence of a fibrous structure called the labrum (9, 29, 47).

The labrum is a dense band of collagen whose fascicles run circumferentially about the glenoid. The insertions of the long heads of the biceps and triceps are also closely related to the labrum superiorly and inferiorly, respectively. The biceps is attached in an intra-articular fashion, and the triceps is attached in an extra-articular less obvious fashion.

The labrum derives its blood supply in common with adjacent ligament or periosteum most often from vessels arising from the subscapular artery. The labrum does not receive vessels from bone.

The ball of the ball and socket joint is the humeral head, which is mainly spherical. The articular surface is angulated approximately 135° from the long axis of the humerus. Its average vertical dimension averages 48 mm, and its transverse arc averages 45 mm. There is a radius of curvature of 25 mm in the vertical arc and 22 mm in the transverse arc. The articular surface of the head covers an arc of about 120–140° with that radius of curvature (38, 39). Of this 120° arc in the vertical dimension, approximately 75–80° are covered by the glenoid, and about 60° are covered in the transverse dimension (38, 39).

The passive stabilizers of the joint include the coracohumeral ligament, the subscapularis muscle, the superior, middle, and inferior glenohumeral ligaments, and the posterior superior and superior capsules (Fig. 1.6). The coracohumeral ligament provides a guide to glenohumeral motion, by producing obligate abduction in forward flexion (13). When taut, it limits external rotation. In addition to closing the rotator interval and restraining the long head of the biceps in the bicipital groove, this ligament produces an anterior translation of the humeral head when the arm is placed into forward flexion (11).

The superior glenohumeral ligament originates off the superior labrum near the attachment of the long head of the biceps (4, 7, 9). In the position of rest, this ligament is taut across the anterior-superior portion of the joint, producing joint compression. It resists inferior displacement of the humerus on the glenoid when the arm is at the side. In abduction the superior glenohumeral ligament is lax.

Below this ligament anteriorly, there is very frequently a gap in the capsule through which the arthroscopist can visualize the tendon of the subscapularis (9). The upper portion of this muscle is so collagen-dense that it functions as a passive stabilizer.

This anterior defect in the capsule above the middle ligament usually connects with a bursa between the subscapularis tendon and the neck of the

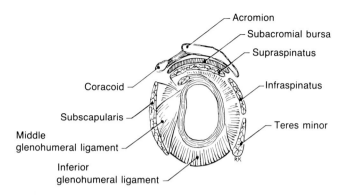

Figure 1.6. Glenohumeral joint: The anterior portion of the joint is to the left. The most important passive stabilizer of the joint is the inferior glenohumeral ligament.

glenoid, referred to as the subscapularis bursa or recess (7, 9). There is occasionally a smaller recess below the middle ligament (7, 9).

Crossing over the front of the subscapularis tendon in an oblique fashion is the middle glenohumeral ligament (7, 9). This ligament is prominent and visible in most specimens, and is made up largely of longitudinal collagen. This contributes to anterior stability when the arm is in about 45° of abduction (30, 42).

The most important part of the capsule, the inferior glenohumeral ligament, amounts to almost all of the lower half of the capsule (7). It originates from the lower half of bony glenoid, passing through the peripheral labrum, and attaches over the inferior portion of the neck of the humerus. The inferior glenohumeral ligament is, in structure, a thicker version of its surrounding capsule, being made up of three layers (30). The inner and thickest layer resembles a normal ligament in that it is made up of longitudinally oriented collagen fascicles running from glenoid to humerus (Fig. 1.7). There is an intermediate layer that is made up of collagen fibers running in a circumferential fashion around the capsule, i.e., perpendicular to the longitudinal fibers of the inner layer. This layer is thinner than the inner layer. The outer layer of this ligament is also quite thin and is largely longitudinal. As might be predicted from its internal fascicle arrangement, these glenohumeral ligaments are less stiff than other ligaments. All of these passive stabilizers are innervated by the passing nerves but most importantly by the suprascapular nerve (12).

The instability of this joint to traumatic forces is predictable from the lack of bony containment and the thinness and normal laxity of the ligaments. Normal stability is less understood and the

subject of much current research. Stability of a joint occurs when the joint resultant vector, i.e., the vector sum of all forces acting across this joint, muscle action, gravity, etc., crosses the joint from bone to bone.

In the ball and socket joints, a considerable portion of the stability of the joint is generated by atmospheric pressure pressing in on the joint (22). When the vacuum within the joint is vented, an inferior subluxation appears in the joint without there having been any damage to the ligaments. Additional tension in the ligaments in vivo is provided by rotator cuff muscles inserting into the capsule. This natural laxity complicates ligamentous reconstruction at the shoulder by making it difficult to judge soft tissue tension. One of the consequences of overly vigorous shortening of the ligaments is loss of range of motion that occurs at the rate of about 25° for every 1 cm deficit in length.

The great range of motion of the joint calls upon the ligaments to act in a variety of directions. Because the capsular ligaments can be tensioned in a number of directions, they can act in concert to prevent a variety of instabilities. Thus, for the two main directions of instability, anterior and posterior, three-quarters of the capsule may function to restrain the head from dislocation (29, 30, 53–55). These two areas of capsule (29–53, 42) overlap, causing many patients with instability in the anterior direction to have some element of posterior instability and vice versa.

Another unique function of glenohumeral capsular ligaments is the containment of a volume of humeral head in positions where the head overhangs the glenoid. A postoperative decrease in this "capacitance" of ligament will displace the humeral head away from the ligament, causing a malalignment of the joint (37). This will lead to eventual joint degen-

Figure 1.7. **A**, The innermost and thickest of the glenohumeral ligament is made up of collagen fascicles running longitudinally from glenoid to humeral head (top to bottom in this picture). **B**, Portions of the thinner intermediate layer the fascicles of which run roughly perpendicular to the longitudinal fascicles of the main layer. (These photos are of different layers of the same specimen in the same orientation and degree of magnification).

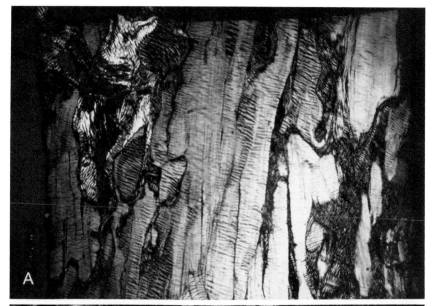

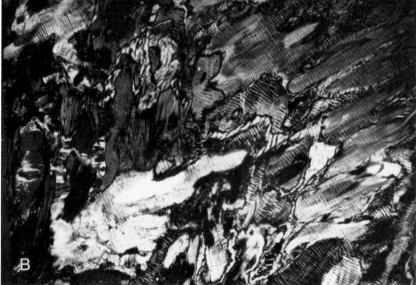

eration as well as immediate loss of range of motion (Fig. 1.8).

This complex arrangement explains how glenohumeral function may be sacrificed by overvigorous shortening of capsular structures on one side of the joint. This can also be caused by overly vigorous "filling" of the glenohumeral space with prosthesis in an attempt to maintain tension of the musculotendinous sleeve, which is also an important consideration (36).

Humerus

The humerus, outside of the glenohumeral articulation, has several important relationships. The attachment of the capsular ligaments is around the anatomic neck, which is less prominent than the articular head (Fig. 1.9). Likewise, the tuberosities are located here, and function for the attachment of muscles.

The prominence of the humeral head relative to the tuberosities is felt to be important to the stabilizing functions of these tendons and muscles, particularly the head-depressing effect of some of the superior musculature (25, 56). These attachments provide an additional stabilizing effect when the prominence of the humeral head is circumscribed by the muscle (25, 56).

The tuberosities are separated by a bicipital

groove, which is located anteriorly about 15° anterior from the main axis of the head (Fig. 1.9). In the transverse plane, the axis of the humeral head is angled in retroversion some 30–45° to meet the anterior angulation of the scapula on the chest wall. The

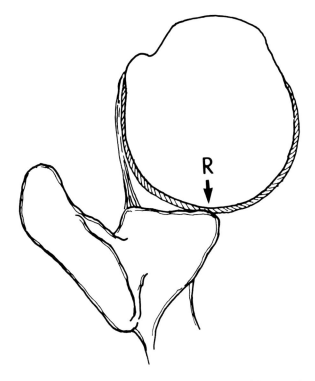

Figure 1.8. Overly aggressive corrective procedures of the capsule limit the range of motion by shortening the length of the ligament. But by decreasing the "capacitance" or the ability of the ligament to accept humeral head overhang, a displacement of the humeral head in the opposite direction may be produced. This leads to a displacement of the joint resultant vector "R" to an undesirable location and secondary arthritis. In this case, the illustration shows a posterior displacement of the humeral head created by overly aggressive reduction in the anterior-inferior capsule.

lesser tuberosity is anterior to the bicipital groove and serves as the attachment of the subscapularis tendon. Posterior to the bicipital groove lies the greater tuberosity, which serves as the attachment of the supraspinatus tendon superiorly, the infraspinatus tendon posterior-superior, and the teres minor posteriorly. The roof of the bicipital groove is made up of a transverse humeral ligament (14, 26), but most importantly by the attachments of the coracohumeral ligament (34, 35, 41).

The blood supply of the humeral head stems from a branch of the anterior humeral circumflex artery ascending in the bicipital groove (23). There are often small vessels entering the head posteromedially, but these are much less important. This anterior artery is a distal extension of the anterior humeral circumflex artery. It can receive several extraosseous collaterals from other arteries about the shoulder. As fractures in this area often involve the bicipital groove, maintenance of this artery in its extraosseous extent is essential.

MUSCLES

Muscles are especially important in this context in that they have several potential sources of complications. Muscles have a higher metabolic rate than the other tissues, making them very susceptible to compromise in circulation. They require intact innervation and depend upon their attachments to bone for proper function. Finally, they undergo atrophy with long-term disuse, from which they may not recover. This has implications for late repairs.

In the shoulder, many of the muscles have broad fleshy attachments to bone. This form of attachment, the indirect insertion, may complicate the reattachment of muscles, detached by injury or sur-

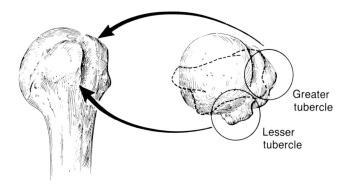

Greater
tubercle

Lesser
tubercle

Figure 1.9. The humeral head from above with the greater and lesser tubercles. Note that the bicipital groove is just lateral to the midline. The dotted line shows an outline of the distal humerus. Note that the humeral head is about 30–45° retroverted with respect to the alignment of the distal humerus.

gery. Surgical reattachment requires careful preservation of sufficient collagen on the muscle for reattachment to bone. We will discuss some of the more important muscles involved with shoulder function.

Trapezius

The trapezius is the largest of the scapulothoracic muscles (Fig. 1.10), taking its origin along the posterior midline from the occiput, the nuchal ligament and the spinous processes of the vertebrae C7–T12. The upper cervical fibers of the muscle insert into the distal clavicle. The lower cervical and upper thoracic fibers attach onto the acromion and spine of the scapula, and the lower fibers into the base of the spine of the scapula. The muscle functions in elevation of the scapula and in retraction of the scapula. Loss of elevating function may result, in time, in the stretching out of sternoclavicular ligaments and a drooping of the shoulder (46, 47). The trapezius's blood supply is via its deep surface and

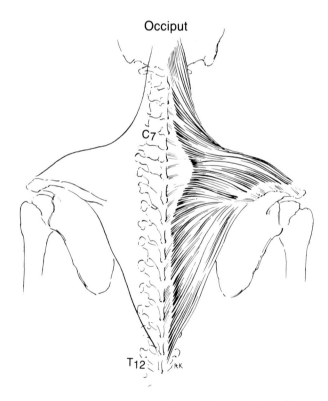

Occiput

C7

T12

Figure 1.10. The trapezius is the largest of the scapulothoracic muscles. It is largely responsible for elevation of the scapula. Its most precarious relationship is its nerve supply, cranial nerve XI, which is in the posterior triangle of the neck. Within the muscle, the nerve runs perpendicular to the muscle fibers and would be endangered by large muscle-splitting incisions in the main bulk of the muscle.

arises from either the transverse cervical artery or the dorsal scapular artery. This supply is infrequently at risk because of the paucity of surgical indications for dissection on the deep surface of the trapezius. The riskier situation exists with respect to its nerve, the 11th cranial nerve, which lies very superficial in the posterior triangle of the neck (57). Here, it runs from sternocleidomastoid to trapezius, and lies immediately deep to the continuation of the muscle fascia of these two muscles (44).

Serratus Anterior

Serratus anterior (Fig. 1.11) another scapulothoracic muscle has three main portions: the first portion is a single slip of muscle originating off of the first rib and intercostal space that inserts into the superior angle of the scapula; the middle portion comes off ribs 2–4 and their interspaces and attaches along the vertebral border of the scapula; the third and major portion of the muscle bulk comes off of ribs 5–9 and inserts on the inferior angle of the scapula. The blood supply of serratus is from three arteries: the lateral thoracic, the thoracodorsal and the supreme thoracic. The size of the contributions from these three arteries varies. Its most precarious relationship is its own nerve supply, the long thoracic nerve, particularly where the nerve runs over the second rib. This nerve can be endangered by surgical dissection on the surface of the muscle as in first rib resection, and may be injured by positioning or traction on the arm during other types of surgery (48, 51–52).

Deltoid

The largest and most constantly functioning glenohumeral muscle is the deltoid (Fig. 1.12) (46, 56). The deltoid muscle seems to function in thirds, the most active portion being the middle-third, which takes origin off the acromion and inserts in the common insertion at the deltoid tubercle on the humerus (45). This portion of the deltoid is active in any elevation of the arm. The anterior third of the deltoid takes its origin off of the lateral third of the clavicle and functions when elevation is in a more anterior direction. The posterior third of the deltoid takes origin off the spine of the scapula and is active when elevation is more in a posterior direction. Innervation is by the axillary nerve, after it exits from the quadrilateral space and has supplied teres minor. Blood supply to the deltoid is mainly from the posterior humeral circumflex artery, but it receives a

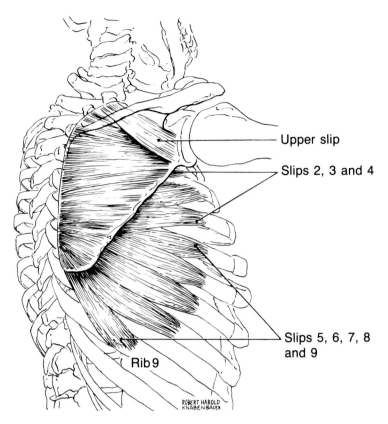

Figure 1.11. The three sections of the serratus anterior muscles: the upper slip inserting into the superior angle of the scapula; the next three slips inserting into the vertebral border, and the last five slips inserting into the inferior angle of the scapula. The most precarious structure is the nerve supply on the muscle's lateral surface, the long thoracic nerve.

number of other collaterals, the most important of which is the deltoid branch of the thoracoacromial axis anteriorly (16). Its venous drainage is also multiple, with the cephalic vein anteriorly being an important auxiliary venous drainage of the anterior third.

The precarious relationships of this muscle include its nerve and its indirect attachment to the clavicle and scapula. The axillary nerve runs transversely to the fibers of the deltoid, in the anterior two-thirds of the muscle. The axillary nerve lies about 2 inches (or 5 cm) below the edge of the acromion and is endangered by muscle-splitting incisions in the anterior two-thirds of the muscle. By shortening the muscle, abduction can decrease the acromion to nerve distance to about 4 cm or less. The posterior branch of the axillary nerve tends to run along the inferior border of the posterior third of the deltoid, and is therefore less endangered by muscle-splitting incisions.

The deltoid's proximal attachment to bone is very broad and fleshy, and the collagen does not insert directly into bone but continues over the surface

of the bone into the insertion of the trapezius muscle. In order to reattach this muscle to bone, care must be taken to preserve a sleeve of this "periosteal" collagen on the muscle so that there will be sufficient collagen to hold sutures. Another potential source of complications has to do with the middle third, which has a multipinnate construction and has heavy intramuscular bands of collagen. This creates a multiple-compartment effect with respect to compartment syndromes, and compartmental releases in the middle third of the deltoid must include multiple fascial incisions.

Supraspinatus

The next most active glenohumeral muscle is the supraspinatus, which takes a fleshy origin off of the supraspinatus fossa. It inserts into the anterior-superior portion of the greater tuberosity. It is also in this area where the high attrition with age occurs (50). Its nerve and artery, the suprascapular nerve and artery, travel on its deep surface adjacent to the scapula. This is the most precarious relationship of

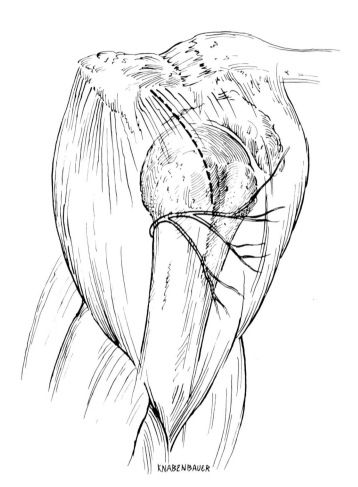

KNABENBAUER

Figure 1.12. An anterolateral view of the deltoid muscle showing its perilous relationship with its major nerve and artery, the axillary nerve and posterior humeral circumflex artery. On the deep surface of the anterior two-thirds of the muscle, they lie approximately 5 cm inferior to the rim of the acromion and clavicle. In this position they are endangered by muscle-splitting incisions. The nerve to the posterior third, the posterior branch of the axillary nerve, goes immediately to the posterior lateral border of the deltoid and is therefore less endangered by muscle-splitting incisions.

the muscle (4, 15). These two structures, the suprascapular nerve and artery, enter at the suprascapular notch with the artery going above the transverse scapular ligament and the nerve going underneath (15). Submuscular dissection may endanger the nerve and vessel, and medial dissection should be limited to about 1 cm from the rim of the glenoid. These two are also tethered at the suprascapular notch so that only about 3 cm of suprascapular muscle slide can be accomplished without compromise.

The supraspinatus along with infraspinatus, teres minor, and subscapularis form an almost continuous cuff of tendon and muscle about the humeral head called the rotator cuff. While it is important to rotation, this cuff might be termed the compressor cuff because its essential function is stabilizing the joint by compression (49). It also has some abducting capacity (58, 59).

Infraspinatus

Infraspinatus provides 60% of the external rotation power of the shoulder (Fig. 1.13). Its origin, off the infraspinatus fossa in a fleshy indirect fashion, is similar to that of supraspinatus and deltoid. It inserts into the greater tuberosity immediately behind and in continuity with the insertion of supraspinatus. Its blood and nerve supply enter on the deep surface via the suprascapular nerve and artery (16) and with a large blood supply from the circumflex scapular artery. Its precarious relationship is with its nerve supply. If the muscle is split along its median raphe, the suprascapular nerve lies little more than 1½ cm medial to the glenoid rim, where it would be endangered (29, 63).

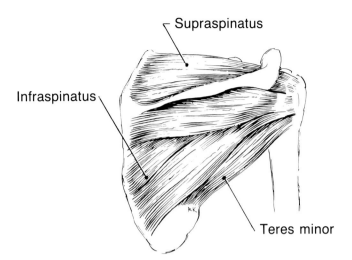

Figure 1.13. Infraspinatus and teres minor. Note the median raphe of the infraspinatus, which may be confused with the internervous plane between teres minor and infraspinatus located more inferior. The most endangered neighbor of the infraspinatus is its own nerve, the suprascapular, which may be as close as 1.5 cm medial to the glenoid on the deep surface of the muscle.

Teres Minor

The next muscle inferiorly is the teres minor (Fig. 1.13), which originates from the middle of the lateral border of the scapula and inserts in the lower part of the greater tuberosity. Teres minor is innervated by the posterior branch of the axillary nerve. It has a multiple blood supply from adjacent blood vessels, including the circumflex scapular and posterior humeral circumflex vessels. Its most dangerous relationship is with the quadrilateral space, of which it is the superior border (62). Here the axillary nerve and posterior humeral circumflex artery will lie within a few mm of the inferior border of this muscle.

Subscapularis

Lying directly anterior to the glenohumeral joint and scapula, the subscapularis (Fig. 1.14) is a large multipinnate muscle, taking its origin off the entire anterior surface of the scapula. It inserts into the lesser tuberosity, and for the upper 70% of its insertion, this is a direct insertion. The lower portion of the muscle is fleshy and has an indirect insertion. As a result, there is little tendinous material in the lowest portion of the muscle for reattachment. The upper portion is so rich in collagen that it functions as a passive stabilizer in cadaveric studies of shoulder stability (42, 60).

There are two nerves to subscapularis, the upper and lower subscapular nerves. Although there is no regular internervous plane by which subscapularis muscle may be split, subscapular denervation does not seem to be a problem. The blood vessels of the subscapularis are somewhat less obvious. There are sometimes vessels accompanying the superior subscapular nerve, but the main vessels come off of the circumflex scapular artery and course on the deep surface of the muscle.

The important relationships for the subscapularis muscle and tendon are the axillary nerve and the coracohumeral ligament and the axillary space. The axillary nerve on its way to the quadrilateral space lies on the anterior surface of the subscapularis muscle. Subscapularis-splitting incisions must be done under direct vision to avoid the axillary nerve. The axillary nerve is tightly wrapped around the inferior border of the muscle, and is actually quite closely applied to the inferior capsule of the shoulder, lateral to the origin of the long head of the triceps. In dissection on the front surface of the inferior portion of the subscapularis, this nerve should be kept in mind.

Multiple Joint Muscles

PECTORALIS MAJOR

One of the more powerful muscles of the shoulder is the pectoralis major (Fig. 1.15). This muscle consists of three portions: the clavicular, the upper sternocostal, and the lower sternocostal portions (54). The clavicular head takes its origin from the clavicle and inserts with its fibers in a parallel fashion along the lateral lip of the bicipital groove. The second portion takes origin from the manubrium, and the upper two-thirds of the body of the

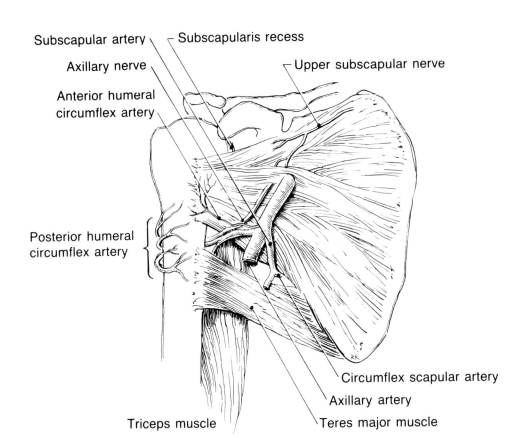

Subscapular artery Subscapularis recess

Axillary nerve

Anterior humeral
circumflex artery

Upper subscapular nerve

Posterior humeral
circumflex artery

Circumflex scapular artery

Axillary artery

Triceps muscle Teres major muscle

Figure 1.14. The subscapularis and the immediately inferior teres major and latissimus dorsi muscles form the posterior wall of the axillary space. As such, they are closely related to the brachial plexus and axillary artery. However, the most frequently visualized structures in shoulder surgery are the two humeral circumflex vessels and the axillary nerve. The arterial supply to this muscle is on its deep surface and is rarely, if ever, encountered in surgery. The upper border of this muscle is marked by the subscapularis recess. This upper border can frequently be visualized intra-articularly, as in arthroscopy.

sternum and ribs 2–4. It inserts into the lateral lip of the bicipital groove, immediately behind the clavicular portion. Its fibers are also parallel in their course. The third portion takes origin from the distal portion of the body of the sternum and ribs 5 and 6, and from the external oblique fascia. In its course, the inferior fibers undergo a 180° rotation and insert behind the other two groups, sometimes somewhat more proximal.

The clavicular head of the pectoralis major is innervated by the lateral pectoral nerve, which carries fibers from spinal nerves C5, C6, and C7. The lower two-thirds of the muscle receives some lateral and some medial pectoral nerve fibers (the medial pectoral nerve carries fibers of spinal nerves C8 and T1). The arterial supply is extensive, with the deltoid artery and pectoral artery supplying most of the muscle. In addition, there are branches coming from the internal mammary artery medially, and at the fourth or fifth intercostal space is a large artery coming off of the intercostal artery (16). This muscle forms the anterior wall of the axillary fossa.

BICEPS BRACHII

Although the biceps muscle has most of its action at the elbow (Fig. 1.16), its two origins at the shoulder are important structures. One of these is off the bicipital tubercle at the top of the glenoid, and the other is off of the coracoid. At the elbow, it inserts into the lacertus fibrosis medially and the biceps tubercle on the radius laterally. It provides about 20% of the supination strength at the elbow but only 8% of the flexion strength (53). Its nerve supply comes from the musculocutaneous nerve. Its arterial supply is quite variable, but comes from a branch or branches off of the brachial artery.

The long heads of the biceps' important relationship at the shoulder is its ability to act as a head depressor, especially in cuff tear or paralysis (61). Some effort is worthwhile in maintaining the long head and its relationship to the bicipital groove. The tendon is restrained in its groove by the transverse humeral ligament (14), but more importantly by a continuation of the coracohumeral ligament. Dis-

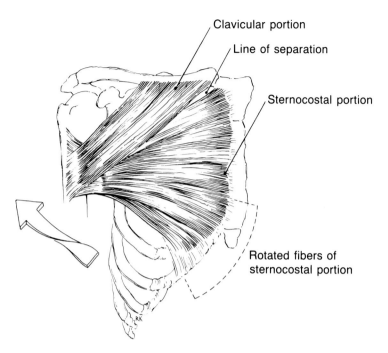

Figure 1.15. The pectoralis major showing the three major sections of the muscle: (1) the clavicular; (2) the upper; and (3) the lower sternocostal portions. The lower portion of the muscle forms the anterior border of the axillary fossa.

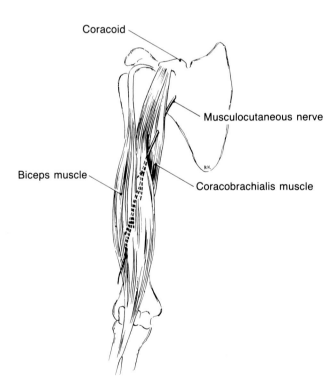

Figure 1.16. Coracobrachialis and biceps muscles and their nerve, the musculocutaneous. The nerve is shown entering the deep surface of the conjoint tendon and muscle formed by the short head of the biceps and the coracobrachialis muscle. The interval is usually 5.5 cm from the tip of the acromion, but three-quarters of shoulders will have one or more nerves entering into the conjoint tendon above this level.

placement of the tendon is rare except in cases where there has been disruption of rotator cuff insertion and with it the coracohumeral ligament (14, 26).

The short head of biceps brachii is part of the conjoint tendon with coracobrachialis. This conjoint tendon is an important landmark in dissection because of its relationship to the musculocutaneous nerve and the brachial plexus.

NERVES

Brachial Plexus

Usually, five roots make up the origin of the brachial plexus (24, 66, 69). These are, in fact, the anterior divisions of the spinal nerves C5–T1 (Fig. 1.17) (15).

First, the nerves form themselves into trunks. The upper trunk is made up of C5 and C6; C7 makes up the middle trunk, and C8 and T1 make up the inferior trunk. These three trunks then divide into anterior and posterior divisions. All of the posterior divisions join as the posterior cord of the brachial plexus. The anterior divisions of the upper and middle trunk produce the lateral cord, and the anterior division of the inferior trunk continues on as the medial cord. All cords are formed before the plexus passes below the clavicle. Above the clavicle, the

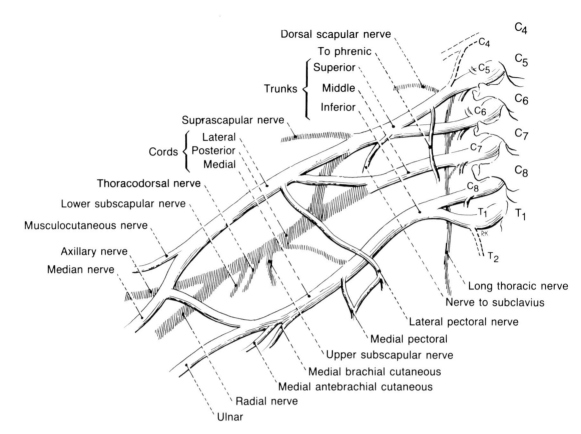

Figure 1.17. The spinal nerves contributing to the formation of the brachial plexus and its organization into trunks, divisions, and cords and finally, peripheral nerves. All of the cords are formed by the time the plexus passes below the level of the clavicle.

plexus passes above the first rib and between the anterior and middle scalene (Fig. 1.18).

Terminal Branches of the Brachial Plexus

The dorsal scapular nerve comes off of C5 before that spinal nerve joins the upper trunk. The dorsal scapular nerve occasionally contains some axons from C4 and is destined for the rhomboids.

The next major nerve is the long thoracic nerve, which is made up of branches from C5, C6, and C7. These contributors come off prior to trunk formation near the intervertebral foramina. This nerve supplies the serratus anterior, and is frequently injured by indirect means. The mechanism remains unclear, but it is believed to be depression of the shoulder, causing stretch of the nerve as it is draped over the prominence of the second rib. The long thoracic nerve is found on the medial wall of the axillary space, and is liable to direct injury in dissection in this area (64).

Fibers of C5 and C6 make up the suprascapular nerve, which comes off of the upper trunk. This nerve travels laterally and passes through the supra-

scapular notch, which is probably its most frequent site of compression (68). The notch is bordered superiorly by the transverse scapular ligament. In addition, the nerve may become entrapped in the spinoglenoid notch at the base of the spine of the scapula (16). At the suprascapular notch, the suprascapular artery travels over the transverse scapular ligament. The notch limits the mobility of the nerve and artery so that the supraspinatus should not be moved more than 3 cm by a muscle repositioning. Its other precarious surgical relationship is with the posterior glenoid. In the upper portion of the posterior glenoid, the nerve may lie only 1.5 cm medial to the rim (4).

The first peripheral nerve arising from the lateral cord is the lateral pectoral nerve. The lateral pectoral nerve contains fibers of C5, C6, and C7. It pierces the clavipectoral fascia, part of the anterior wall of the axillary space, and arises, ironically, more medial than the medial pectoral nerve.

The second branch off the lateral cord is the musculocutaneous nerve, which in the majority of the cases is supplemented by one or more unnamed nerves off the lateral cord. These nerves go to the conjoint muscle made up of the coracobrachialis and the short head of biceps. As a general rule, it penetrates into this muscle tendon unit 5–6 cm below the tip of the coracoid, but the range is 1½–9 cm below the tip of the coracoid. Taking into account the extra nerve, 74% of the shoulders will have one or more nerves entering within 5 cm of the tip of the coracoid (65).

The final branch off the lateral cord is the lateral root to the median nerve.

Five branches originate from the posterior cord. Two of the more proximal of these are the upper and lower subscapular nerves. The upper nerve is made up of C5 fibers and always innervates the upper half of the subscapularis muscle. The lower subscapular nerve is made up of C5–C6 and innervates only the lower 20% of the muscle and the teres major.

The thoracodorsal nerve usually originates from the posterior cord between the two subscapular nerves. It is longer, and contains fibers of C7–C8. The thoracodorsal nerve innervates latissimus dorsi.

The axillary nerve, containing fibers of C5 and C6, penetrates the quadrilateral space accompanied by the posterior humeral circumflex artery into the back of the shoulder. Its precarious relationships are numerous. The nerve lies across the anterior surface

of the subscapularis muscle perpendicular to the fibers of the muscle and may be endangered by muscle-splitting incisions here. It wraps along the inferior border of the subscapularis and may be at risk here. The axillary nerve passes through the quadrilateral space, which is bounded medially by the long head of the triceps and laterally by the shaft of the humerus and above by the glenohumeral joint capsule (62, 67). The space and nerve are also bounded above by the teres minor and subscapularis, and below by the teres major. Finally, the nerve lies perpendicular to the fibers of the deltoid about 5 cm below the rim of the acromion. Here it may be injured by muscle-splitting incisions. The nerve is brought closer to the acromion by abduction. The final branch of the posterior cord is the radial nerve, containing fibers of C5–C8. The first muscle that it innervates is the triceps.

Also having five terminal branches in the medial cord, whose most proximal branch is the medial pectoral nerve, containing fibers of C8 and T1. This nerve innervates the pectoralis minor and penetrates through pectoralis minor to innervate some of pectoralis major.

Two cutaneous nerves arise next. The first is the medial brachial cutaneous nerve, containing fi-

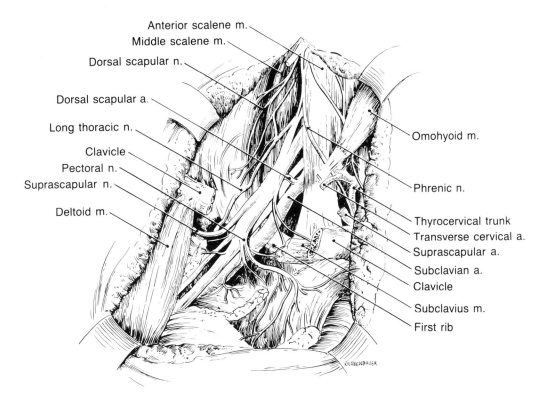

Figure 1.18. The appearance of the brachial plexus at surgery and the important adjacent structures.

bers of T1. The second is the medial antebrachial cutaneous nerve, containing fibers of C8 and T1. This nerve continues farther on down the arm, innervating the ulnar side of the forearm.

Finally, the medial cord gives off the medial root of the median nerve, containing fibers of C8 and T1 and the ulnar nerve, containing fibers from C8 and T1 and quite frequently fibers of C7.

BLOOD VESSELS

The main arterial axis of the upper limb is a subclavian artery and its continuation, the axillary artery (Fig. 1.19) (16).

Fortunately, the subclavian artery is well protected from surgical complications unless this particular area is sought by the surgeon, as in a first rib resection (Fig. 1.18) (70, 72). In this area, the artery and vein are draped over the first rib. They are protected in front by the clavicle and muscles. The important branches from the subclavian artery for the

shoulder surgeon are the suprascapular artery, the vertebral artery, and the blood supply to trapezius and rhomboids. This last supply is variable, being either a transverse cervical artery off the thyrocervical trunk or a dorsal scapular artery directly off of the subclavian.

The suprascapular artery originates from the thyrocervical trunk. It crosses laterally and into the supraspinatus muscle just over the top of the transverse suprascapular ligament, and travels thereafter with the suprascapular nerve.

As a direct branch of the subclavian artery, the vertebral artery makes a small S-curve and enters into the transverse process of C6. From that point on, it travels through the transverse processes superiorly. The artery has a very close relationship with the spinal nerves as they exit. The portion of the vertebral artery before it enters C6 is subject to damage from surgery or needle puncture. The vertebral artery supplies much of the proximal brachial plexus.

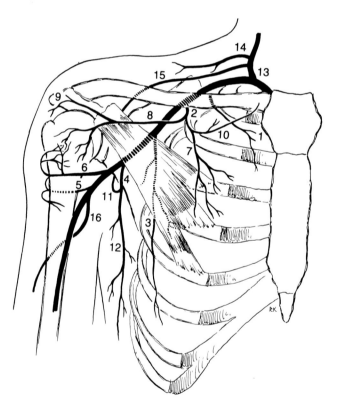

Figure 1.19. The major source artery of the upper limb, the subclavian and axillary arteries. This drawing shows the important anterior relationships between the clavicle and the pectoralis minor. Note also that the thoracoacromial axis is shown originating, as it frequently does, at a more superior level. Vessel Nos.: (1) Supreme thoracic artery; (2) Thoracoacromial axis; (3) Lateral thoracic artery; (4) Subscapular artery; (5) Posterior humeral circumflex artery; (6) Anterior humeral circumflex artery; (7) Pectoral artery; (8) Deltoid artery; (9) Acromial artery; (10) Clavicular artery; (11) Circumflex scapular artery; (12) Thoracodorsal artery; (13) Thyrocervical trunk; (14) Transverse cervical artery; (15) Suprascapular artery; (16) Profunda brachii artery.

Careful attention must also be given to the regions of the axillary artery. They are numbered with respect to their position relative to the pectoralis minor muscle and tendon (71). Proximal to pectoralis minor, starting at the lateral edge of the first rib, is the first region. Deep to pectoralis minor is the second, and distal to pectoralis minor is the third. The first region gives off the supreme thoracic artery, which supplies the first two intercostal spaces and muscles and some of serratus.

The second portion of the axillary artery gives off the thoracoacromial axis (73), which has four major branches: (a) the pectoral artery goes to the pectoralis major; (b) the deltoid artery goes to the pectoralis major and the anterior portion of the deltoid and to some skin over the deltopectoral groove; (c) the acromial artery, routinely a branch of the deltoid, lies just medial to the coracoacromial ligament and supplies the area of the acromion; and (d) the clavicular branch has a variable exit from the trunk or one of its branches and supplies the skin over the proximal part of the clavicle and some of the bone in this area. The other second zone branch is the lateral thoracic artery, which may be missing in as many as 25% of patients. It supplies the serratus anterior muscle and some of the pectoralis minor.

Providing the largest branch of the axillary artery, the subscapular artery is its third portion. The subscapular artery divides into two major branches. The first, the circumflex scapular artery, disappears through the triangular space and supplies the skin over the posterior portion of the shoulder and much of the arterial supply to muscles on the back side of the scapula. The other branch, the thoracodorsal, goes to the latissimus dorsi with contributions to the teres major muscles.

The posterior humeral circumflex artery also comes off in the third region and accompanies the axillary nerve through the quadrilateral space. The posterior humeral circumflex artery has a contribution to bone in the posterior inferior portion of the humeral head, but is mainly destined for the deltoid muscle.

Likewise from the third region of the axillary artery, the anterior humeral circumflex artery continues laterally along the inferior border of subscapularis muscle and sends important branches to the subscapularis tendon, but its most important branch continues up through the bicipital groove and enters into the humeral head as the arcuate artery. This ascending artery to the head has numerous extraosseous anastomoses. Intraosseously, it is connected only with those osseous branches that come off the posterior humeral circumflex artery, which are not present in all cases. Damage to the artery ascending in the bicipital groove may compromise blood flow to the humeral head, especially if the collaterals are not sufficient.

The veins accompany the arteries and drain into the axillary vein. In addition, a large superficial vein, the cephalic vein, enters into the deltopectoral groove and makes an important contribution to the drainage of the anterior deltoid.

The lymphatics of the limb drain according to the same pattern as the veins, mainly into nodes in the axilla. The extra-axillary drainage along the cephalic vein is cited by cancer surgeons to account for those patients who do not develop lymphedema following radical mastectomy.

SKIN

Surgical complications with respect to skin are usually one of three types: the most important of these is circulation problems, arterial or venous. The second is loss of sensation, and the third is problems with cosmesis.

The skin of the shoulder is blessed with an abundant circulation, and consequently, sloughing of large areas of skin or even wound edges is rare except in radical surgery or irradiated skin (Fig. 1.20). The skin in most areas of the shoulder is relatively mobile, particularly over pectoralis major, and carries with it an auxiliary blood supply in the subcutaneous fascia. These vessels enter this level close to the axilla and travel in the subcutaneous fascia so that there is relatively little motion between vessel and skin. This allows a great deal of bloodless dissection adjacent to the deep fascia. Additional sources of blood entering the skin come from the cutaneous continuation of the circumflex scapular artery, and a branch of the posterior humeral circumflex coming around the posterior border of the deltoid muscle. Where skin is tightly adherent to the underlying muscle, as it is over the deltoid, additional circulation comes from direct arteries that penetrate the muscle, but these areas may also be less forgiving in extensive subcutaneous dissection.

Sensation is, oddly enough, rarely a complaint at the shoulder even though patients will often be found to have numbness if it is sought. Few of the nerves innervating the deep structures of the shoulder have a cutaneous representation. The main exception is the axillary nerve, which has a branch coming off the posterior portion of the axillary nerve and wraps around the posterior third of the deltoid

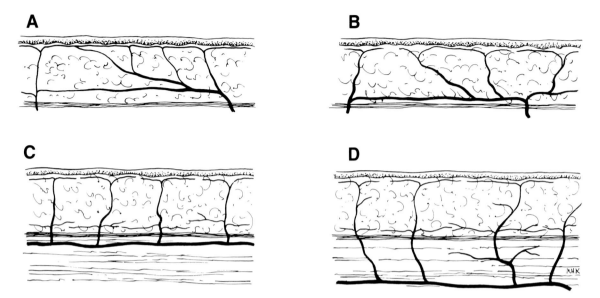

Figure 1.20. **A**, Skin circulation in the areas of the body where there is considerable motion between the skin and the deep fascia, as is seen over pectoralis major. The accessory blood vessels enter adjacent to the sternum and at the axilla and travel in the subcutaneous fascia. In these areas of the body there can be relatively bloodless dissection at the level of the deep fascia. **B**, This circulation occurs in areas where the relative motion occurs between muscle and the overlying deep fascia. This would be seen over the biceps. Here the accessory vessels of the skin lie on the deep fascia and dissection deep to deep fascia has the advantage of being relatively bloodless. **C**, This occurs only in the hand and foot where the accessory blood supply is deep to the palmar or plantar fascia. The vessels ascend vertically to the skin. **D**, This occurs where the skin is attached to the underlying deep fascia and muscle as over gluteus maximus. In these areas, the extra blood supply travels deep to the muscle and sends ascending vessels to the skin.

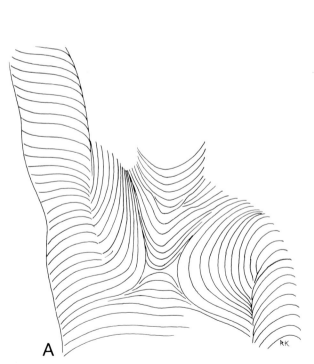

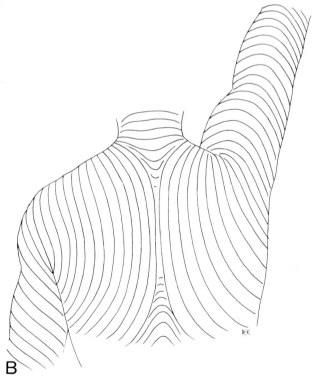

Figure 1.21.   Relaxed skin tension lines. The lines in the drawing indicate the typical location of the lines of tension in the skin. As these are determined by the shape of the underlying structures and by motion, they will differ between sexes and between individuals (75).

and becomes the upper lateral brachial cutaneous nerve. This innervates the skin over the area of the deltoid. Most of the shoulder innervation superiorly comes from the supraclavicular nerves lower down on the chest anterior, and posterior innervation comes from intercostal nerves. Down the inside of the arm, there is some innervation from medial antebrachial cutaneous and medial brachial cutaneous. The intercostal brachial nerve, from T2, mixes with the medial brachial cutaneous, yielding a mixed pattern on the inside of the arm with respect to which area of the skin is innervated by which nerve (the intercostal brachial or the medial brachial cutaneous). In this area of the intercostal brachial nerve, there may be some postoperative problems with lack of sensation and pain. This latter complication is not infrequent in mastectomy.

Cosmesis, often the final consideration in the design of a surgical procedure, is becoming more emphasized in surgery. For over 100 years, surgeons have recognized that there is a dominant pattern to the alignment of the collagen fibers in the skin (Fig. 1.21). Incisions made parallel to the dominant pattern in the skin tend to stretch less during the course of healing and are, therefore, cosmetically more acceptable. These lines were found by Langer to be related to the shape of the underlying structures and to motion of the underlying structures (76, 77).

The shoulder is an often visible area of the body and is a very prominent and mobile portion of the body. Not surprisingly, then, incision orientation plays a large role in the cosmetic result. Current recommendations are: to be aware that the tension lines vary between sexes and between individuals, and to use the thumb and index finger to relax the tension in the skin, and observe for the appearance of parallel lines. When the skin lines are parallel, this is felt to be the optimum alignment for incision (74, 75).

References

BONE AND JOINTS

1. Abbott LS, Lucas DB: The function of the clavicle. Its surgical significance. Ann Surg 1954;140:583–597.
2. Bearn JG: Direct observations on the function of the capsule of the sternoclavicular joint in clavicular support. J Anat 1967;101:159–170.
3. Bigliani LU, Morrison DS, April EW: The morphology of the acromion in its relationship to rotator cuff tears. Orthop Trans 1986;10:228.
4. Bigliani LU, McCann PD, Dalsey RM: An anatomic study of the suprascapular nerve. Orthop Trans 1989;13:232–233.
5. Brookes M: The blood supply of irregular and flat bones. In: Blood supply of the bone. New York: Appleton-Century-Crofts, 1971:47–66.
6. Cave AJE: The nature and morphology of the costoclavicular ligament. J Anat 1961;95:170–179.
7. DePalma AF, Callery G, Bennett GA: Variational anatomy and degenerative lesions of the shoulder joint. Am Acad Orthop Surgeons Instructional Course Lectures 1949;6:255–281.
8. DePalma AF: Surgical anatomy of acromioclavicular and sternoclavicular joints. Surg Clin North Am 1963;43:1541–1550.
9. Detrisac DA, Johnson LL: Arthroscopic shoulder anatomy. Pathologic and surgical implications. Thorofare, NJ: Slack Inc., 1986.
10. Fukuda K, Craig EV, An K, et al: Biomechanical study of the ligamentous system of the acromioclavicular joint. J Bone Joint Surg 1986;68A:434–439.
11. Gagey O, Bonfair H, Gillot C: Anatomic basis of ligamentous control of elevation. Surg Radiol Anat 1987;9:19–26.
12. Gardner E: The innervation of the shoulder joint. Anat Rec 1948;102:1–18.
13. Harryman DI, II, Sidles JA, Clark JM, McQuade KJ, Gibb TD, Matsen FA, III: Humeral head translation on the glenoid occurs with passive glenohumeral motions. J Bone Joint Surg (In press).
14. Hitchcock HH, Bechtol CO: Painful shoulder. Observations of the role of the tendon of the long head of the biceps brachii in its causation. J Bone Joint Surg 1948;30A:263–273.
15. Hollinshead WH: Textbook of anatomy. 2nd ed. New York: Harper & Row, 1967.
16. Hollinshead WH: Anatomy for surgeons, vol. 3. 3rd ed. New York: Harper & Row, 1982.
17. Howard FM, Shafer SJ: Injuries to the clavicle with neurovascular complications: a study of fourteen cases. J Bone Joint Surg 1956;47A:1335–1346.
18. Inman VT, Saunders JBDCM, Abbott LC: Observations on the function of the shoulder joint. J Bone Joint Surg 1944;26:1–30.
19. Jobe CM: Real and apparent motion of the glenohumeral joint—its significance for glenohumeral ligament function. Paper presented at the American Shoulder and Elbow Surgeons annual meeting, Chicago, November 8, 1990.
20. Johnson EW, Jr, Collins HR: Nonunion of the clavicle. Arch Surg 1963;87:963–966.
21. Kennedy JC: Retrosternal dislocation of the clavicle. J Bone Joint Surg 1949;31B:74–75.
22. Kumar VP, Balasubramanian P: The role of atmospheric pressure in stabilizing the glenohumeral joint: an experimental study. J Bone Joint Surg 1985;67B:719.
23. Laing PG: The arterial supply of the adult humerus. J Bone Joint Surg 1956;38A:1105–1116.
24. Laumann U: Kinesiology of the shoulder joint. In: Kolbel R et al. eds. Shoulder replacement. Berlin: Springer-Verlag, 1987.
25. Matsen FA: Biomechanics of the shoulder. In: Frankel VH, Nordin M, eds. Basic biomechanics of the skeletal system. Philadelphia: Lea & Febiger, 1980:221–242.
26. Meyer AW: Chronic functional lesions of the shoulder. Arch Surg 1937;35:646–674.
27. Neer CJ: Anterior acromioplasty for chronic impingement syndrome of the shoulder. J Bone Joint Surg 1972;54A:41–50.
28. Neer CS, Poppen NK: Supraspinatus outlet. Orthop Trans 1987;11:234.
29. O'Brien SJ, Warren RF, Schwartz E: Anterior shoulder instability. Orthop Clin North Am 1987;18:395–408.
30. O'Brien SJ, Arnoczky SP, Warren RF, Rozbuch RS: Developmental anatomy of the shoulder and anatomy of the glenohu-

meral joint. In: Rockwood CA, Matsen F eds. The shoulder. Philadelphia: WB Saunders, 1990:1–33.

31. Ovesen JO, Nielsen S: Stability of the shoulder joint. Cadaver study of stabilizing structures. Acta Orthop Scand 1985; 56:149–151.

32. Ovesen J, Nielsen S: Anterior and posterior shoulder instability. Acta Orthop Scand 1986;57:324–327.

33. Ovesen J, Nielsen S: Posterior instability of the shoulder. Acta Orthop Scand 1986;57:436–439.

34. Paavolainen P, Slatis P, Aalto K: Surgical pathology in chronic shoulder pain. In: Bateman JE, Welsh RP, eds: Surgery of the shoulder. St. Louis: CV Mosby, 1984:313–318.

35. Petersson CJ: Spontaneous medial dislocation of the tendon of the long biceps brachii. An anatomic study of prevalence and pathomechanics. Clin Orthop 1986;211:224–227.

36. Rietveld ABM, Daanan HAM, Rozing PM, Obermann WR: The lever arm in gleno-humeral abduction and after hemiarthroplasty. J Bone Joint Surg 1988;70B:561–565.

37. Rockwood CA, and Green DP: Fractures in adults, vol. 1, part II: Subluxations and dislocations about the shoulder. Philadelphia: JB Lippincott, 1984:722–947.

38. Saha AK: Dynamic stability of the glenohumeral joint. Acta Orthop Scand 1971;42:491.

39. Saha AK: Mechanism of shoulder movements and a plea for the recognition of "zero position" of the glenohumeral joint. Clin Orthop 1983;173:3–10.

40. Schwartz RE, O'Brien SJ, Warren RF, et al: Capsular restraints to anterior posterior motion of the abducted shoulder: A biomechanical study. Orthop Trans 1988;12:727.

41. Slatis P, Aalto K: Medial dislocation of the tendon of the long head of the biceps brachii. Acta Orthop Scand 1979;50:73–77.

42. Turkel SJ, Panio MW, Marshall JL, Girgis FG: Stabilizing mechanisms preventing anterior dislocation of the glenohumeral joint. J Bone Joint Surg 1981;63A:1208–1217.

43. Urist MR: Follow-up notes on articles previously published in the journal: complete dislocation of the acromioclavicular joint. J Bone Joint Surg 1963;45A:1750–1753.

44. Woodward JW: Congenital elevation of the scapula: correction by release and transplantation of muscle origins. A preliminary report. J Bone Joint Surg 1961;43A:219–228.

MUSCLES

45. Abbott LC, Lucas DB: The tripartite deltoid and its surgical significance in exposure of the scapulohumeral joint. Ann Surg 1952;136:392–402.

46. Basmajian JV: Muscles alive. Their functions revealed by electromyography. 4th ed. Baltimore: Williams & Wilkins, 1979.

47. Dewar FP, Harris RI: Restoration of function of the shoulder following paralysis of the trapezius by fascial sling fixation and transplantation of the levator scapulae. Ann Surg 1950;132:1111–1115.

48. Durman DC: An operation for paralysis of the serratus anterior. J Bone Joint Surg 1945;27:380–382.

49. Franklin JL, Barrett WP, Jackins SE, Matsen FA: Glenoid loosening in total shoulder arthroplasty. Association with rotator cuff deficiency. J Arthroplasty 1988;3:39–46.

50. Grant JCB, Smith CG: Age incidence of rupture of the supraspinatus tendon. Anat Rec 1948;100:666.

51. Horwitz MT, Tocantins LM: Isolated paralysis of the serratus anterior (magnus) muscle. J Bone Joint Surg 1938b; 20A:720–725.

52. Lorhan PH: Isolated paralysis of the serratus magnus following surgical procedures. Report of a case. Arch Surg 1947;54:656–659.

53. Mariani EM, Cofield RH, Askew LJ, et al: Rupture of the tendon of the long head of the biceps brachii. Surgical vs. nonsurgical treatment. Clin Orthop 1988;228:233–239.

54. Marmor L, Bechtol CO, Hall CB: Pectoralis major muscle. J Bone Joint Surg 1961;43A:81–87.

55. Nuber GW, Jobe FW, Perry J, et al: Fine wire electromyography analysis of muscles of the shoulder during swimming. Am J Sports Med 1986;14:7–11.

56. Perry J: Biomechanics of the shoulder. In: Rockwood C ed. The shoulder. New York: Churchill Livingstone, 1988.

57. Sakellarides HT: Injury to spinal accessory nerve with paralysis of trapezius muscle and treatment by tendon transfer. Orthop Trans 1986;10:449.

58. Staples OS, Watkins AL: Full active abduction in traumatic paralysis of the deltoid. J Bone Joint Surg 1943;25:85–89.

59. Strohm BR: Shoulder dysfunction following injury to suprascapular nerve. J Am Phys Ther Assoc 1965;45:106–111.

60. Symeonides PP: The significance of the subscapularis muscle in pathogenesis of recurrent anterior dislocation of the shoulder. J Bone Joint Surg 1972;54B:476–483.

61. Ting A, Jobe FW, Barto P, et al: An EMG analysis of the lateral biceps in shoulders with rotator cuff tears. Orthop Trans 1987;11:237.

NERVES

62. Cahill BR, Palmer RE: Quadrilateral space syndrome. J Hand Surg 1983;8:65–69.

63. Flatow EL, Bigliani LU, April EW: An anatomical study of the musculocutaneous nerve and its relationship to the coracoid. Clin Orthop Rel Res 1989;244:166–171.

64. Horwitz MT, Tocantins LM: An anatomical study of the role of the long thoracic nerve and the related scapular bursae in the pathogenesis of local paralysis of the serratus anterior muscle. Anat Rec 1938a;71:375–385.

65. Jobe CM: Unpublished data from dissections carried out at A.A.O.S. Summer Institute, 1986.

66. Kerr AT: The brachial plexus of nerves in man: the variations in its formation and branches. Am J Anat 1918;23:285–394.

67. Loo RL, Graham B: Anatomy of the axillary nerve and its relation to inferior capsular shift. Orthop Trans 1987;11:245.

68. Rengachary SS, Neff JP, Singer PA, Brackett CE: Suprascapular entrapment neuropathy. A clinical, anatomic and comparative study. Part I. Neurosurg 1979;5:441–446.

69. Walsh JF: The anatomy of the brachial plexus. Am J Med Sci 1887;74:387–399.

BLOOD VESSELS

70. Daseler EH, Anson BJ: Surgical anatomy of the subclavian artery and its branches. Surg Gynecol Obstet 1959; 108:149–174.

71. Huelke DF: Variation in the origins of the branches of the axillary artery. Anat Rec 1959;135:33–41.

72. Radke HM: Arterial circulation of the upper extremity. In: Strandness DE Jr, ed. Collateral circulation in clinical surgery. Philadelphia: WB Saunders, 1969:294–307.

73. Reid CD, and Taylor GI: The vascular territory of the acromiothoracic axis. Br J Plast Surg 1984;37:194–212.

SKIN

74. Borges AF: The relaxed skin tension lines (RSTL) vs. other skin lines. Plast Reconstr Surg 1984;73:144–150.

75. Kraissel CJ: Selection of appropriate lines for elective surgical incisions. Plast Reconstr Surg 1951;8:1–28.

76. Langer K: On the anatomy and physiology of the skin: I. The cleavability of the skin. Br J Plast Surg 1978;31:3.

77. Langer K: On the anatomy and physiology of the skin: II. Skin tension. Br J Plast Surg 1978;31:93.

2
Evaluation of Shoulder Problems

Peter D. McCann

INTRODUCTION

The essential goal in the evaluation of shoulder problems is to obtain the correct diagnosis. Once determined, the diagnosis will require the appropriate management for complications following shoulder surgery. This chapter focuses on a general approach to the patient with a surgical complication, identifying the characteristics of the particular problem, and reviewing the practical points that help to establish a diagnosis. Finally, specific diagnostic tests that aid in identifying the correct diagnosis following failed procedures for shoulder instability, subacromial impingement, proximal humeral fractures, and glenohumeral arthritis will be reviewed. The details of the management of specific surgical complications will be discussed in subsequent chapters.

The initial history and physical examination are the most important factors in the assessment of complications following shoulder surgery. The importance of this initial evaluation cannot be overemphasized. Routine ancillary tests such as roentenograms, blood tests, and specific injections as well as more sophisticated procedures including computerized tomography and magnetic resonance imaging are helpful in confirming the initial clinical impression based on history and physical examination.

HISTORY

Two broad categories may account for complications following shoulder surgery: physician factors and patient factors. Both issues must be addressed at the initial history to evaluation surgical failures. Physician factors include improper patient selection, misdiagnosis, and compromised technique. Patient factors include unrealistic expectations, poor compliance with postoperative rehabilitation protocols, and active litigation or compensation cases.

Review of the patient's preoperative symptoms and physical findings as well as preoperative diagnostic tests help to assess the degree of disability and the accuracy of the initial diagnosis. Original office and/or hospital records and the actual preoperative tests are essential for this evaluation. Review of the operative record and postoperative roentenograms may indicate errors in technique (Fig. 2.1). Review of the patient's initial degree of disability, specifics of the postoperative rehabilitation including types of exercises as well as frequency and duration of physical therapy may expose factors that contribute to surgical failures.

Historical points important during the initial evaluation following previous surgery include the length of the postoperative pain-free interval, any intervening traumatic events, and the manifestation of other coexistent pathologic conditions. Such conditions might include the constant pain associated with infected prosthetic arthroplasties or the shoulder pain that may be secondary to a cervical radiculopathy. A thorough review of the patient's pain and functional disability is summarized in the American Shoulder and Elbow Surgeons' evaluation form (Table 2.1).

PHYSICAL EXAMINATION

A complete shoulder examination is summarized in the American Shoulder and Elbow Surgeons' patient form (Table 2.1) and includes active and passive range of motion in forward elevation in the scapular plane, as well as internal and external rotation with the humerus at both 0° and 90° of abduction. The patient is examined with the entire upper torso exposed and seated on a table that permits the physician access both in front of and behind the patient. Initially, the patient is asked to identify the location of pain and to perform the activity that elicits discomfort.

Evaluation of Shoulder Problems   25

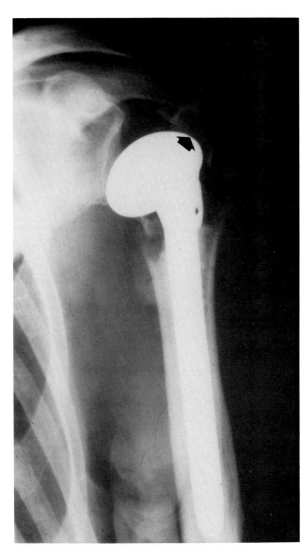

Figure 2.1. AP radiograph of the left shoulder demonstrating greater tuberosity displacement (*arrow*) following humeral head replacement for a 4-part fracture of the left proximal humerus. Active exercises were instituted before healing of the tuberosity to the shaft, leading to loss of tuberosity fixation.

Following the recording of range of motion both active and passive in the sitting and supine positions, the exam proceeds with inspection of the patient from behind where testing of the neck and scapular muscles can be performed. While standing behind the patient, the physician continues the physical examination in a systematic manner. Range of motion of the neck and palpation of the thoracic and parascapular areas is followed by palpation anteriorly of the sternoclavicular joint and acromial clavicular joint. Palpation of the subacromial space anteriorly may indicate the presence of an impingement syndrome. Certain conditions such as atrophy of the infraspinatus muscle in patients with rotator cuff tears

can be appreciated only by the physician behind the patient (Fig. 2.2). From this position, certain maneuvers such as to elicit the impingement sign, shoulder apprehension tests, and other findings of shoulder instabilities such as the sulcus sign (indentation of the lateral subacromial space with inferior traction on the humerus) or the Fukuda test (excessive posterior translation of the humeral head) can be performed (12).

With the physician now in front of the patient, notation of prior incisions and inspection of anatomic landmarks from the front may indicate underlying pathology (Fig. 2.3). A detailed neurological assessment is crucial to exclude other pathologic states such as C5–C6 cervical root dysfunction in patients with cervical radiculopathy or intrinsic hand dysfunction in a patient with ipsilateral glenohumeral joint destruction, which may indicate cervical syringomyelia.

The data collected from a thorough history and physical examination is then used to establish a preliminary diagnosis, to be confirmed with appropriate ancillary tests.

ANCILLARY TESTS

Routine blood tests including CBC, ESR, SMAC 20, and serology should be reviewed to exclude systemic causes of shoulder pain such as infection, inflammatory arthritis, metastatic disease, and liver disease. The following ancillary tests are more helpful in delineating specific shoulder pathology and the particular advantages of each test will be reviewed.

ROENTGENOGRAMS

A standard shoulder series is essential to evaluate shoulder problems following failed surgery. The series consists of three anterior-posterior views of the scapula with the humerus in neutral, internal, and external rotations. The three rotational AP views help to demonstrate shoulder lesions such as calcific tendinitis, Hill-Sachs defect associated with shoulder instability, and impingement findings that may not be apparent on a single AP view (Fig. 2.4). The scapular plane is used to give a more accurate image of the glenohumeral articulation (Fig. 2.5). The final two views of the shoulder include the lateral scapula and axillary views.

The true lateral view of the scapula is obtained with a 5–10° caudal tilt to give better detail of the acromion and region of the supraspinatus tendon,

Table 2.1.　American Shoulder and Elbow Surgeons' Shoulder Evaluation Form

NAME _____ HOSP.# _____ DATE _____ SHOULDER: R/L

I.　PAIN: (5 = none, 4 = slight, 3 = after unusual activity, 2 = moderate, 1 = marked,
　　　0 = complete disability, NA = not available)_____

II.　MOTION:
　　A.　Patient sitting
　　　　1.　Active total elevation of arm:_____ degrees[a]
　　　　2.　Passive internal rotation:
　　　　　　(Circle segment of posterior anatomy reached by thumb)
　　　　　　(Note if reach restricted by limited elbow flexion)

1 = Less than trochanter	5 = L5	9 = L1	13 = T9	17 = T5
2 = Trochanter	6 = L4	10 = T12	14 = T8	18 = T4
3 = Gluteal	7 = L3	11 = T11	15 = T7	19 = T3
4 = Sacrum	8 = L2	12 = T10	16 = T6	20 = T2

　　　　3.　Active external rotation with arm at side: _____ degrees
　　　　4.　Active external rotation at 90° abduction:_____ degrees
　　　　　　(Enter "NA" if cannot achieve 90° of abduction)
　　B.　Patient supine
　　　　1.　Passive total elevation of arm:　　　　_____ degrees[a]
　　　　2.　Pasive external rotation with arm at side _____ degrees

III.　STRENGTH:
　　　　(5 = normal, 4 = good, 3 = fair, 2 = poor, 1 = trace, 0 = paralysis)
　　A.　Anterior deltoid _____　　C.　External rotation _____
　　B.　Middle deltoid _____　　D.　Internal rotation _____

IV.　STABILITY:
　　　　(5 = normal, 4 = apprehension, 3 = rare subluxation, 2 = recurrent subluxation, 1 = recurrent dislocation,
　　　　0 = fixed dislocation, NA = not available)
　　A.　Anterior_____　　B.　Posterior_____　　C.　Inferior_____

V.　FUNCTION:
　　　　(4 = normal, 3 = mild compromise, 2 = difficulty, 1 = with aid, 0 = unable, NA = not available)
　　A.　Use back pocket ...._____　　I.　Sleep on affected side..........._____
　　B.　Perineal care............................_____　　J.　Pulling ...._____
　　C.　Wash opposite axilla..............._____　　K.　Use hand overhead................._____
　　D.　Eat with utensil......................._____　　L.　Throwing ...._____
　　E.　Comb hair ...._____　　M.　Lifting ...._____
　　F.　Use hand with arm at
　　　　shoulder level ...._____　　N.　Do usual work........................._____
　　G.　Carry 10–15 lbs. with arm
　　　　at side ...._____
　　H.　Dress.._____　　O.　Do usual sport ...._____

[a]Total elevation of arm measured by viewing patient from side and using goniometer to determine angle between arm and thorax.

and has been termed the supraspinatus outlet view by Neer (11). This view has also been helpful in assessing the acromial morphology, which has been related to the incidence of rotator cuff tears (1). In addition, the supraspinatus outlet view is useful in assessing the adequacy of subacromial decompression for impingement lesions (Fig. 2.6). Finally, the axillary view, performed with the patient supine and the arm slightly abducted and externally rotated, is helpful in accessing the glenohumeral articulation in fracture and instability cases (Fig. 2.7). The trauma shoulder series is mandatory for the Neer classification of proximal humeral fractures and includes a single AP scapula, lateral scapula, and axillary views (9).

COMPUTERIZED TOMOGRAPHY (CT)

The CT scan has specific but limited use in the evaluation of shoulder pathology. The CT without contrast is useful in delineating the type of severe proximal humerus fractures. It is especially useful in

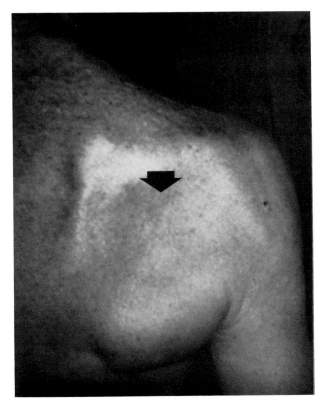

Figure 2.2. Posterior view of the right shoulder of a patient with an arthrogram-documented full-thickness rotator cuff tear. The concavity inferior to the spine of the scapula (*arrow*) demonstrates infraspinatus atrophy.

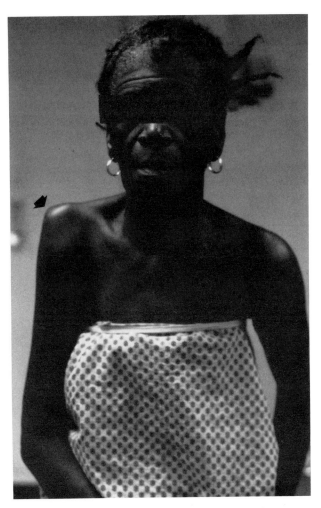

Figure 2.3. Frontal view of a patient status post-right hemiplegia secondary to a stroke with persistent right shoulder pain. Loss of the rounded contour of the right shoulder (*arrow*), along with prominence of the humeral head anteriorly on physical exam, suggest a chronic anterior dislocation of the right shoulder, which was confirmed by radiographs.

detailing tuberosity displacement and occult fractures of the humeral head, which may not be apparent in plain roentgenograms (Fig. 2.8). CT without contrast is also helpful in the evaluation of the glenoid in patients with shoulder instability or glenohumeral arthritis.

The CT may offer more accurate rendering of the contour of the anterior glenoid in the patient with primarily anterior instability. Patients with osteoarthritis often demonstrate excessive wear of the posterior glenoid, thereby increasing the normal retroversion of the glenoid articular surface relative to the glenoid neck. Excessive posterior glenoid wear may necessitate the use of a bone graft to ensure appropriate version of the glenoid component in patients requiring total shoulder arthroplasty.

The CT scan with contrast provides excellent detailing of the labrum and capsular attachments and is especially useful in the evaluation of shoulder instability (2). The use of a contrast agent enhances the ability of the CT to identify Bankart lesions (Fig. 2.9).

MAGNETIC RESONANCE IMAGING (MRI)

The MR image offers the most detailed imaging of the rotator cuff. T2-weighted images provide evidence of inflammation and partial thickness tears of the rotator cuff tendons (Fig. 2.10), as well as full-thickness rotator cuff tears (14). MR is an extremely sensitive technique and, accordingly, may overread pathology of the rotator cuff. Nevertheless, as clinical experience with MR develops, this technique may supplant the shoulder arthrogram as the definitive test for documenting full-thickness rotator cuff tears.

A recent report has described the use of a saline-enhanced MRI to give improved definition of

Figure 2.4. AP radiograph with internal humeral rotation of a patient with recurrent dislocations of the left shoulder. The internal rotation view best demonstrates the Hill-Sachs lesion of the anterolateral portion of the humeral head (*arrow*).

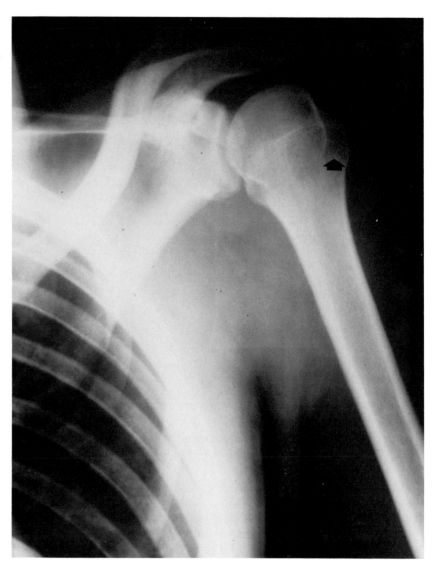

the labrum and glenohumeral joint capsule (13). MR alone gives poor detailing of the labrum and anterior ligaments crucial in the evaluation of shoulder instability. The advantage of the saline MR is that both the rotator cuff and labrocapsular complex may be imaged with a single test, especially in patients with a differential diagnosis of impingement and shoulder instability. Further evaluation will be required to determine whether or not this promising technique will have widespread clinical usefulness.

SHOULDER ARTHROGRAM

The shoulder arthrogram (Fig. 2.11) remains the gold standard for the evaluation of full-thickness tears of the rotator cuff (5). The arthrogram is less sensitive than the MRI for assessing partial-thickness tears of the rotator cuff and cannot identify inflammation of the rotator cuff tendons. The advantages of its lower cost and proven reliability outweigh its disadvantage as an invasive procedure when compared with the MRI for the evaluation of suspected full-thickness tears of the rotator cuff. However, as clinical experience with the MRI expands, the MRI may well become the definitive test for evaluation of the rotator cuff.

ULTRASOUND

Ultrasonography of the shoulder has been advocated by some authors as a noninvasive means of imaging the rotator cuff (7). The technique requires a special adapter to image the shoulder and a sonog-

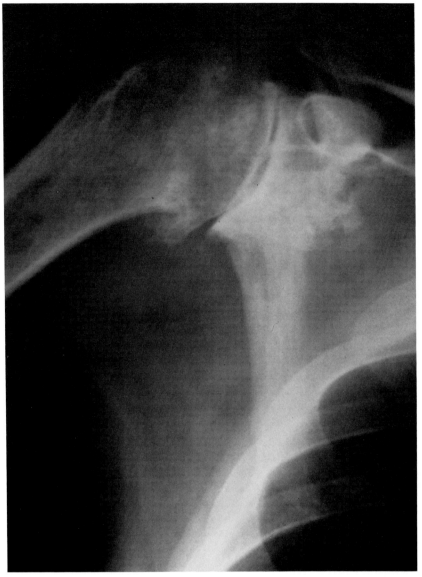

Figure 2.5. An AP radiograph of the right shoulder in the scapular plane demonstrating severe osteoarthritis of the glenohumeral joint. This is characterized by joint space narrowing, subchondral sclerosis, and ostrophyte formation on the inferior aspect of the humeral head.

rapher with considerable experience. Consequently, this test has not gained widespread use.

Ultrasonography of the shoulder is of limited usefulness in the evaluation of complications following rotator cuff surgery because scarred tendons sonographically may resemble degenerated tendons or partial and small rotator cuff tears (3). Therefore, ultrasonography may not provide additional information that cannot be obtained with a shoulder arthrogram or MRI.

ELECTROMYOGRAPHY (EMG)

EMG and nerve conduction studies are especially useful in the assessment of suspected neurologic pathology following failed shoulder surgery. They are particularly helpful in identifying lesions of the brachial plexus and the cervical spinal roots.

Shoulder pain may be referred from the neck in patients with cervical radiculopathy. While some reports have indicated relief of neck and radicular symptoms following rotator cuff surgery (8), persistent cervical radiculopathy may account for persistent shoulder pain in patients with shoulder pain following shoulder surgery. Occult brachial plexus injuries may coexist with additional shoulder pathology following trauma such as dislocations, proximal humeral fractures, or acute extensions of chronic rotator cuff tears. The EMG will help localize lesions of the brachial plexus that may account for persistent shoulder symptoms (6).

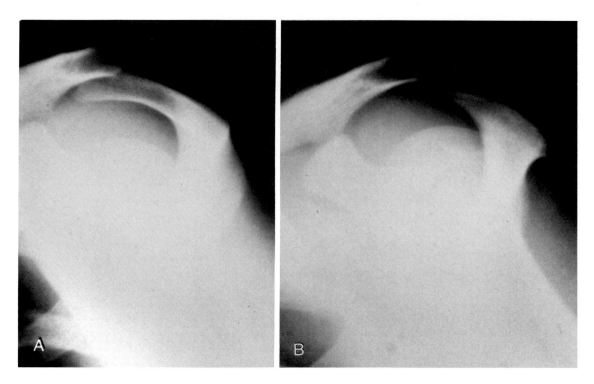

Figure 2.6.   **A**, Preoperative and **B**, Postoperative supraspinatus outlet views of the supraspinatus outlet following anterior acromioplasty.

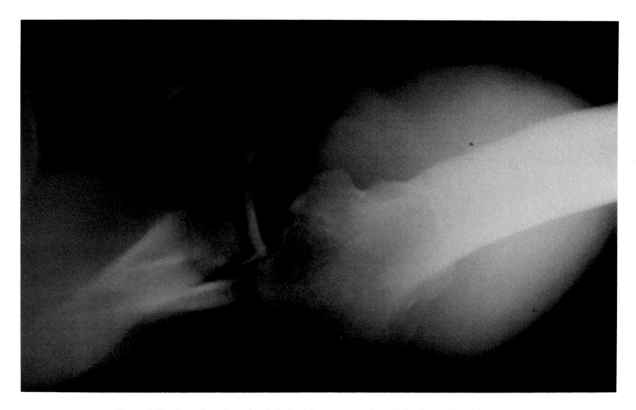

Figure 2.7.   An axillary view of the left shoulder demonstrating a locked posterior dislocation of the left glenohumeral joint.

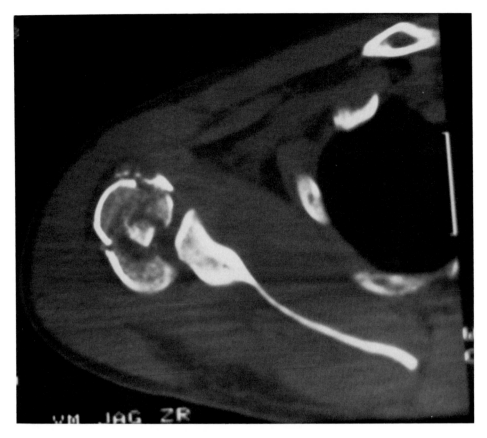

Figure 2.8. CT scan of the right shoulder demonstrating humeral head impaction in a patient with a 4-part fracture of the right proximal humerus.

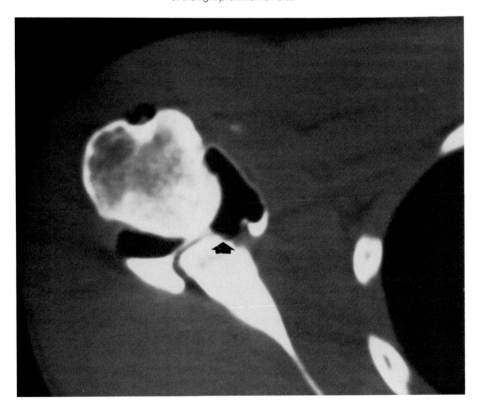

Figure 2.9. CT arthrogram of the right shoulder demonstrating anterior labral detachment (Bankart lesion) as well as bony erosion of the anteri-or glenoid margin (*arrow*) consistent with recurrent anterior dislocations of the right shoulder.

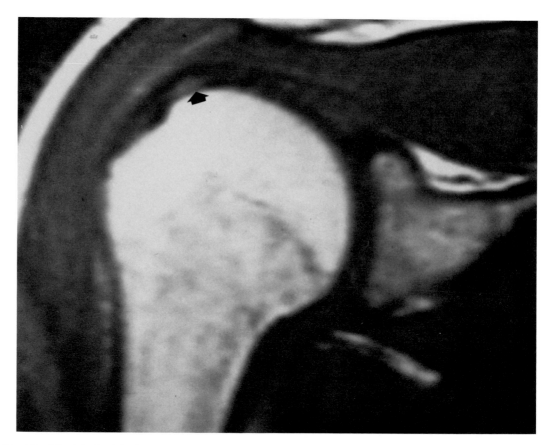

Figure 2.10. MRI of the right shoulder demonstrating a focus of high-density signal within the substance of the supraspinatus tendon (*arrow*). Preservation of the high-intensity subdeltoid fat line suggests this is a partial and not a full-thickness rotator cuff tear.

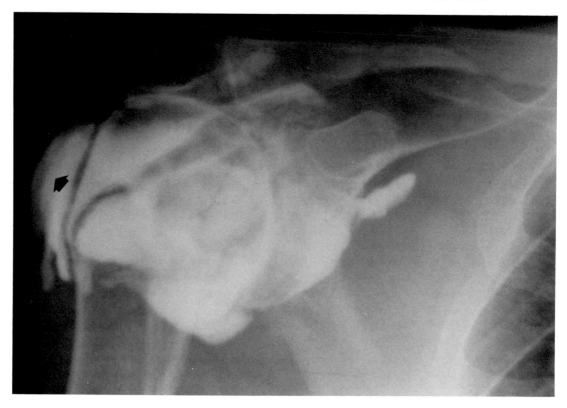

Figure 2.11. Arthrogram of the right shoulder demonstrating contrast material in the subdeltoid bursa lateral to the greater tuberosity (*arrow*) consistent with a full-thickness rotator cuff tear.

INJECTION TESTS

The installation of lidocaine with immediate relief of pain is extremely helpful in localizing the site of shoulder pathology. Neer described the positive injection test when shoulder pain and the impingement sign were completely relieved following the subacromial injection of lidocaine, thereby localizing pathology in the shoulder to the subacromial space (10). Similarly, the installation of lidocaine into the acromioclavicular joint with prompt relief of pain may localize pathology to the acromioclavicular joint, as in acromioclavicular arthritis. Failure to resolve pain with specific lidocaine injections indicates a remote site of pathology such as shoulder instability or cervical radiculopathy in patients with suspected impingement syndrome. In such cases, a poor result to a specific lidocaine injection is extremely helpful in excluding a certain diagnosis.

EXAMINATION UNDER ANESTHESIA AND SHOULDER ARTHROSCOPY

In most cases, an adequate history and physical examination as well as review of appropriate tests will result in the correct diagnosis. In some instances, examination under anesthesia and diagnostic shoulder arthroscopy can be extremely useful. The principal use for these procedures is in differentiating between impingement syndrome and shoulder instability, especially in the overhead-throwing athlete. Jobe has described the syndrome of shoulder instability associated with subacromial impingement in patients engaged in repetitive overhead activities (4). Examination under anesthesia can be extremely helpful in documenting a dislocating shoulder. It may be inadequate, however, in the assessment of subtle instabilities associated with symptomatic shoulder subluxations. Comparison of the stability of the contralateral shoulder is helpful in the assessment of significant shoulder instability.

Documentation of a Bankart lesion by shoulder arthroscopy may indicate instability as the primary pathology in patients with pain during overhead activities. Examination of the subacromial bursa may reveal significant thickening of the bursa and inflammation of the rotator cuff tendon that may respond to subacromial decompression.

SUMMARY

The evaluation of shoulder problems following shoulder surgery requires a systematic approach. The most important aspects are the initial history and physical examination, which will help to distinguish the patient factors and physician factors that may account for the particular complications. Ancillary tests are used to confirm initial impressions gained from the history and physical exam. Following this systematic approach, the appropriate diagnosis can be established, which will then dictate the appropriate treatment.

References

1. Bigliani LU, Morrison DS, April EW. The morphology of the acromion and its relationship to rotator cuff tears. Orthopaedic Transactions 1986;10:228.
2. Bigliani LU, Singson R, Feldman F, Flatow EL. Double contrast CT arthrography of shoulder instability. Surgical Rounds in Orthopaedics 1987;1:37-45.
3. Craig EV, Fritts HM, Crass JR. Noninvasive imaging of the rotator cuff. In: Post M, Morrey BF, Hawkins RJ, eds. Surgery of the shoulder. St. Louis: CV Mosby Year Book, 1990:6-10.
4. Jobe FW, Kvitne RS. Shoulder pain in the overhead or throwing athlete—The relationship of anterior instability and rotator cuff impingement. Orthop Rev 1989;18:963-975.
5. Kay JJ, Schneider R. Positive contrast shoulder arthrography I. In: Freiberger RH, Kay JJ, eds. Arthrography. East Norwalk, CT: Appleton-Century-Crofts, 1979:137-164.
6. Leffert RD. Brachial plexus injuries. Orthop Clin North Am 1970;1:399-417.
7. Mack LA, Matsen FA III, Kilkoyne RF, Davies PK, Sickler ME. Ultrasonographic evaluation of the rotator cuff. Radiology 1985;157:207-209.
8. McCann PD, Weiss RA, Bigliani LU. Results of anterior acromioplasty and rotator cuff repair in patients with impingement and cervical radiculopathy. In: Post M, Morrey BF, Hawkings BJ, eds. Surgery of the shoulder. St. Louis: CV Mosby Year Book, 1990:321-324.
9. Neer CS II. Displaced proximal humeral fractures. Part 1. J Bone Joint Surg 1970;52A:1077-1089.
10. Neer CS II. Impingement lesions. Clin Orthop 1983; 173:70-77.
11. Neer CS II, Popper NK. Supraspinatus outlet. Orthopaedic Transactions 1987;11:234.
12. Neer CS II. Shoulder reconstruction. Philadelphia: WB Saunders, 1990.
13. Schobert W, Nottage WM, Stauffer A. Saline magnetic resonance imaging of the shoulder. Presented at 17th Annual Meeting—American Orthopaedic Society for Sports Medicine. July 11, 1991; Orlando, Florida.
14. Seeger LL. Magnetic resonance imaging of the shoulder. Clin Orthop 1989;244:48-59.

3
Complications Following Anterior Acromioplasty and Rotator Cuff Repair

Melvin Post

INTRODUCTION

Impingement syndrome and rotator cuff tear are among the most common conditions causing shoulder pain and loss of function. Failure of surgical treatment for these conditions and the attendant complications can be minimized if the surgeon has a correct diagnosis, knows the cause and extent of the impingement and rotator cuff tear, the duration of symptoms, the condition of the glenohumeral joint, the quality of the rotator cuff tissues, and the strength of the shoulder girdle muscles. All these factors are important in determining the result of a surgical procedure. Moreover, the first operation gives the greatest hope of correcting the condition, while each succeeding procedure lessens the chance of success (2, 9, 12).

DIAGNOSIS

Impingement syndrome is often associated with a rotator cuff tear (7, 10, 11). The chief causes of tear are traumatic and degenerative (7, 12). It is important to know if other conditions associated with rotator cuff tear are present. These include arthritic joint disease, pseudogout, rheumatoid arthritis, and cuff tear arthropathy. These conditions require special treatment considerations, discussed elsewhere, and not mere repair of a torn rotator cuff and acromioplasty.

The surgeon should establish a careful physical examination data base to determine if future treatment goals have been reached and to what degree. For example, if advanced atrophy of external rotator muscles is present, it is unlikely that a complete recovery will be reached. The surgeon should exclude all other conditions as possible causes of the patient's shoulder pain, and not assume anything. A carefully recorded history and physical examination and laboratory testing as needed may help to differentiate a rotator cuff tear from an entrapment of the suprascapular nerve. The examination should include both upper extremities including the entire shoulder girdle, as well as the cervical spine. Even systemic conditions may affect the shoulder and need to be differentiated.

PHYSIOLOGICAL CONSIDERATIONS

Good function of a glenohumeral joint requires congruous articular surfaces. The shoulder muscles and tendons must be capable of creating normal tensions and compression forces to allow active motions (12). The size of a rotator cuff tear alone does not determine the outcome following a repair. Accordingly, a well-repaired extensive tear, as an example, will not give a good result if atrophied muscles are not contracting adequately, or if there is excessive tension placed upon a repaired attenuated torn rotator cuff. Thus, in comparing an acute tear of good-quality rotator cuff tissue versus a similar size tear in attenuated, poor rotator cuff tissue, the former is more likely to demonstrate a much better result. It is also necessary to restore adequate tension in the rotator cuff structures rather than achieving a water-tight seal alone. It follows that a repair of attenuated, frayed, scarred, and fibrillated cuff tissue contributes to the risk for failure regardless of the adequacy of the cuff closure. Similarly, using fascia lata grafts or other inert materials to close a defect, in my opinion, does not improve the chance for success in most cases because a stable fulcrum for the humeral head upon its glenoid is not achieved (10). In these cases, the normal compression and tension forces in the shoulder joint are lost. When this occurs, there is a corresponding decrease in active elevation of the arm. Impingement and associated pain may increase as the humeral head subluxes superiorly.

REHABILITATION

Postoperative muscle power of the deltoid and external rotator muscles help to determine the success of any repair. The initiation and extent of the physical therapy program must be individualized and will vary with each patient. A recent study of a comparison of muscle power by clinical examination and an evaluation by Cybex muscle testing of external rotator and deltoid muscle power during flexion motion showed that the deltoid is more important in creating active arm elevation and determining which patients return to work rather than external rotation muscle power (13). This finding may explain why acromioplasty alone for severe impingement, even in the presence of an irreparable large rotator cuff tear permits good postoperative active function. The deltoid muscle provides strength to elevate the extremity in this case (Fig. 3.1). This should not be interpreted that it is unimportant to repair a torn rotator cuff because normal shoulder function does require a functioning rotator cuff mechanism. Moreover, the more normal the rotator cuff mechanism is, the better the function will be. Lastly, good scapular function is needed to stabilize the shoulder.

ROENTGENOGRAM FINDINGS AND THEIR SIGNIFICANCE

When superior subluxation of the humeral head exists, this usually indicates poor rotator cuff function, a highly attenuated rotator cuff, or a large tear of the rotator cuff. The surgeon should look for significant degenerative changes in the glenohumeral joint, the acromioclavicular joint, or erosion of the undersurface of the acromion. If a geyser sign is present following an arthrogram, the surgeon should examine the acromioclavicular joint for tenderness and if present should consider resecting the lateral end of the clavicle as a part of the operation in repairing a rotator cuff tear in addition to performing an acromioplasty (12).

PRINCIPLES OF SURGICAL TREATMENT

Mechanical impingement is relieved by decompressing the subacromial space. This means thinning but not shortening the acromion, and removing all osteophytes including those on the undersurface of the acromioclavicular joint. Prominent distal clavicular osteophytes should be removed and the undersurface of the distal clavicle beveled. If the joint is

Figure 3.1. **A** and **B**, An elderly concert violinist had a painful, irreparable tear of the rotator cuff. An acromioplasty was performed. Excellent pain relief and improved active motion were achieved. He had poor muscle endurance and zero external rotator muscle power. The result was excellent. (Reprinted with permission from Post M. Complications of rotator cuff surgery. Clin Orthop, 1990;254:97–104.)

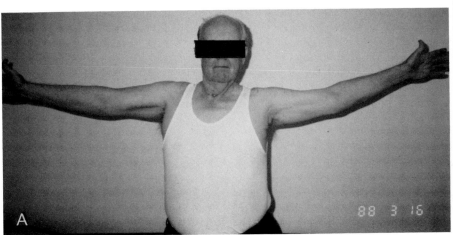
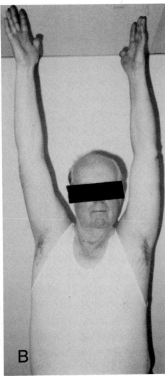

tender or painful, the lateral end of the clavicle should be resected. I do not recommend routine resection of lateral clavicle in every case. Moreover, if the shoulder muscles remain weak, thereby allowing superior subluxation, a dynamic impingement will persist.

OPERATIVE TECHNIQUE

Only a small length of deltoid tendon is detached from the anterior acromion and then split longitudinally for no more than 4–5 cm in order to repair the rotator cuff and avoid injury to the axillary nerve. A repair of a larger tear of the cuff can be achieved through a small deltoid muscle split if the surgeon passively elevates and rotates the arm in or out as needed to achieve complete cuff exposure for the repair. Occasionally, the deltoid must be detached from the lateral anterior clavicle. Lateral and posterior detachment of the deltoid origin should be avoided. It may be necessary to swing flaps of rotator cuff tissue including the upper half of the subscapularis tendon, the supraspinatus and infraspinatus as needed to effect closure of a large defect (8, 12). I do not recommend fascia lata or interposed synthetic grafts as they do not generally provide improved function.

In suturing a fresh edge of rotator cuff tissue to raw bone, or reattaching the deltoid to the raw acromial bone edge, the arm should be passively elevated while the sutures are tied to avoid excessive tension of the suture on the soft tissue and the bone, if the suture is placed through the bone. Arm elevation permits easy closure, avoids weakening of the suture material when it is pulled taut, or even tearing of the tissues as the suture is tied. It is axiomatic that whenever possible the repaired rotator cuff tissue should be attached directly to raw humeral bone surfaces. I do not recommend making a large trough into the cancellous bone, especially when the bone is demineralized. I prefer to achieve raw bleeding bone on the surfaces of intact subchondral bone (12).

In addition, the integrity of the deltotrapezius aponeurosis must be restored (12). Very small os acromiale lesions can be resected and the origin of the deltoid tendon and muscle reattached to the raw edge of the acromion using #1 synthetic nonabsorbable sutures (5). In the past, extensive acromionectomy was advocated (1, 4). The acromion should not be shortened during an acromioplasty operation for fear of permanently decreasing the fulcrum of the deltoid (6). Accordingly, for larger os acromiale lesions I prefer to internally fix the unstable bone lesion with two Steinmann pins and bone grafting with autogenous bone. In my experience, when a stabilization of an os acromiale lesion is done during an

acromioplasty procedure, there is a high rate of nonunion and persistent impingement primarily because the blood supply to the acromion is decreased during the acromioplasty. I recommend bone grafting the larger os acromiale lesions in an initial operation followed by the acromioplasty 2 months later.

Complications

Some commonly and uncommonly encountered painful shoulder complications associated with operations for rotator cuff and impingement syndrome are listed in Table 3.1.

NONFUNCTIONING DELTOID

The deltoid tendon and muscle that are reattached to the raw acromial bone edge may pull away because they are improperly reattached, or there may be a true traumatic postoperative avulsion. Often the surgeon may reattach the muscle fibers to the acromion alone while failing to reattach the underlying deltoid tendon as well. Even when the deltoid is properly reattached too early, vigorous muscle exercises or trauma may cause a true avulsion of the deltoid. It is difficult to diagnose these complications early because of associated swelling and pain. Surgical repair must be done in the first 2 weeks following these complications because retraction of the deltoid and scarring often prevent an adequate repair later (Fig. 3.2). Rarely, a portion of the acromion and deltoid may be avulsed during active stressful arm use against resistance. In these unusual cases, I

Table 3.1.   Complications of Surgery for Rotator Cuff and Impingement Syndromes

Nonfunctioning deltoid—postoperative
   Detached deltoid
   Avulsed deltoid
   Axillary nerve injury
Unrecognized, unstable acromion
   Os acromiale lesion
   Iatrogenic fracture
Inadequate subacromial decompression
   Osteophytes at acromioclavicular joint
   Inadequate acromioplasty
   Formation of postoperative osteophytes and ectopic bone
   Unrecognized thickened acromion (diffused idiopathic skeletal hypertrophy-DISH syndrome)
Suprascapular nerve injury
Failed rotator cuff repair
   Closure of thickened bursal tissue
   Avulsion of repaired rotator cuff
   Failure to close rotator cuff defect
   Unrecognized partial and intimal tears
   Failure to repair torn glenohumeral ligaments
Infection

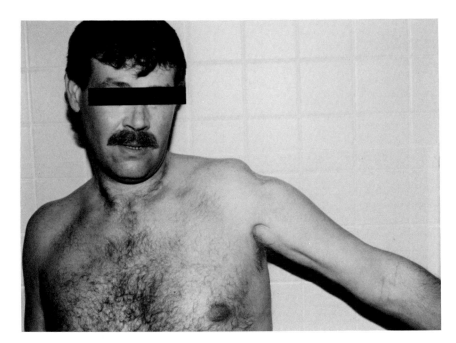

Figure 3.2. Following a rotator cuff repair and acromioplasty, the deltoid avulsed from its acromial origin several weeks postoperatively during vigorous physical therapy exercises. There was a failed attempt to repair the avulsed deltoid several months later. The result was poor.

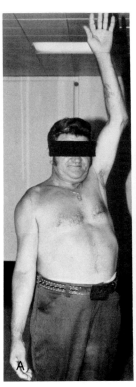

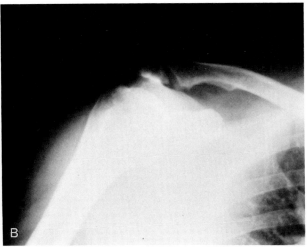

Figure 3.3. **A**, An adult male complained of pain and loss of active elevation following a rotator cuff repair and acromioplasty. **B**, Most of the acromion had been resected. The result was poor.

recommend reattachment of the bone fragment early if it is more than a few millimeters in width. In any event, proper reattachment of the deltoid is essential for effective deltoid function. Longitudinal splits in the anterior deltoid should be closed. I prefer 2–0 absorbable synthetic suture.

If the deltoid muscle is split anteriorly for more than a length of 5 cm, branches of the axillary nerve will be damaged, rendering a corresponding portion of the deltoid muscle ineffective. The smallest possible split in the deltoid should be made that permits a good exposure of the rotator cuff. To achieve adequate exposure through a small deltoid split, the arm may be moved passively in various positions in forward flexion and rotation, as stated.

The acromion must not be surgically shortened in order to prevent loss of the deltoid fulcrum (Fig. 3.3) (6, 12). Even when a well-performed closure of a rotator cuff tear is accomplished, the loss of deltoid action will cause a severe loss of shoulder function. It cannot be emphasized too strongly that acromial shortening is to be avoided.

UNRECOGNIZED, UNSTABLE ACROMION

Preoperatively, a true axillary roentgenogram will show an os acromiale lesion (Fig. 3.4C). If the lesion is missed and the os acromiale fragment is unstable, the loose lateral bone segment can be the cause of persistent pain in the shoulder. Small os acromiale fragments can be resected and the deltoid reattached to the residual raw acromial bone edge. I routinely look for os acromiale lesions preoperatively, in the axillary film, and avoid resection of larger lesions. I recommend internal fixation and autogenous bone grafting in a first-stage operation and perform an acromioplasty 2 months later when

healing of the defect in the acromion is well on the way to union. This avoids the risk of a painful nonunion if both operations are done in one sitting.

Lastly, whenever the acromioplasty procedure is done and the rotator cuff inspected and repaired, care must be taken to avoid excessive torque on the thinned bone with a retractor, especially if the bone is demineralized for fear of creating an iatrogenic fracture of the acromion (Fig. 3.5).

INADEQUATE SUBACROMIAL DECOMPRESSION

In performing an acromioplasty for subacromial decompression, the acromion must be ade-

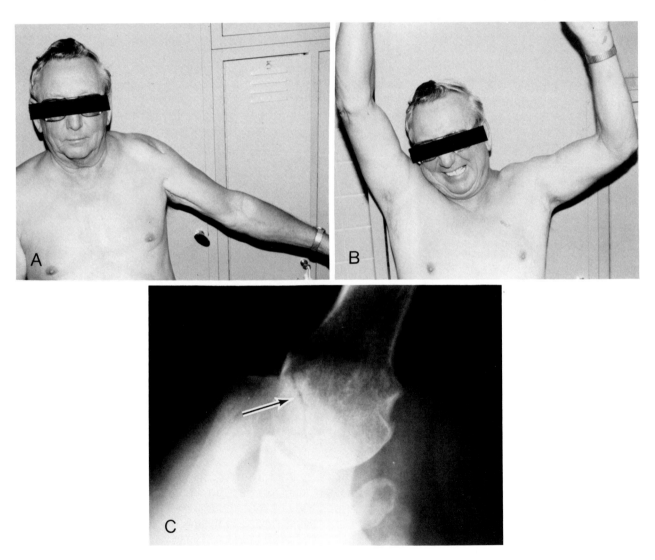

Figure 3.4.   A, A middle-aged man had a rotator cuff repair. The deltoid was excessively split, causing an injury to the axillary nerve. **B,** The patient had poor active elevation. In addition, he had severe pain that was associated with a persistent postoperative impingement. **C,** The patient had had a surgical resection of much of the acromion, thereby causing a loss of the deltoid fulcrum. Moreover, an unstable os acromial lesion had been missed (*arrow*). The result was poor. (Reprinted with permission from Post M. Complications of rotator cuff surgery. Clin Orthop, 1990;254:97–104.)

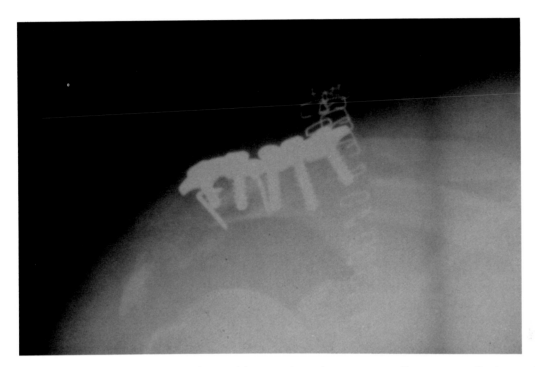

Figure 3.5. An adult male had an acromioplasty. The remaining acromion fractured. A second operation consisting of Steinmann pin fixation failed and resulted in a nonunion. A third operation included pin fixation and autogenous bone graft and failed. In a final fourth operation, a plate and screws were used to secure a new iliac bone graft onto the fragmented ununited fractured acromion. The operation failed. The patient complained of pain and severe limitation of shoulder motion.

quately thinned from its anterior edge as the bone is cut and tapered to the apex on the undersurface of the bone. It should not be shortened in any direction. Osteophytes and sharp edges of bone are removed. Large osteophytes are also removed from the undersurface of the lateral clavicle and medial acromion. If pain symptoms and findings referable to the acromioclavicular joint are present, the lateral clavicle and any osteophytes are resected.

In some rare cases, ectopic bone and osteophytes may form following an acromioplasty with recurring symptoms. In these cases, a revision acromioplasty may be required (Fig. 3.6).

Forestier and Rotes-Querol (3) described a type of ankylosing hyperostosis of the spine (14). Particularly in the thoracic region, there may be bony outgrowths in extraspinal locations. It must be differentiated from ankylosing spondylitis and osteoarthritis.

A thickened acromion or diffuse idiopathic skeletal hypertrophy (DISH syndrome) may be an extra-axial manifestation of this disorder. Thickened acromia (Fig. 3.7) must be adequately thinned and even tapered, extending posteriorly to avoid rough bone edges and later attrition of the rotator cuff. Failure to thin the acromion has been noted in re-

ferred cases who have had an attempt at an inadequate arthroscopic subacromial decompression. This is best done in an open procedure, in my opinion.

SUPRASCAPULAR NERVE INJURY

Occasionally, when the supraspinatus tendon is advanced by opening the superior capsule above the origin of the long head of the biceps, the suprascapular nerve can be damaged as it courses about the base of scapular spine. Accordingly, surgeons should recognize that the supraspinatus and its muscle tendon should not be dissected more than a distance of 2 cm medial to the superior glenoid rim for fear of causing nerve injury and additional weakening of the external rotator muscles.

FAILED ROTATOR CUFF REPAIR

In second reoperations it has been found that thickened, hypertrophied bursal tissue resembling diseased rotator cuff tissue has been closed over a rotator cuff defect in the mistaken belief that true rotator cuff tissue was being repaired. Scarred bursal tissue that may have filled the defect must be peeled back and resected from the underlying rotator cuff before an adequate closure can be performed. If the

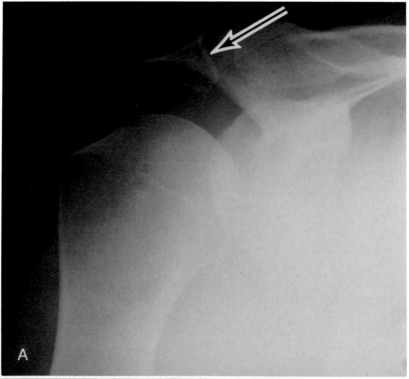

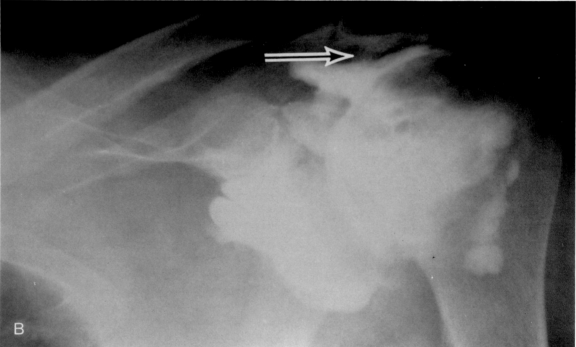

Figure 3.6.   **A**, A patient had a routine acromioplasty and seemed to make an uneventful recovery. Several months later, he developed increasing pain and a positive impingement sign in his shoulder. A roentgenogram showed ectopic bone formation (*arrow*) along the site of the resected coracoacromial ligament. A revision arthroplasty is being considered to relieve pain. **B**, An adult male underwent a repair of the rotator cuff and an acromioplasty and did well postoperatively for several months. Thereafter, the patient developed increasing weakness in the external rotators and a positive impingement sign. A new arthrogram showed a new tear of the cuff and an osteophyte that developed postoperatively on the undersurface of the acromion (*arrow*). Revision surgery was performed with good results.

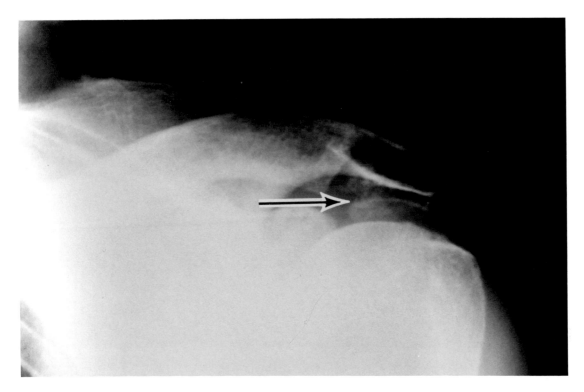

Figure 3.7. A middle-aged woman had a failed rotator cuff repair and an acromioplasty when the surgeon failed to recognize a thickened acromion and did not remove enough of the undersurface of the acromion (*arrow*). A sharp edge of acromion had been left on the undersurface of the acromion. An open revision arthroplasty and repair were done with good results.

defect cannot be closed primarily with ease, rotator cuff tissue may need to be mobilized by transposing the upper one-half of the subscapularis tendon, utilizing the long head of the biceps as an anchor point for rotator cuff edges, especially if it degenerated and dislocated from its groove, or advancing the infraspinatus or supraspinatus, if necessary (8, 12). I do not believe that synthetic grafts add to increasing rotator cuff function in very large defects. I have found that when massive tears cannot be closed in the presence of a good deltoid, subacromial decompression alone will permit active elevation because pain is relieved (Fig. 3.1). This is ordinarily adequate for activities of daily living.

The surgeon should not rely on a positive arthrogram as the only reason to repair a torn rotator cuff. Even in the presence of a normal arthrogram, weakened external rotator muscles may be more important in determining the need for an operation since the tear may be incomplete. When a significant surface or intimal tear is present, the diseased tissue should be resected and a primary repair performed. Similarly, if there is a thinned area of the rotator cuff, this may be detected by palpation or by injecting diluted methylene blue intra-articularly. If the blue dye

shows the extent of a thinned area, the diseased area should be resected and the cuff edges repaired.

Before repairing the torn rotator cuff edges, the inner surface of the cuff should be inspected to determine if intimal tears are present. Such tears of the cuff tissue should be differentiated from glenohumeral ligaments that occasionally may mimic true intimal tears. In any event, intimal tears should be repaired and the whole cuff edge treated as an unit during the repair. If the glenohumeral ligaments are torn, they should be carefully repaired if enough good tissue is present.

Tendons that are advanced during a repair should not be overstretched for fear of injuring the muscle tissues. Thus, excessive tension on these tissues must be avoided.

INFECTION

Should a postoperative infection occur, it must be eradicated as soon as possible to avoid serious damage to the rotator cuff structures and the joint itself. Sinus tracts must be entirely excised, even if it means excision of the deeper soft tissues. The function will depend upon residual muscle power. Preop-

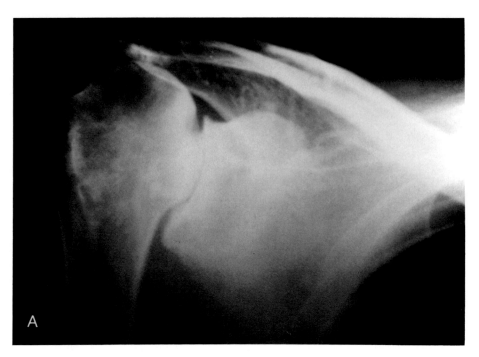

Figure 3.8. **A**, A 40-year-old man developed a postoperative infection following a rotator cuff repair. There were several failed surgical attempts to eradicate the infection. Function was poor. There was pain with joint motion. Eighteen months postoperatively, an extensive debridement of a sinus tract was performed after injection of dilute methylene blue. **B**, The sinus tract entered the joint and involved the entire rotator cuff, necessitating excision of the infected rotator cuff (*arrow*). **C**, **D**, There was excellent healing and excellent motion. The deltoid was strong. External rotator power was absent. The result was excellent. **E**, There was painless motion 2 years later in spite of the fact that severe joint degeneration had been present as a result of the infection. (Reprinted with permission from Post M. Complications of rotator cuff surgery. Clin Orthop, 1990;254:97–104.)

eratively, a sinus tract should be injected with radio-opaque dye and roentgenograms taken to demonstrate the extent of the tracts. The surgeon must not rely on this alone because closed soft tissue pockets may harbor infected material and not show on the film. Intra-operatively, dilute methylene blue is injected into the sinus tract before an incision is made. This makes it easy for the surgeon to resect all infected tissues. A meticulous resection of the involved tissues must be carried out if the infection is to be eradicated (Fig. 3.8).

Many complications can be avoided if the tissues are not damaged, a correct diagnosis is known, and careful surgical principles are followed. Once a complication arises, it should be treated adequately to lessen the sequelae.

References

1. Armstrong JR. Excision of the acromion in treatment of the supraspinatus syndrome. J Bone Joint Surg 1949;31B:436–442.
2. DeOrio JK, Cofield RH. Results of a second attempt at surgical repair of a failed initial rotator cuff repair. J Bone Joint Surg 1984;66A:563–567.
3. Forestier J, Rotes-Querol J. Senile ankylosing hyperstosis of the spine. Ann Rheum Dis 1950;9:321–330.
4. Hammond G. Complete acrominoectomy in the treatment of chronic tendinitis of the shoulder. A follow-up study of 90 patients. J Bone Joint Surg 1971;53A:173–200.
5. Mudge MK, Wood VE, Frykman GK. Rotator cuff tears associated with os acromiale. J Bone Joint Surg 1984;66A:427–429.
6. Neer CS II, Marberry TA. On the disadvantages of total acromionectomy. J Bone Joint Surg 1981;63A:416.
7. Neer CS. Anterior acromioplasty for the chronic impingement syndrome in the shoulder. A preliminary report. J Bone Joint Surg 1972;54A:41–50.
8. Neviaser RJ, Neviaser TJ. Transfer of subscapularis and teres minor for massive defects of rotator cuff. In: Bayley IB, Kessel L, eds. Shoulder surgery. Berlin: Springer-Verlag, 1982:60–69.
9. Post M, Silver R, Singh M. Rotator cuff tear—diagnosis and treatment. Clin Orthop 1983;173:78–91.
10. Post M. Roataor cuff repair with carbon filament polyactic acid. Clin Orthop 1985;196:154–158.
11. Post M, Cohen J. Impingement syndrome—diagnosis and management. Clin Orthop 1986;207:90–96.
12. Post M. The shoulder—surgical and nonsurgical management. 2nd ed. Philadelphia: Lea & Febiger, 1988.
13. Post M, Rabin SI. A comparative study of clinical muscle testing and Cybex evaluation following shoulder operations. In: Post M, Morrey B, Hawkins R, eds. Surgery of the shoulder. Chicago: Year Book, 1990:40–43.
14. Resnicke D, Shaul SR, Robins JM. Diffuse idiopathic skeletal hyperosis (DISH): Forestier's disease with extraspinal manifestations. Diag Radiol 1976;115:513–524.

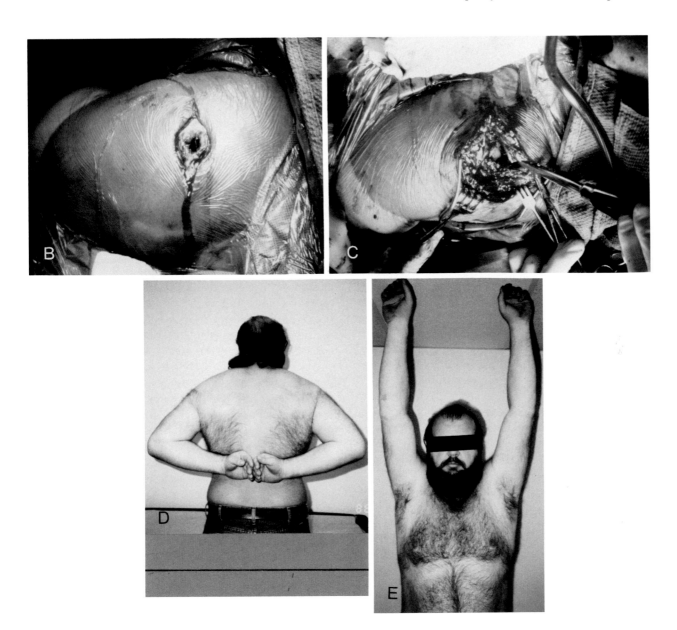

4

Rotator Cuff Tear Arthropathy

Frederick A. Matsen, III, Craig T. Arntz, and Douglas T. Harryman, II

INTRODUCTION

In 1983, Neer, Craig, and Fukuda (19) coined the term "cuff tear arthropathy" to denote the collapse the humeral articular surface in association with a massive rotator cuff defect. Their report described 26 cases; 75% were in females, with an average age of 69 years. These authors hypothesized that the arthropathy resulted from mechanical factors (such as anterior-posterior instability and superior migration of the humeral head) and nutritional factors, such as loss of a closed joint space, lack of normal diffusion of nutrients to the joint surface, and disuse.

In this chapter, we have taken the liberty of extending the definition of cuff tear arthropathy as follows: a degenerative condition of the glenohumeral joint characterized by (*a*) a massive rotator cuff defect; (*b*) upward displacement of the humeral head so that it articulates with the undersurface of the acromion; and (*c*) substantial loss of articular cartilage from the humeral head and upper glenoid (Fig. 4.1).

GLENOHUMERAL STABILITY

A primary feature of cuff tear arthropathy is the upward displacement of the humeral head with respect to the glenoid. It is thus important to consider the mechanisms by which the humeral head is normally stabilized in the glenoid. These considerations are paramount in the choice of options for treating this condition.

The rotator cuff is a major stabilizer of the humeral head in the shallow glenoid fossa. While it is frequently stated that the supraspinatus functions as a humeral head "depressor," the supraspinatus is not positioned to apply a significant inferiorly directed force to the humeral head. Even the infraspinatus and subscapularis are not well oriented to

provide humeral head depression. Thus, the stabilization of the humeral head by the rotator cuff seems more likely to occur by *compression* of the head of the humerus into the concave glenoid. This is analogous to the action of gravity stabilizing a golf ball on a concave golf tee. In the normal shoulder, this "concavity-compression" stabilizes the head of the humerus against displacing forces, such as the upward pull of the deltoid. One can demonstrate the concavity-compression effect with a simple experiment. In the relaxed normal shoulder, an examiner can passively translate the humeral head in an anterior, posterior, or inferior direction. However, the slightest contraction of the rotator cuff musculature makes it virtually impossible to passively translate the humeral head on the glenoid. Some recent experiments in our laboratory demonstrate that this mechanism is highly effective: a glenohumeral compressive force of 100 units can resist a superiorly directed force of over 66 units, if the glenoid articular cartilage and labrum are intact. Lesions of the glenoid labrum or loss of concavity of the glenoid articular surface compromise the concavity-compression mechanism, just as a chip in the lip of a golf tee renders the ball unstable.

It is interesting to note that this concavity-compression mechanism does not require an intact supraspinatus: it only requires that there is sufficient muscle action available to compress the humeral head into the glenoid. This is consistent with the observation that many patients with sizeable supraspinatus defects can center their humeral heads in the glenoid during active elevation of their arm. In these situations, it appears that the contraction of the remaining muscles compresses the humeral head into the glenoid concavity so that it is stabilized against the upward pull of the deltoid. In this chapter, we will refer to the stabilization of the humeral head in the glenoid fossa by factors such as

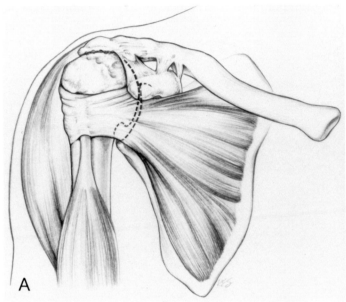

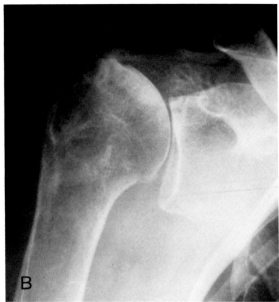

Figure 4.1. **A**, Anatomical changes typical of cuff tear arthropathy: A massive rotator cuff defect, upward displacement of the humeral head resulting in nonphysiologic contact of the humeral head with the coracoacromial arch, and substantial loss of the articular cartilage from the humeral head and upper glenoid. **B**, Roentgenogram showing some of these changes. The upward displacement of the humeral head that accompanies massive cuff deficiency results in localized contact between the head of the humerus and the superior rim of the glenoid.

concavity-compression as primary stabilization of the head of the humerus.

The anatomy of the shoulder also provides a backup or secondary stabilizing system when the primary mechanism is not functional (e.g., in severe rotator cuff deficiency) or overwhelmed (e.g., when a sudden large force is directed upward along the axis of the humerus). This secondary stability is provided by the acromion, the coracoid, and the coracoacromial ligament: the coracoacromial arch. This arch forms a backstop to the primary stabilization of the shoulder. As we will see subsequently, when one is considering an acromioplasty and coracoacromial ligament section, it is very important to first understand the degree to which the humerus is stabilized by this secondary mechanism. If the shoulder is dependent on the secondary stabilizing mechanism, the humeral head can be rendered unstable by acromioplasty and coracoacromial ligament section.

PATHOGENESIS

Rotator cuff failure appears to be an age-related degenerative disease. As patients get older, they have a higher risk of rotator cuff fiber failure, larger tears, poor-quality tissue, bilateral involvement, and a higher chance of retear after repair (4, 5, 9, 17, 21). These degenerative tears typically begin as partial-thickness tears in the anterior supraspinatus and then progress to full-thickness lesions of the supraspinatus. The infraspinatus is next in the succession, followed by the subscapularis. As the cuff defect becomes greater, the ability of the cuff musculature to stabilize the humeral head against the upward pull of the deltoid becomes less. As a result, the head of the humerus and any intervening residual cuff tissue are squeezed against the undersurface of the coracoacromial arch. The undersurface of the acromion, now under load, may become sclerotic (Fig. 4.2 A, B). The coracoacromial ligament is placed under tension, and a traction spur may develop in it (18). The impingement of the acromion on residual cuff tissues hastens their dissolution. The more the cuff fails, the less the head is stabilized and the more the humeral head rides upwards (Fig. 4.2 C, D). The upwardly displaced humeral head may sculpt a concavity in the undersurface of the acromion. This sculpting may continue until the acromioclavicular joint is involved.

When the humeral head comes in contact with the coracoacromial arch, it becomes secondarily stabilized against the deltoid pull. This may allow a surprising degree of function for a shoulder with little remaining cuff tissue. However, secondary stabilization may take its toll: nonphysiologic contact of the humeral articular surface with the acromion leads to

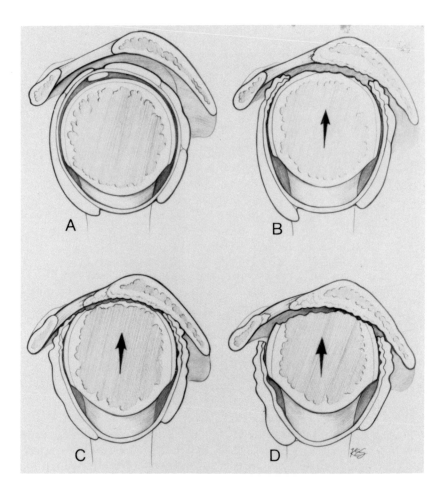

Figure 4.2.   The pathogenesis of rotator cuff tear arthropathy. **A**, Normal anatomy. **B**, Progressive cuff fiber failure accompanied by upward displacement of the humeral head "loading" the undersurface of the acromion. The coracoacromial ligament is placed under tension, and a traction spur may develop in it. The impingement of the acromion on residual cuff tissue hastens its dissolution (**C** and **D**). The more the cuff fails, the less the head is stabilized and the more the humeral head rides upwards, causing progressive arthropathy.

abrasion of the hyaline cartilage. The result is an arthropathy that starts at the superior lateral aspect of the humeral head and extends to involve more and more of the humeral articular surface. Thus, while the secondary stabilizing mechanism may provide stability against which the deltoid can function to elevate the arm, this stability comes at the cost of wear of the articular cartilage on the head of the humerus.

Wear also tends to occur in another location. Because the humeral head and the glenoid have essentially the same radius of curvature, displacement of the humerus relative to the glenoid will result in a sharply narrowed contact area at the glenoid rim. Thus, the upward displacement of the humeral head that commonly accompanies massive cuff deficiency results in concentrated contact pressures between the head of the humerus and the superior rim of the glenoid. The effect of this localized contact is not only accelerated wear of the articular surface of the humerus, but also wear of the superior lip of the glenoid (Fig. 4.1B). This superior glenoid wear lessens even further the stability of the glenohumeral joint by depriving the glenoid of its superior concavity.

Repeated abrasion of the tuberosities (no longer protected by rotator cuff) under the coracoacromial arch smooths them off, making the proximal humerus progressively more round, like a femoral head ("femoralization") (Fig. 4.3A). Erosion of the superior aspect of the glenoid and the undersurface of the acromion, along with the formation of a traction osteophyte in the coracoacromial ligament, can progress to form a deep, acetabulum-like socket for the head of the humerus ("acetabularization") (Fig. 4.3B).

In summary, we base our management on the following concept of pathogenesis:

- Cuff fiber failure is predominantly a degenerative process; chronic, massive cuff defects in older people may not be amenable to durable cuff repair;
- Loss of the normal strength of the rotator cuff mechanism may jeopardize the primary stability from dynamic compression of the humeral head into the concave glenoid;
- When this primary stabilizing mechanism is absent, secondary stability may be provided by contact between the head of the humerus and the coracoacromial arch;
- Contact between the head of the humerus and the coracoacromial arch may result in traction spurring in the coracoacromial ligament;
- Prolonged compression of the uncovered humeral articular cartilage against the undersurface of the coracoacromial arch and against the upper lip of the glenoid may shear off the articular cartilage, producing an arthropathy.

DIAGNOSIS

Cuff tear arthropathy is the end stage of cuff degeneration, where the loss of cuff function leads to the destruction of the glenohumeral joint. It usually occurs in patients over 60 years of age. The history reveals progressive, atraumatic loss of strength, comfort, and function of the shoulder. The physical examination shows weakness of external rotation, atrophy of the spinatus muscles, a mild to moderate effusion, and glenohumeral crepitance. Standard radiographs (an anteroposterior view in the plane of the scapula, a 35° external rotation view of the proximal humerus, and an axillary view) are usually the only imaging modalities required. Magnetic resonance imaging, arthrograms, and ultrasonography are not necessary in diagnosing this end-stage process.

We suspect the diagnosis of cuff tear arthrop-

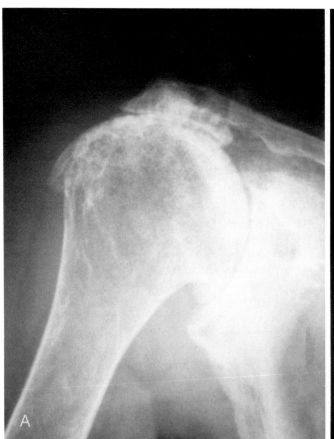
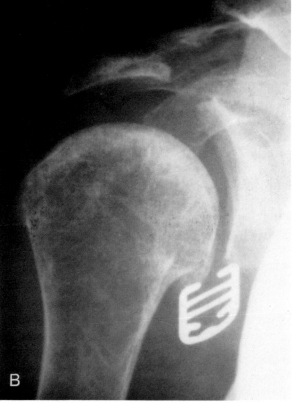

Figure 4.3. **A**, Roentgenographic features of cuff tear arthropathy: upward displacement of the humeral head with respect to the glenoid, bone-on-bone contact at the undersurface of the acromion, erosion of the upper glenoid fossa, "femoralization" of the proximal humerus, and "acetabularization" of the coracoacromial arch. **B**, These changes are particularly well seen on a traction view.

athy when the following are present: (*a*) chronic, massive cuff deficiency; (*b*) upward displacement of the humeral head with respect to the glenoid; and (*c*) bone-on-bone contact between the humeral head and the undersurface of the acromion.

Other features that may accompany this diagnosis include:

• Erosion of the upper glenoid fossa;
• Rounding off of the tuberosities ("femoralization" of the proximal humerus); and
• Formation of a socket from the acromion, coracoacromial ligament, and upper glenoid ("acetabularization")

It is important to take a thorough history. Previous surgery that may have affected the integrity of the deltoid or the acromion, how many steroid injections the patient has had into the shoulder, and whether the patient has had any evidence of shoulder joint sepsis, are all critical factors in the diagnosis and management.

DIFFERENTIAL DIAGNOSIS

Recognizing this end-stage condition with all of its characteristic manifestations is not difficult. There are, however, some other conditions that need to be excluded from the differential diagnosis, including Milwaukee shoulder, neuropathic arthropathy, and septic arthropathy. Milwaukee shoulder (11, 12, 14–16) may actually be the same condition as cuff tear arthropathy. It is reported to be characterized by synovial crystals of calcium hydroxyapatite. Neuropathic arthropathy is most commonly due to syringomyelia (13, 20), which characteristically is associated with loss of temperature and pain sensibility in the hands. An MRI of the cervical spine is usually diagnostic. Septic arthritis (1, 3) most often occurs in someone who has diminished defenses. It is diagnosed by a Gram's stain, culture, and sensitivity of the joint aspirate.

NONOPERATIVE TREATMENT

The presence of characteristic radiographic findings of cuff tear arthropathy does not mandate surgical treatment. Some patients with striking x-rays also have strikingly functional shoulders. If pain is not a substantial problem, nonoperative management with gentle strengthening of the anterior deltoid muscle may increase the functionality of the joint.

SURGICAL MANAGEMENT

There is no perfect surgical treatment for this condition. Every method of surgical reconstruction has substantial disadvantages. Nevertheless, in certain circumstances, surgery can be beneficial. The following guidelines are helpful in determining the various surgical alternatives.

Debridement/Acromioplasty

In cuff tear arthropathy, by definition, the joint surface of the glenohumeral joint is lost. Thus, it is unlikely that debridement or acromioplasty is likely to be of benefit in relieving symptoms or improving function. Furthermore, acromioplasty with resection of the coracoacromial ligament may deprive the humeral head of its secondary stabilizing mechanism. In fact, we have seen patients whose cuff tear arthropathic shoulders were rendered less functional and less comfortable by acromioplasty (Fig. 4.4A). This is even more true if the quality of the deltoid attachment to the acromion or the innervation of part of this muscle is compromised.

Arthrodesis

Arthrodesis achieves a stable glenohumeral joint, but sacrifices deltoid function. Equally important, arthrodesis deprives the glenohumeral joint of rotation that is crucial to activities of daily living, such as perineal care. Recognizing that cuff degeneration is often a bilateral process, the shoulder contralateral to one involved with cuff tear arthropathy is frequently abnormal as well. A final argument against arthrodesis is that the patient with cuff tear arthropathy is often elderly, a fact that creates concern about both the quality of the bone and the tolerance for cast immobilization.

Arthrodesis becomes an important consideration in shoulders with a deltoid that has been damaged, detached, or denervated by previous surgical attempts. In this situation, there may be insufficient muscle about the glenohumeral joint to empower or stabilize an arthroplasty.

TECHNIQUE

Arthrodesis for cuff tear arthropathy requires several special considerations. If the patient has any degree of pulmonary compromise, his/her tolerance for spica cast immobilization must be assessed preoperatively. Elderly bone may make rigid internal

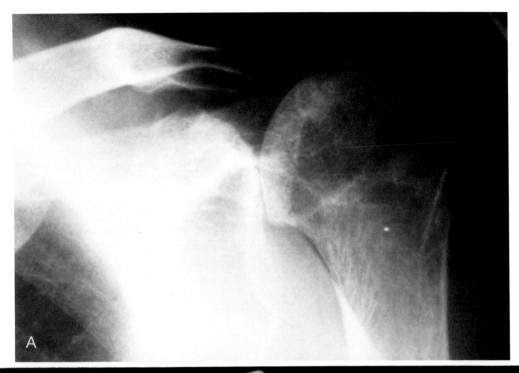

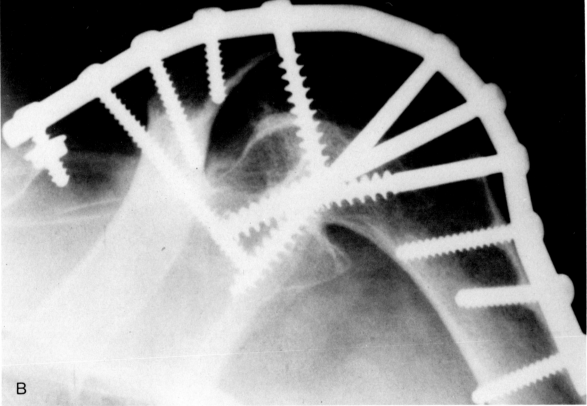

Figure 4.4. **A**, Anteroposterior radiograph of a 57-year-old male with disabling left shoulder pain after two failed rotator cuff repair attempts. Deltoid function and secondary stability had been significantly compro-mised after acromioplasty. **B**, Anteroposterior roentgenogram 4½ years after successful glenohumeral arthrodesis. This patient reported pain only after unusual activity.

fixation more difficult. Patients with abnormal function of the opposite shoulder may have difficulty with the loss of function attendant to a shoulder arthrodesis. The position of fusion must consider the functional demands on the specific extremity being treated in light of the overall functional requirements of the patient. We have found that a fusion position of 15° of flexion, 15° of abduction, and 45° of internal rotation allows performance of some of the important activities of daily living, such as reaching the mouth and the opposite axilla. However, reaching the perineum is difficult with this position unless there is great flexibility at the scapulothoracic joint. This relatively low position of fusion has the additional advantage of not requiring retraction of the scapula to put the arm at the side. In more flexed and abducted positions, the retraction required for putting the arm at the side can make sitting in a straight-backed chair or lying supine difficult.

Even though the deltoid cannot move the shoulder after an arthrodesis, it is desirable to preserve as much of its integrity as possible. A reattached, innervated and vascularized deltoid provides important soft tissue coverage and improved cosmetics for a fused shoulder.

Internal fixation may consist of three humeroglenoid and one acromiohumeral cancellous screws, if the quality of the bone is good. If the quality of fixation is in doubt, a neutralization plate may be added across the scapular spine and down the humeral shaft (Fig. 4.4B).

RESULTS

The literature reveals that fusion for patients with chronic cuff disease yields some improvements in comfort and function, but that the results are not always predictable (6–8). We had the opportunity to review 10 of our patients who had shoulder arthrodesis for the combination of massive cuff deficiency and loss of glenohumeral articular cartilage. None of them was known to have rheumatoid arthritis, neuropathic arthropathy, or metabolic abnormalities. Nine of the ten had at least one prior unsuccessful attempt at cuff repair. Six of these had undergone two or more previous repair attempts. One of these shoulders had developed a staphylococcus infection after a second rotator cuff repair; there was no evidence of residual infection at the time of shoulder arthrodesis 8 months later. Significant deltoid deficiency was a characteristic of many of these shoulders.

Spica casting was used for an average of 3 months in the six shoulders with compression screw

fixation alone. The five shoulders with tension band plate fixation were protected only with an abduction bolster.

Results were judged by the American Shoulder and Elbow Surgeons evaluation protocol (2). Preoperatively, pain was marked in five and disabling in five. Postoperatively, five patients had slight to no pain and three had pain after unusual activities; two had moderate to marked pain early in the postoperative period related in a delayed union. One had been initially treated with compression screws and spica casting for 3 months; the other patient had compression screws and a tension band plate with no cast postoperatively. These patients underwent subsequent bone graft and repeat fixation at 2 and 5 months after their initial procedures, respectively.

On final follow-up these patients had no significant pain and a solid clinical and radiographic arthrodesis. One patient with disabling pain preoperatively reported moderate pain in follow-up. Two patients required additional surgery to remove prominent fixation hardware after achieving solid shoulder arthrodesis.

Radiographically, nine shoulders showed evidence of a solid fusion at final follow-up with bony trabecula bridging the glenohumeral joint space. One shoulder showed dense periarticular bone with persistence of a radiolucent line at the joint space.

Active range of flexion improved an average of 15° from 51 to 66° (range 35–75° degrees). Not surprisingly, passive flexion decreased from a preoperative average of 88° to a postoperative average of 76° (range 52–94°). Active external rotation remained unchanged at −10°.

Four patients were able to wash the opposite axilla before surgery; eight were able to do so after surgery. Preoperatively, no patients could comb their hair, whereas seven could perform this function after surgery. No patients were able to sleep on their side before surgery, whereas six could do this after surgery. Preoperatively, three patients could perform perineal care, while only only two patients could perform this function after surgery. No patients could use their hand above shoulder level, either before or after their shoulder fusion.

Of the 10 patients available for follow-up, four rated their shoulders as much better than before surgery, five as better, and one as unchanged.

Total Shoulder Arthroplasty

In theory, total shoulder arthroplasty presents to the patient with loss of glenohumeral articular cartilage an excellent opportunity for a comfortable and functional shoulder. In a mechanically sound total shoulder, there is contact only between the prosthetic head and the prosthetic glenoid so that metal on bone contact is avoided. In cuff tear arthropathy, however, normal mechanics are compromised by the lack of stabilization of the humeral head in its normal relation to the glenoid. Characteristically, the shoulder is stabilized only by the secondary mechanism of contact between the humeral head and coracoacrominal arch. In shoulder arthroplasty, this creates a variety of biomechanical problems. In the first place, there is no proven method for durable resurfacing of the acromiohumeral "joint." Even though attempts have been made to insert prostheses in this interval or to use glenoid components with an exaggerated upper lip, no long-term follow-up of substantial numbers of successful cases have been reported. Secondly, with upward riding of the head of the humerus relative to the glenoid, a glenoid component placed in the standard location is at

risk for rim contact with the attendant problems of cold flow of the polyethylene, loosening of the glenoid component via the "rocking horse" mechanism (2, 10) and rim wear (Figs. 4.5 and 4.6). These problems are particularly severe when the glenoid and humeral components are of identical radius. In this situation, no superior translation can occur without having rim contact at the glenoid. Although some glenoid components are designed to allow for a certain amount of humeral head translation, the effectiveness of these component systems in managing cuff tear arthropathy has not been demonstrated.

The surgeon has the option to place the glenoid component in a higher than normal position so that the humeral head stabilized by the secondary mechanism will come to lie against the center of the glenoid component. The problem here is that the bony glenoid becomes narrower and more anteriorly inclined at its superior extent. Therefore, the fixation of the glenoid component is jeopardized by the minimal

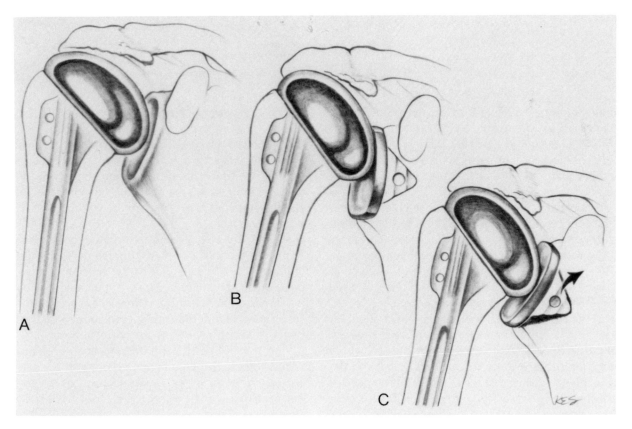

Figure 4.5. Biomechanical problems associated with the use of shoulder arthroplasty in the management of cuff tear arthropathy. **A**, The humeral component rides upwards to contact the acromion. **B**, The incidence of glenoid component loosening is high when total shoulder arthroplasty is used in shoulders where chronic rotator cuff insufficiency allows upward displacement of the head with respect to the glenoid. **C**, This upward displacement results in rim contact with the attendant problems of cold flow, rim wear, and loosening of the glenoid component via the "rocking horse" mechanism.

Figure   4.6. Roentgenogram demonstrating rocking horse loosening.

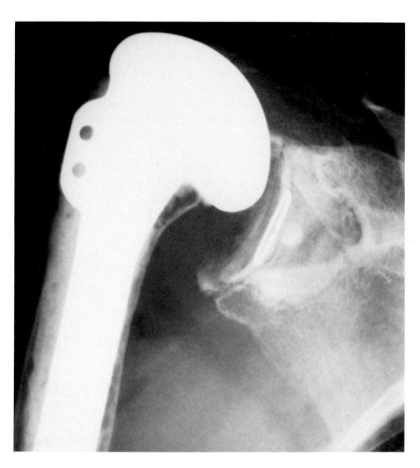

amount of bone available for securing it in this elevated position.

It has been observed that the incidence of glenoid component loosening is high when total shoulder arthroplasty is performed in the presence of a substantial rotator cuff defect (2, 10). Therefore, in this situation, the surgeon needs to judge whether or not there is sufficient potential for recreating concavity-compression. In our experience it is quite rare for the rotator cuff to be reconstructible in cases of cuff tear arthropathy. Thus, it remains likely that the head will translate superiorly until it is stabilized by contact with the coracoacromial arch.

Our current practice is to use total shoulder arthroplasty in the management of cuff tear arthropathy only in the relatively rare patient where the cuff is either reconstructible or where the residual cuff looks strong enough to stabilize the head of the humerus by concavity-compression. In this situation, the patient needs to be aware of the increased risk of glenoid component loosening. Particular care must be taken to optimize the position of the glenoid component both to the bone stock available and to the position assumed by the head of the humerus.

Special Hemiarthroplasty

For the surgical treatment of most shoulders with cuff tear arthropathy and a functionally intact deltoid, we prefer a special hemiarthroplasty. This procedure does not require the "down time" of a shoulder fusion. It is usually more comfortable than a shoulder fusion and has superior cosmetics. Rather than a prosthetic glenoid, it utilizes the "acetabulum" scupted in the coracoacromial glenoid arch for stability; thus, it does not carry the risk of glenoid component loosening. Most importantly, special hemiarthroplasty has the potential for a substantial restoration of function and does not eliminate the internal rotation necessary for perineal care.

Conventionally, hemiarthroplasty is used in situations where the glenoid and rotator cuff are intact, such as in fractures, avascular necrosis, or in certain patterns of arthrosis where the glenoid articular cartilage is relatively spared. In the situation of cuff tear arthropathy, this is truly a "special" hemiarthroplasty because the surgeon is attempting to resurface the humeral aspects of not only the glenohumeral joint but also the "acromial humeral" joint (Fig. 4.7A, B). Since the socket is already fashioned

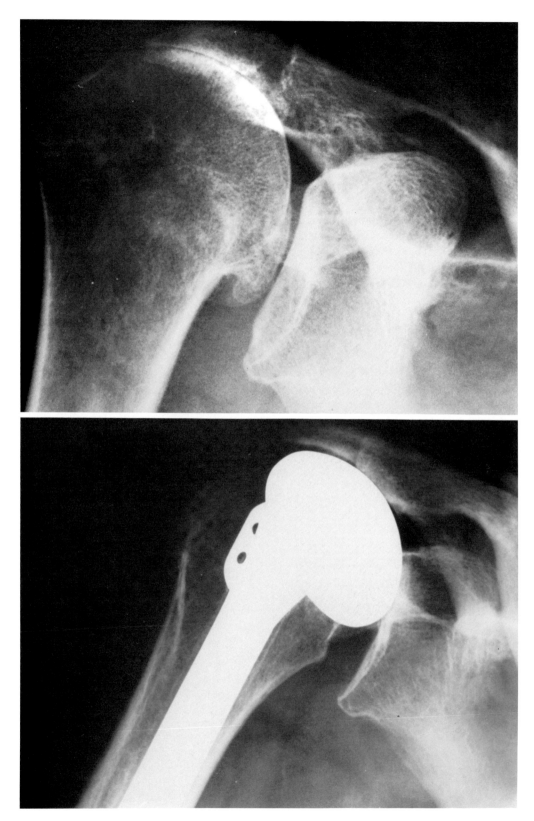

Figure 4.7.   A, Cuff tear arthropathy. **B**, Glenohumeral and acromiohumeral resurfacing using special hemiarthroplasty.

by the previous wear of the biologic humeral head, there is usually no need for further sculpting of this area. Even though the glenoid is not resurfaced, the surface area available for articulation of the humeral head is expanded over the physiologic situation to include the acromion, coracoacromial ligament, and the upper part of the glenoid. This broad contact area reduces the force per unit area. We suspect that this reduced contact pressure enhances the comfort and the quality of the result in special hemiarthroplasty.

Contraindications to special hemiarthroplasty include: (a) sepsis; (b) a deficient, damaged, or denervated deltoid; or (c) a coracoacromial "socket" that has been compromised by an extensive acromioplasty and coracoacromial ligament section. Deficiency of the anterior acromion and coracoacromial ligament can give rise to an anterosuperior instability that defunctionalizes the shoulder. In the situation of serious deltoid compromise or anterosuperior instability, a glenohumeral arthrodesis becomes a more attractive surgical alternative.

TECHNIQUE

We prefer a brachial plexus block as the anesthetic. In older, less robust patients, it has particular value in minimizing the need for systemic medication and ventilatory support. It also provides about 18 hours of postoperative analgesia during which the patient can see how smoothly and easily the new joint can be moved. Hemiarthroplasty is performed through a standard anterior dectopectoral incision. During this procedure, the deltoid is protected with extreme vigilance. The thickened walls of the subacromial-subdeltoid bursa are excised. The humeral head is resected in 35° of retroversion at an angle of 45° with the long axis of the humeral shaft. The canal is reamed to provide the best prosthetic stem fit. The prosthesis head and neck that come closest to duplicating the location of the humeral joint surface are selected (Fig. 4.8 A, B). In this position, the prosthetic joint surface will neither tighten nor loosen the soft tissues about the glenohumeral joint. Furthermore, a humeral prosthesis that duplicates the size of the resected head will come closest to fitting the coracoacromio-glenoid socket. Excessive tightness is to be avoided in this procedure. The temptation to use oversized or bipolar components is to be avoided. As we were going through the learning curve on this procedure, we used a prosthesis with a 15-mm head and neck thickness in two cases, a prosthesis with a 22-mm head and neck thickness in seven cases, and a prosthesis with a 28-mm head and neck thickness in three cases. More recently, we have recognized the importance of adequate soft tissue

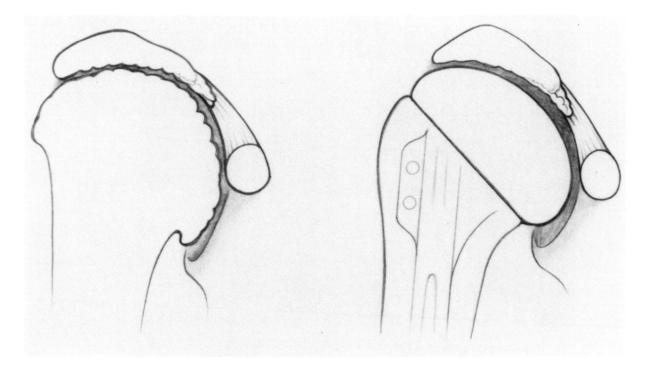

Figure 4.8.   A special hemiarthroplasty resurfaces, but does not tense or extend the joint.

laxity and have tended toward the lower end of the head and neck size spectrum. A number of checks are helpful in making sure the humeral component is not too big: (a) the surgeon should be able to posteriorly translate the humeral prosthesis on the glenoid by 50% of its head diameter; and (b) the surgeon should be able to internally rotate the abducted arm to 90°.

We have not found reparable rotator cuffs in our patients with cuff tear arthropathy. We have not performed rotator cuff tendon transfers, interpositional grafts, latissimus dorsi, teres major or trapezius transfers, or other types of attempted cuff reconstruction in conjunction with special hemiarthroplasty.

Prior to the final insertion of the humeral component, it is desirable to assure smoothness of the coracoacromio-glenoid socket. It is also advisable to resect any prominent parts of the greater tuberosity that impinge against the acromion. Any potentially interfering debris, scar, sutures from previous cuff repair attempts, and other nonfunctional tissues are removed as well.

At the time of closure, the security of the deltoid is assured. Drains are placed and brought out through long soft tissue tracks. In patients that had substantial joint and bursal effusions preoperatively, it is critical to place large drains and to leave them in position until the production of fluid is minimal.

POSTOPERATIVE MANAGEMENT:

In the routine case, we institute immediate postoperative continuous passive motion (CPM). We use an eccentric cam/overhead pulley system to raise the arm from 0 to 90° of flexion. CPM is started while the patient is in the recovery room and continued for 20 of the next 36 hours. The patient can discontinue CPM at any time to get out of bed or to perform activities of daily living or early assisted range of motion exercises. The early exercise program includes assisted elevation and assisted external rotation. Because there is virtually nothing to heal about this operation except the skin, these patients can start using the hand and arm for activities of daily living as soon as they wish after the procedure. A sling is not used after day 2. We usually keep the patients hospitalized until they can demonstrate assisted forward evaluation of 140°, assisted external rotation to 40°, and internal rotation to the perineum. Hand gripping and deltoid isometric exercises are started immediately after surgery. One of the nice things about this procedure is that it is not necessary to instruct these patients to avoid activities

nor to immobilize their shoulders. Because these patients are often elderly and may have compromise of the contralateral extremity, the benefit that this "early function" program offers is apparent.

In our initial series of 10 patients having hemiarthroplasty for cuff tear arthroplasty, our average follow-up was 41 months (range 21–120 months). Preoperatively, eight of these patients had marked or disabling pain. Postoperatively six had only slight pain, and four patients had pain only after unusual activities (Fig. 4.9).

Active range of flexion improved from a preoperative average of 71° (range 50–100°) to a postoperative average of 115° (range 50–160°). Passive range of forward flexion improved an average of 18°. The range of passive external rotation improved from an average of 30 to 41°; the range of internal rotation improved by four body segments, that is, from being able to touch the spine of L5 to reaching L1.

The patients' ability to perform five activities of daily living (comb hair, wash opposite axilla, perform perennial care, use hand above shoulder level, and sleep on the affective side) were compared before and after surgery. With respect to perineal care, only two could perform this function before surgery and

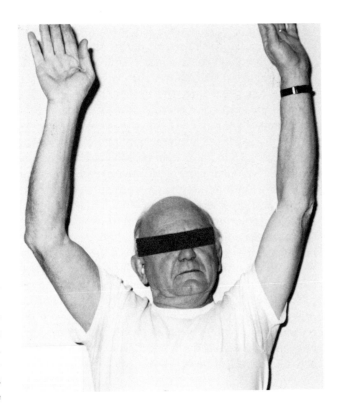

Figure 4.9. A 69-year-old man successfully returned to competitive horseshoe pitching after a special hemiarthroplasty of his right shoulder.

nine could do so after surgery. The ability to reach the opposite axilla improved from three to 10 shoulders. Preoperatively, only two patients could comb their hair, whereas eight could do so after surgery. The ability to sleep on the affected side improved from two to nine shoulders. The ability to use the affected shoulder above shoulder level improved from zero to six. While this series was not prospectively matched to that of shoulder fusions described above, the difference in comfort and function between these two groups is striking.

One patient with disabling pain preoperatively reported marked pain at follow-up and underwent revision surgery, as described below. Another patient who attained a superb result with respect to comfort and function fell 7 months after surgery, sustaining a displaced acromial fracture (Fig. 4.10). Despite open reduction and internal fixation of the shoulder, she failed to recover the function demonstrated prior to the fall.

All the patients felt they benefited from the procedure. Eight described the results as "much better" than before the surgery, and two as "better." The radiographic evaluation indicated no evidence of humeral component loosening at follow-up. In addition to the patient requiring open reduction internal fixation of a fractured acromion, one additional patient required surgery. This was a 79-year-old woman, who was treated with humeral hemiarthroplasty for marked shoulder pain resulting from a massive cuff defect and classic cuff tear arthropathy. Three years prior to her procedure, the patient had undergone surgical and radiation therapy for ipsilateral breast carcinoma. Pain relief and function were rated as excellent 1 year after humeral hemiarthroplasty. Approximately 15 months postoperatively, however, the patient developed a problem with progressive pain and loss of motion associated with substantial erosion of the superior half the glenoid. The patient's previous radiation therapy may have contributed to the problem of glenoid erosion. Nineteen months after the initial procedure, we revised the hemiarthroplasty in an attempt to loosen the glenoid humeral joint by releasing scar tissue, mobilization of the remaining cuff tissues, and recessing the humeral articular surface. At final follow-up, 17 months after revision, the patient was improved, reporting pain only after unusual activities and demonstrating 85° of active and 135° of passive forward elevation.

CONCLUSION

Cuff tear arthropathy is an end-stage result of the mechanical instability seen in the presence of massive degeneration of the rotator cuff. In the presence of a working deltoid muscle and secondary stabilization of the humeral head by the coracoacromial arch, substantial comfort and function can be restored by resurfacing (but not enlarging) the humeral articular surface with a special hemiarthroplasty. In this procedure, preservation of the coracoacromio-glenoid socket is essential to the stability of the articulation. The deltoid must also be preserved: "If you have a deltoid, you have a shoulder".

References

1. Baker GL, Oddis CV, Medsger TA, Jr. Pasteurella multocida polyarticular septic arthritis. J Rheumatol 1987;14:355–357.
2. Barrett WP, Franklin JL, Jackins SE, et al. Total shoulder arthroplasty. J Bone Joint Surg 1987;69A:865–872.
3. Burdge DR, Reid GD, Reeve CE, et al. Septic arthritis due to dual infection with mycoplasma hominis and ureaplasma urealyticum. J Rheumatol 1988;15:366–368.
4. Codman EA. Complete rupture of the supraspinatus tendon. Operative treatment with report of two successful cases. Boston Med Surg J 1911;164:708–710.
5. Codman EA. The shoulder, rupture of the supraspinatus tendon and other lesions in or about the subacromial bursa. Boston: Thomas Todd, 1934.
6. Cofield RH. Arthrodesis and resection arthroplasty of the shoulder. In: McCollister Evarts C, ed. Surgery of the musculosketal system. New York: Churchill Livingstone, 1983: 109–124.
7. Cofield RH. Total shoulder arthroplasty with the Neer prosthesis. J Bone Joint Surg 1984;66A:899–906.
8. Cofield RH. Shoulder arthrodesis and resection arthroplasty. AAOS Instruct Course Lecture 1985;34:268–277.
9. DePalma AF. Surgery of the shoulder. 2nd ed. Philadelphia: JB Lippincott, 1973.
10. Franklin JL, Barrett WP, Jackins SE, Matsen FA, III. Glenoid loosening in the total shoulder arthroplasty. J Arthroplasty 1988;3:39–46.
11. Garancis JC, Cheung HS, Halverson PB, McCarty DJ. Milwaukee shoulder—association of microspheroids containing hydroxyapatite crystals, active collagenase, and neutral protease with rotator cuff defects. Arthritis Rheum 1981;24:484–491.
12. Halverson PB, Cheung HS, McCarty DJ, et al. Milwaukee shoulder—association of microspheroids containing hydroxyapatite crystals, active collagenase, and neutral protease with rotator cuff defects, II. Synovial fluid studies. Arthritis Rheum 1981;24:474–483.
13. Maui H, Nebinger G. Arthropathy of the shoulder joint in syringomyeila. J Orthop 1986;124:157–164.
14. McCarty DJ, Halverson PB, Carrera GF, et al. Milwaukee shoulder—association of microspheroids containing hydroxyapatite crystals, active collagenase, and neutral protease with rotator cuff defects. I. Clinical aspects. Arthritis Rheum 1981;24:464–473.
15. McCarty DJ, Halverson PB, Carrera GF, et al. Milwaukee shoulder—association of microspheroids containing hydroxyapatite crystals, active collagenase, and neutral protease with rotator cuff defects. I. Clinical aspects. Arthritis Rheum 1981;24:353–354.

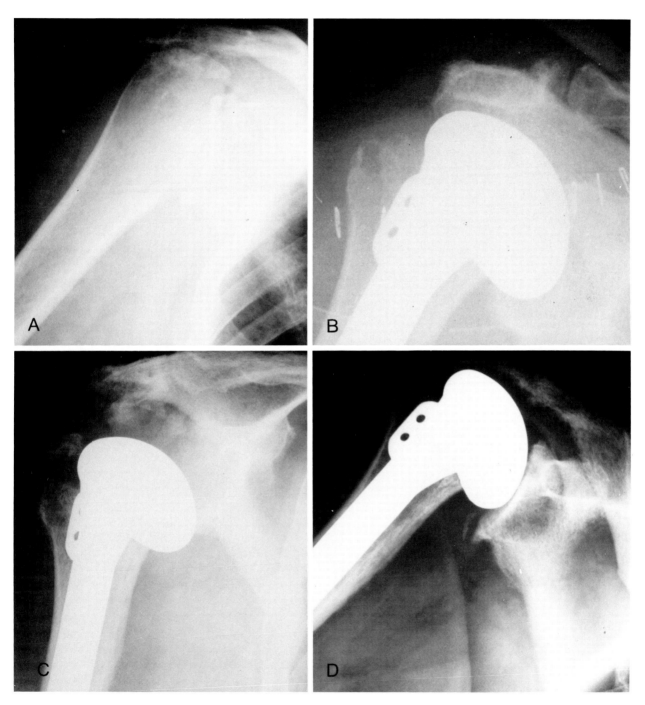

Figure 4.10. **A**, Anteroposterior roentgenogram of a 79-year-old woman with cuff tear arthropathy. **B**, Postoperative roentgenogram. **C**, 7 months after a successful arthroplasty, the patient fell, fracturing her acromion. **D**, Despite an anatomic reduction and secure fixation, the shoulder failed to recover the function demonstrated prior to the fall.

16. McCarty DJ. Crystals, joints and consternation. Ann Rheum Dis 1983;42:243–253.

17. Meyer AW. Further evidence of attrition in the human body. Am J Anat 1924;34:241–267.

18. Neer CS, II. Anterior acromioplasty for the chronic impingement syndrome in the shoulder. J Bone Joint Surg 1972;54A:41.

19. Neer CS, II, Craig EV, Fukuda H. Cuff-tear arthropathy. J Bone Joint Surg 1983;65A:1232–1244.

20. Tully JG, Jr, Latteri A. Paraplegia, syringomydia tarda and neuropathic arthrosis of the shoulder: a triad. Clin Orthop 1978;134:244–248.

21. Watson M. Major ruptures of the rotator cuff. The results of surgical repair in 89 patients. J Bone Joint Surg 1985;67B:618–624.

5
Complications of Total Shoulder Replacement

Seth R. Miller and Louis U. Bigliani

INTRODUCTION

The French surgeon Pean performed the first reported prosthetic arthroplasty of the shoulder in 1893 for tuberculosis (17). Although this platinum and rubber prosthesis required removal 2 years later for uncontrolled infection, today the success of unconstrained total shoulder replacement is well established. Five recent series of nonconstrained total shoulder replacements totalling 329 arthroplasties with an average follow-up of 46 months had only a 8.2% overall revision rate (3–5, 7, 11). One additional series, including 615 total shoulder replacements of which more than half of the patients were under 60 years of age, reported a 3.6% revision rate (22). This is quite favorable since these series represented first-generation total shoulder replacements and included more complex reconstructive problems as well as primary degenerative disease. The techniques and indications for total shoulder replacement have evolved to the point that glenohumeral arthrodesis or resection is now rarely required.

The initial total shoulder arthroplasties were of the constrained design (14, 16, 25, 26). The stability achieved by a "fixed fulcrum" design was considered important to substitute for a deficient rotator cuff. However, these implants have been associated with a high rate of mechanical failure and do not reliably reproduce cuff function. Furthermore, the rotator cuff is intact or able to be repaired in most situations requiring a total shoulder arthroplasty. There are very few large series reporting clinical results of constrained arthroplasty and in these series with limited follow-up, the results are not encouraging (14, 16, 25). Thus, today constrained replacements and their inherent complications are rarely indicated (26). In 1973, Neer redesigned his original humeral fracture prosthesis and added a polyethylene glenoid component to create an unconstrained total shoulder replacement (21). This prosthesis was developed to maintain near normal anatomy and had no mechanical constraints. Kenmore, et al. also reported on the use of a polyethylene glenoid liner with the Neer humeral prosthesis in 1974 (13). Today, the Neer unconstrained design is the most commonly used total shoulder arthroplasty. It is fortunate during this early period of total shoulder replacement that the incidence of complications has been less common than for other major joints. However, when they occur, the sequel can be profound. Complications encompass a wide range and can be specific to certain diagnosis.

EVALUATION

The evaluation of complications following a total shoulder replacement should be as thorough as the initial workup for a primary replacement. A complete history, including previous operative notes and physical examination, is essential. Pain, tenderness, and loss of function must be determined. The presence of deformity, neurological injury, infection, instability, and loss of motion must be clearly outlined. If infection is being considered, diagnostic laboratory tests including a CBC and ESR, as well as an aspiration should be considered.

Also, a complete shoulder series is needed including an AP in the plane of the scapula in internal rotation, neutral, external rotation, a scapular lateral or outlet view, and an axillary view. The AP views help delineate the relationship of the humeral head prosthesis to the shaft and tuberosities as well as the superior and inferior position in reference to the glenoid. Also, glenoid loosening can be evaluated on the AP views. Rotational views are helpful to outline tuberosity displacement or ectopic bone formation. The axillary view will detect anterior or posterior dislocation of the humeral head as well as displacement of the glenoid prosthesis (Fig. 5.1). The

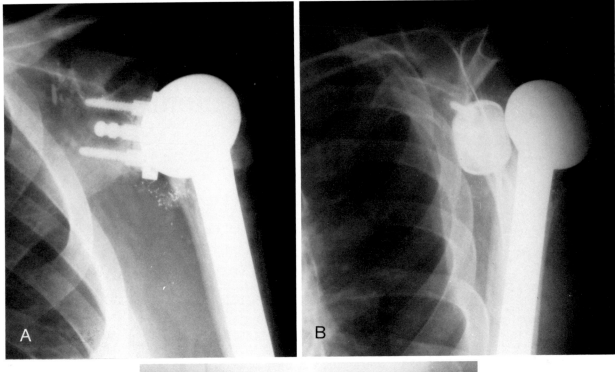

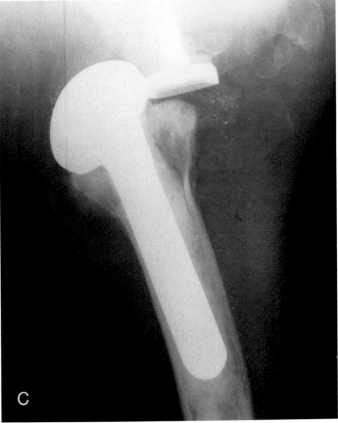

Figure 5.1. The patient sustained a posterior dislocation of the humeral prosthesis secondary to excessive retroversion of the humeral component. **A,** The AP radiograph is not diagnostic. **B,** The lateral x-ray taken in the plane of the scapula demonstrates the posterior dislocation. **C,** However, the axillary clearly shows the posterior dislocation. The humeral component was revised and placed in less retroversion, and a stable prosthesis resulted.

supraspinatus outlet view, a lateral in the scapula plane, will reveal any subacromial impingement lesion.

An arthrogram is useful to evaluate the rotator cuff for complete-thickness rotator cuff tears (Fig. 5.2). Also, loosening may be appreciated if the dye leaks between the cement bone interface. A CT scan may also be helpful to evaluate bone stock and component loosening, but special techniques must be used to decrease metal scatter. Bone scanning is useful to differentiate between aseptic loosening and infection. At present, standard MRI is not as useful as these other diagnostic procedures in the evaluation of total shoulder replacements. Arthroscopy may prove useful, especially to determine glenoid component loosening, but this is still developmental.

TYPES OF PROBLEMS

Infection

The incidence of infection after total shoulder arthroplasty is extremely low; only four infections have been reported in 1168 cases, an incidence of 0.34%. This compares very favorably with reported infection rates following other major joint replacements. Neer reported only two infections in his personal series of 776 unconstrained arthroplasties (22). Both infections occurred in patients with positive cultures at the time of surgery, which grew out later from enrichment medium. This favorable infection rate is due in part to careful preoperative screening, but also, the shoulder joint has excellent vascularity and abundant soft tissue coverage. If there is a high suspicion for infection at the time of primary revision surgery, the usual screening blood tests, CBC and ESR, can be supplemented with nuclear scans, aspiration, frozen sections, or imprints at the time of surgery to aid in the identification of an infection. The compromised host is an especially vulnerable target for a bacterial infection. These patients can be defined as anyone with impaired resistance to infection, secondary to a disease such as rheumatoid arthritis, or therapy for the disease process.

Since there are so few cases reported, the treatment of a septic shoulder arthroplasty should follow the same principles as other large joints. The treatment is related to the timing of the infection. An early infection can potentially be managed by thorough debridement, wound closure with closed drainage, and appropriate antibiotics. Initially, the antibiotic should be a broad-spectrum drug with a high sensitivity to Gram-positive organisms, which are the most common. Delayed infections require removal of the prosthesis and all cement, foreign bodies, or sequestra as well as antibiotic therapy. The shoulder is immobilized for approximately 3 months to allow fibrous healing. The patient in Figure 5.3 has an infected total shoulder replacement and has severe rheumatoid arthritis. Because this patient is a compromised host and on chronic corticosteroid medication, the prosthesis was removed and not exchanged. She has a fibrous union with adequate pain relief and limited function. If the patient is dissatisfied at approximately 12 months, a fusion can be considered if there are no signs of osteomyelitis. Amstutz et al. reported a primary exchange procedure in one patient with septic loosening of the glenoid (2). We have exchanged several hemiarthroplasties that are infected for a total shoulder with antibiotic impregnated cement (Tobramycin). The short term results are acceptable and this procedure should be performed with caution. It is preferable when the organism is Gram-positive and sensitive to antibiotics. In addition, osteomyelitis should not be present.

Nerve Injuries

Nerve injury during total shoulder arthroplasty is uncommon. Fortunately, these injuries most often represent a neuropraxia, which can be treated expectantly. Electromyography and nerve conduction studies can be useful in documenting the extent of injury as well as any serial improvement in nerve function. The axillary nerve is the most likely to be injured as it runs on the inferior aspect of the capsule and then curves posteriorly on the undersurface of the deltoid muscle. If there is a suspicion that the axillary nerve was lacerated at surgery and the electromyograph at 6 weeks reveals a complete lesion with no improvement at 12 weeks, early exploration and repair are suggested. If the initial lesion is partial and improving, observation is indicated.

Careful localization or palpation of the axillary nerve, particularly in revision or posttraumatic surgeries, is essential. If an intraoperative injury is identified, microsurgical repair should be performed at that time. Unfortunately, the muscle transfers presently available for deltoid paralysis are not satisfactory.

Fractures

Intraoperative fractures are uncommon but may occur, especially in osteoporotic or rhematoid

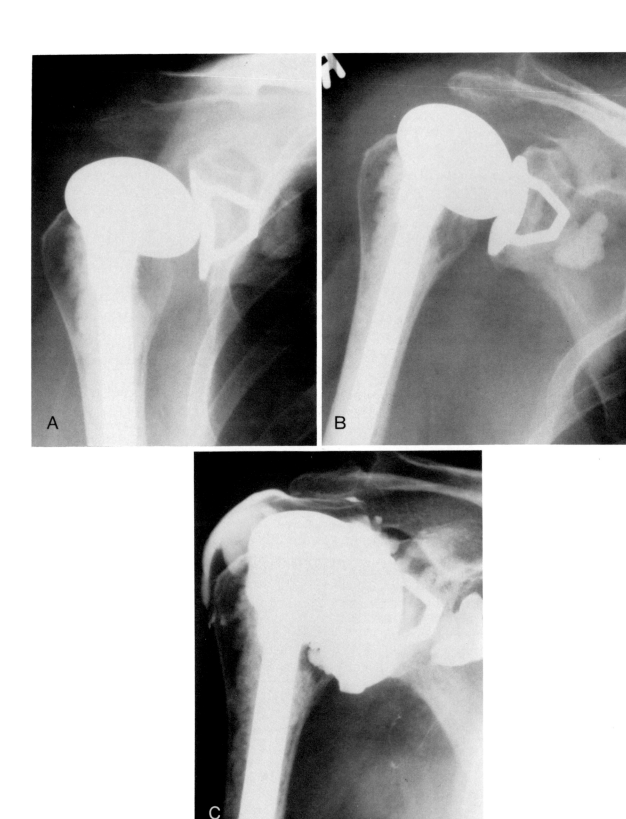

Figure 5.2. The patient fell and sustained a posterior dislocation. The humeral prosthesis was stable following closed reduction, but there was significant weakness in forward elevation and external rotation. **A**, An AP prior to the fall. **B**, An AP after the fall, showing superior migration of the head. **C**, An arthrogram revealing the full-thickness rotator cuff tear. The tear was repaired, and the patient has a satisfactory result with 160° forward elevation and 40° of external rotation.

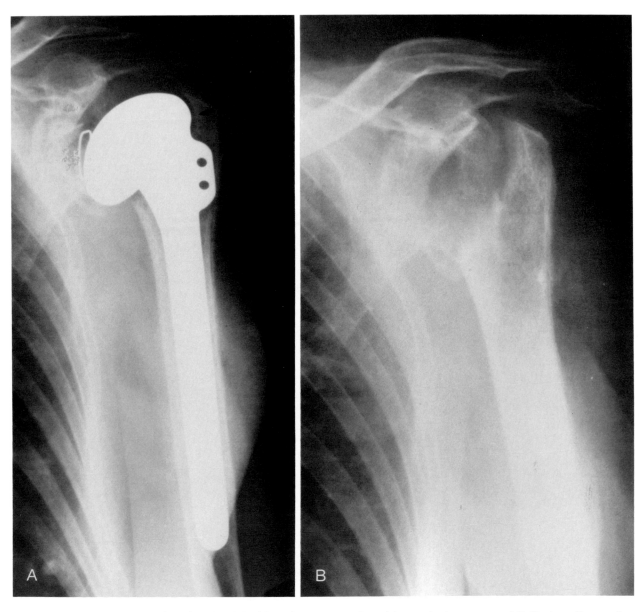

Figure 5.3. **A**, An AP radiograph of an infected total shoulder replacement in a patient with severe rheumatoid arthritis. Note the lucent lines between the prosthesis and the bone. The patient had severe osteoporosis, and the prosthesis was removed. **B**, She has a fibrous union with adequate pain relief and limited function.

bone. The bone is extremely soft and the cortices are thin. Fracture commonly occurs either with reaming, dislocation of the humeral head, or reduction of the prosthesis. It is important while reaming the shaft to keep the reamers in the longitudinal direction of the humeral shaft. If there has been a previous prosthesis, the track of the previous stem may guide the reamers out of the cortex. Therefore, it is important to break through the most inferior part of the previous stem track with a small drill. If the hole in the shaft is near the tip of the prosthesis, a long-stemmed prosthesis may be required to bridge the gap. A rubber sheet should be placed on the outside part of the shaft to avoid extravasation of cement into the soft tissue and possible radial nerve injury. The patient in Figure 5.4 had the humeral shaft penetrated because the reamer followed the path of a previous prosthesis. An uncemented long-stemmed prosthesis was used to bridge the gap. Healing occurred, and the patient has a functional extremity at 6-year follow-up. Oblique fractures of the shaft that occur with rotation are treated in a similar fashion.

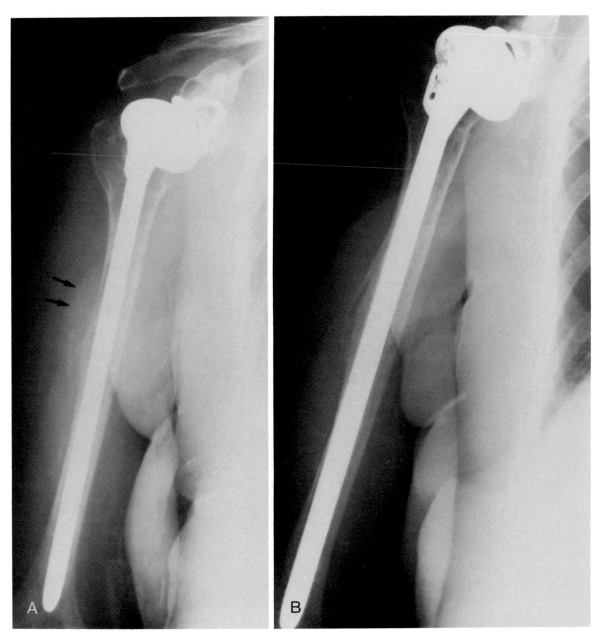

Figure 5.4. **A**, The patient sustained a penetration of the humeral shaft by the reamer following the path of a previous prosthesis. An uncement- ed long-stemmed prosthesis was used to bridge the gap. **B**, Healing occurred, and the patient has a functional extremity at 6-year follow-up.

However, sometimes the prosthesis will allow for a secure, stable fit. In this instance, the rehabilitation should be modified in the postoperative period to avoid active exercises for an 8–12-week period of time to allow sufficient fracture healing. The patient in Figure 5.5 sustained an oblique fracture of the shaft during reduction of the humeral prosthesis. The fracture was stable. The patient was protected with a plastic coaptation splint and passive exercises for 8 weeks until there was sufficient healing. He has progressed to an excellent result.

Postoperative fractures can be treated conservatively if the fracture is stable. The patient in Figure 5.6 had a fracture of the shaft 2 years after insertion of the prosthesis and was treated with a plastic coaptation splint with a successful outcome. He had excellent healing around the prosthesis and cement and did not require operative intervention. If the fracture is unstable, further surgery is required. Internal fixation may be extremely difficult, and in most instances a custom, long-stemmed prosthesis is indicated. Neer reported a case in which a patient fell off a ladder, fracturing a humerus, causing rotation of the prosthesis and posterior dislocation. In this instance, the fracture was unstable and required prosthesis revision. Both components were replaced as the glenoid prosthesis was deformed by the fin of the displaced humeral component.

Tuberosity fractures can also occur in soft osteoporotic bone. Fortunately, these can be managed the same way as a four-part fracture with nonabsorbable nylon sutures through the tuberosities. These should be attached to both the fin of the prosthesis

as well as to the proximal shaft. The patient in Figure 5.7 sustained a fracture of the greater tuberosity and surgical neck area during the dislocation of the head. Fixation with several nylon sutures created a stable situation.

Loosening

Revision surgery for component loosening following total shoulder replacement is rare (7, 10, 11, 14, 21, 27). Very few cases of humeral component

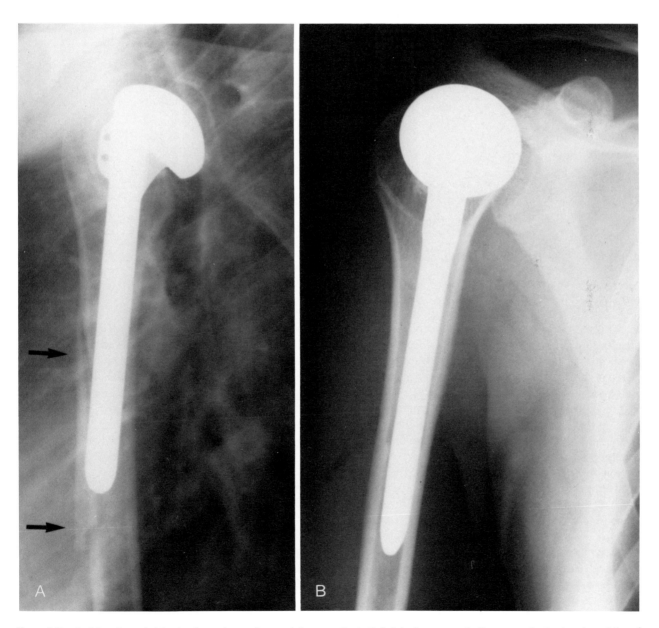

Figure 5.5. **A**, A transthoracic lateral radiograph revealing an oblique fracture of the shaft that occurred during reduction of the humeral pros- thesis. **B**, Solid union occurred with conservative treatment consisting of a plastic coaptation splint.

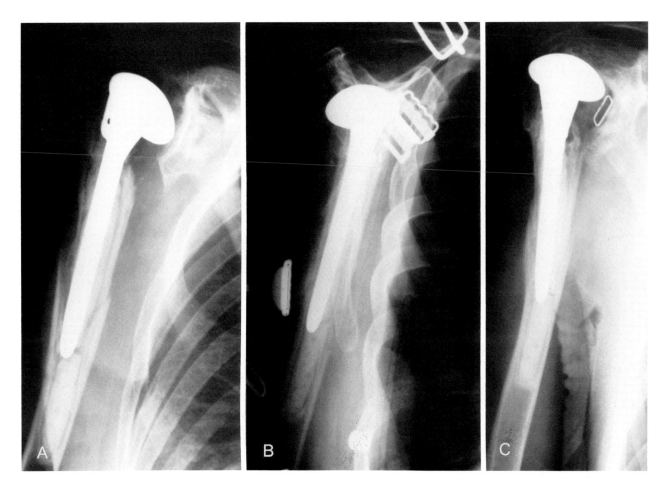

Figure 5.6. **A,** AP radiograph showing a fracture around the humeral prosthesis 2 years after surgery. **B,** The fracture was stable and treated with a plastic coaptation splint. **C,** Union occurred, and the patient achieved a stable humerus.

loosening have been reported. Neer reported no significant loosening in the humeral component in his personal series of 776 cases (21). However, some cases of humeral head subsidence do occur, especially if there is osteoporotic soft bone. In this instance, it is probably wise to use cement to avoid subsidence. A press fit is indicated only when there is sufficient bone stock, usually in the younger patient, to support the prosthesis.

Although radiolucent lines around the glenoid are common (30–83%), there has not been a direct correlation between radiolucent lines and clinical loosening (5, 6, 11, 12). A radiographic follow-up study of 69 total shoulder replacements found that 48 patients had lucent lines present before hospital discharge (6). However, only six of these progressed, and one was symptomatic after an average follow-up of 5 years. A recent series of 70 total shoulder replacements followed for 5–11 years noted a complete lucent line of 1.5 mm or more around one-third of glenoids, yet only three revisions were necessary for

glenoid loosening (11). Barrett reviewed 140 total shoulder replacements in patients with rheumatoid arthritis; he noted 82% glenoid radiolucent lines. Only 1% were definitely loose, and 8% were considered probably loose (5). No glenoid revisions were performed in this series. The overall glenoid loosening rate in reported series is 4.3%.

The clinical relevance of radiolucent zones at the glenoid bone interface is difficult to interpret. Since these lucent lines are frequently noted in the immediate postoperative period, they may reflect cementing technique or the poor quality of glenoid bone stock. Neer attributed these radiolucencies to a variety of factors, including inconsistent radiographic technique, variable density and strength of bone, stress shielding by the glenoid component, and disuse osteoporosis (22). The patient in Figure 5.8 has rheumatoid arthritis and lucent glenoid lines. However, the patient has a pain-free result at this time and has excellent functional use of the arm.

Neer and Brems both reported a higher incidence of complete cement lines in the earlier cases in their series performed during the learning curve (6, 21). Careful preparation of the glenoid slot with thorough lavage and adequate hemostasis will decrease the incidence of lucent lines. Also, the amount of cement used in the glenoid should be minimal. Basically, only enough to fill the slot should be used. We have found that pressure lavage has been extremely helpful in removing debris and achieving hemostasis in the glenoid vault.

Despite the significant incidence of radiolucent zones at the glenoid cement-bone interface, there are only 12 reported cases of revision surgery for glenoid loosening. Reinsertion of the glenoid component should be performed only if sufficient bone stock is available, allowing for secure fixation.

Instability

Fortunately, postoperative subluxation or dislocation has been reported to occur in only 1–2% of cases. Stability of an unconstrained implant depends on preservation of humeral length, proper version of the components, and balance of the soft tissue repair. Also, an intact rotator cuff is essential for superior stability. Careful attention to maintaining humeral length will help to prevent inferior subluxation, since it is important to maintain the myofascial sleeve. Dr. Neer reported on 194 total shoulder replacements with an average of 37 months follow-up (24). There were four dislocations—two anterior, two posterior, and all occurred within 3 weeks of surgery. All were reduced, closed, and immobilized for 3–6 weeks and then rehabili-

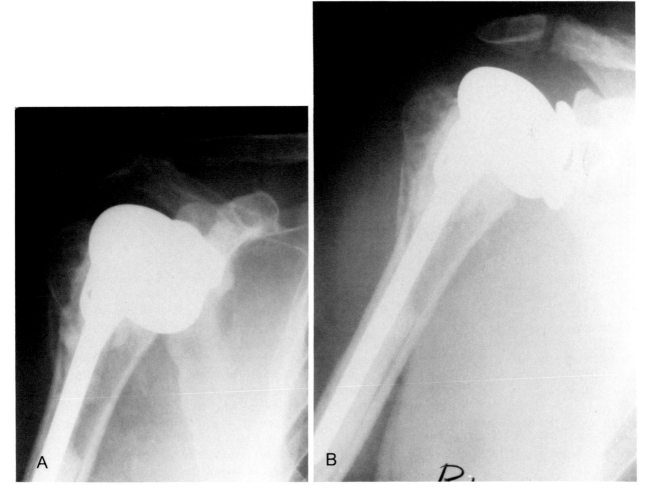

Figure 5.7. **A**, An AP radiograph showing a fracture of the greater tuberosity sustained during dislocation of the head. **B**, Adequate healing occurred after fixation with several nylon sutures to the shaft of the humerus and the fin of the prosthesis.

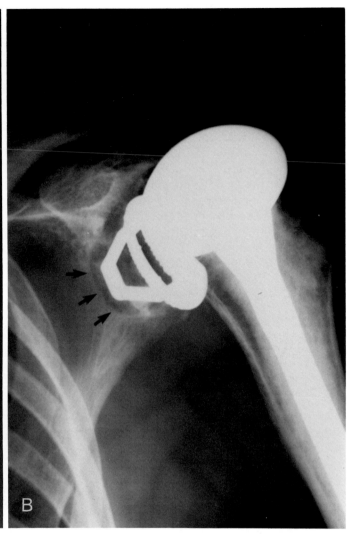

Figure 5.8. **A**, AP radiograph in the immediate postoperative period of a patient with rheumatoid arthritis. **B**, Lucent lines are apparent 5 years postoperatively. The patient is asymptomatic and has excellent function despite the lucent lines.

tated. None required further surgery, although one had recurrent subluxations.

The humeral component should be inserted in 30–40° of retroversion unless there is uneven glenoid wear. If there is significant posterior glenoid wear, then less retroversion is needed. However, the decrease in retroversion should not be excessive, as anterior dislocation may occur. The patient in Figure 5.9 had too great a reduction in the retroversion and subsequently has anterior dislocation of the humeral prosthesis. There was a significant amount of posterior glenoid wear, and the decrease retroversion was needed to accommodate the glenoid prosthesis, which was facing more posteriorly. Glenoid wear can be corrected by either a combination of lowering the

prominent side or altering the amount of head retroversion. Bone grafting may be required for those cases with severe glenoid deficiency. A recent series of 20 large internally fixed bone grafts reported this to be a valuable method for providing additional support for the glenoid with a glenoid implant (23). Also, if there is insufficient glenoid bone stock, it may be prudent to not replace the glenoid. The patient in Figure 5.10 had excessive glenoid bone loss, and another prosthesis could not be implanted. The patient has done well without a glenoid component and only a humeral head that is not unstable. Also, the prosthesis should be placed at the proper height to be at the level of the tuberosity or higher. This modular prosthesis (Fig. 5.11) was inserted too low, and impingement of the greater tuberosity against the acromion occurred. Also, this can lead to inferior subluxation.

The patient in Figure 5.1 sustained a posterior dislocation of the prosthesis secondary to excessive retroversion of the humeral component. An axillary view is important to demonstrate the posterior dislocation, as this may be missed on the AP radiograph. The patient also had significant limitation and was locked in 15° of internal rotation. Revision of a dislocated prosthesis generally entails a correction of prosthesis malposition as well as soft tissue procedures of both the capsule and the muscles about the shoulder to achieve soft tissue equilibrium.

Heterotopic Bone

Clinically significant formation of heterotopic bone following total shoulder replacement has been uncommon. However, a recent series from Denmark reported that 10% of their cases had ossifications bridging the glenohumeral and/or glenoacromial space and were associated with limited range of motion (14). However, ectopic bone formation has not been clinically significant in most series. These authors reported no correlation between shoulder pain and the development of ossification.

Rotator Cuff Tears

Postoperative tearing of the rotator cuff is one of the more frequent complications following total shoulder arthroplasty, with an incidence of 3–4%. Neer reported five traumatic cuff tears in his initial report on 194 total shoulder replacements (19). Two underwent surgical repair, two remained weak but without symptoms, and one had intermittent pain but refused further surgery. Cofield analyzed 73 shoulder arthroplasties and noted rotator cuff tears in five patients postoperatively (7). One patient had significant pain and was considering further surgery. The other four patients had anterosuperior subluxation and weakness, but only minimal discomfort, and they refused reoperation. The patient in Fig. 5.2 fell and sustained a posterior dislocation. The patient was stable following closed reduction, but there was significant weakness in elevation and external rotation. Also, the AP radiograph revealed superior migration of the head. An arthrogram revealed a full-thickness rotator cuff tear that was repaired. The patient now has 160° of forward elevation with 40° of external rotation and no instability.

Although patients with rotator cuff tears show some functional limitation, significant pain has not been an associated problem in the majority of re-

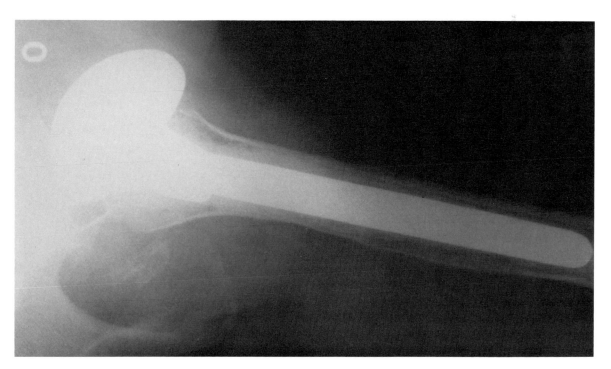

Figure 5.9. Axillary radiograph demonstrating a anterior dislocation of a humeral prosthesis that had too great a reduction in the amount of retroversion.

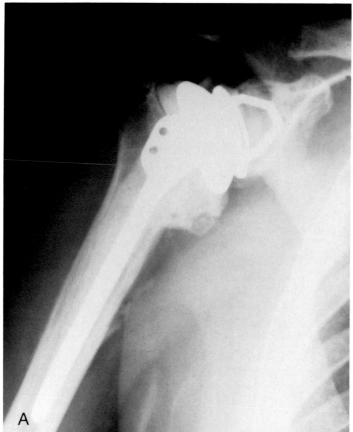

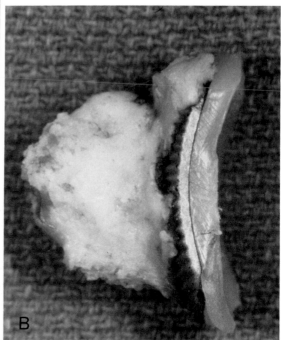

Figure 5.10. **A**, AP radiograph showing significant glenoid loosening. **B**, Glenoid prosthesis, revealing significant plastic deformation. **C**, Revision was performed without the use of a glenoid component because of the extensive bone loss, and the patient has done well with only a large humeral head prosthesis.

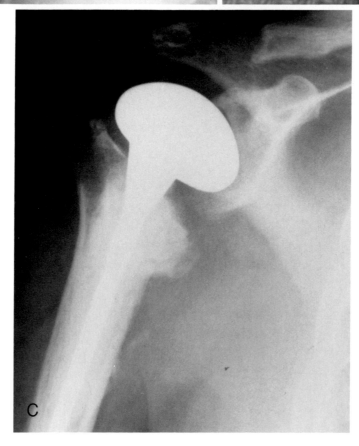

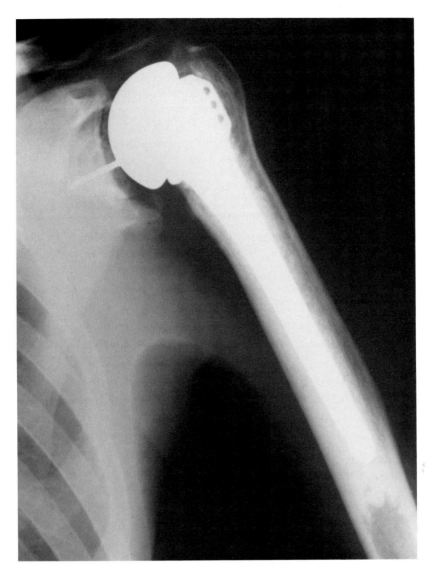

Figure 5.11.   A modular prosthesis that was inserted too low, revealing impingement of the greater tuberosity against the acromion.

ports. While further repair is not always required, the report by Franklin concerning glenoid loosening and large cuff tears may support repairing large, postop rotator cuff tears, as suggested by Cofield (8).

RESULTS/REVISION

The results of total shoulder arthroplasty are, overall, as good or better than other joint replacements. Fortunately, revision rates are low, ranging from 0–9% (4, 7, 19, 21). Neer and Kirby reported on the revision of 40 shoulder arthroplasties (20). They noted two significant problems with fixed-fulcrum prostheses; loss of external rotator and mechanical failure. This design requires excision of the rotator

cuff for proper placement. Also, because there are several moveable parts, mechanical failure can occur. Other causes of failure for constrained and total arthroplasties include deltoid scarring and detachment, subscapularis shortening, subacromial scarring and adhesions between cuff and deltoid, prominent or retracted greater tuberosity, loss of humeral length, uneven or central glenoid wear, and lack of a supervised rehabilitation program (22). The authors revised 34 patients and achieved satisfactory pain relief and function in all but five of these cases. However, they stated that revision total shoulder arthroplasty was extremely difficult technically, due to the combination of bone loss, muscle weakness, scar, and the increased risk of infection. Clearly, the results of version are not as good as primary surgery. Therefore, prevention of complications is still the best treatment.

References

1. Adams MA, Weiland AJ, Moore JR. Nonconstrainted total shoulder arthroplasty: An eight-year experience. Orthop Trans 1986;10:232–233.

2. Amstutz HC, Thomas BJ, Kabo JM, et al. The Dana total shoulder arthroplasty. J Bone Joint Surg 1988;70A: 1174–1182.

3. Bade HA III, Warren RF, Ranawat C, Inglis AE. Long term results of Neer total shoulder replacement. In: Bateman JE, Welsh RP, eds. Surgery of the shoulder. St. Louis: CV Mosby, 1984;294–302.

4. Barrett WP, Franklin JL, Jackins SE, et al. Total shoulder arthroplasty. J Bone Joint Surg 1987;69A:865–872.

5. Barrett WP, Thornhill TS, Thomas WH, et al. Nonconstrainted total shoulder arthroplasty in patients with polyarticular rheumatoid arthritis. J Arthrop 1989;4:91–96.

6. Brems JJ, Wilde AH, Borden LS, et al. Glenoid lucent lines. Orthop Trans 1986;10:231.

7. Cofield RH. Total shoulder arthroplasty with the Neer prosthesis. J Bone Joint Surg 1984;66A:899–906.

8. Cofield RH. Degenerative and arthritic problems of the glenohumeral joint. In: Rockwood CA, Matsen FA III, eds. The shoulder. Philadelphia: WB Saunders, 1990;678–749.

9. Franklin JL, Barrett WP, Jackins SE, et al. Glenoid loosening in total shoulder arthroplasty: association with rotator cuff deficiency. J Arthrop 1988;3:9–46.

10. Frich LJ, Moller BN, Sneppen O. Shoulder arthroplasty with the Neer Mark-II prosthesis. Arch Orthop Trauma Surg 1988;107:110–113.

11. Hawkins RJ, Bell RH, Jallay B. Experience with the Neer total shoulder arthroplasty: a review of 70 cases. Orthop Trans 1986;10:232.

12. Kelly IG, Foster RS, Fischer WD. Neer total shoulder replacement in rheumatoid arthritis. J Bone Joint Surg 1987;69B:723–726.

13. Kenmore PI, MacCartee C, Vitek B. A simple shoulder replacement. J Biomed Mater Res 1974;5:329–330.

14. Kessel L, Bayley J. Prosthetic replacement of the shoulder joint: preliminary communication. J Roy Soc Med 1979; 72:748–752.

15. Kjaersgaard AP, Frich LH, Sjbjerg JD, et al. Heterotopic bone formation following total shoulder arthroplasty. J Arthrop 1989;4:99–104.

16. Lettin A, Copeland SA, Scales T. The Stanmore total shoulder replacement. J Bone Joint Surg 1982;64B:47–51.

17. Lugli T. Artificial shoulder joint by Pean (1893). The facts of an exceptional intervention and the prosthetic method. Clin Orthop 1978;133:215–218.

18. Neer CS II. Articular replacement for the humeral head. J Bone Joint Surg 1955;37A:215–228.

19. Neer CS II. Replacement arthroplasty for glenohumeral osteoarthritis. J Bone Joint Surg 1974;56A:1–13.

20. Neer CS II, Kirby RM. Revision of the humeral head and total shoulder arthroplasties. Clin Orthop 1982;170:189–195.

21. Neer CS II, Watson KC, Stanton FJ. Recent experience in total shoulder replacement. J Bone Joint Surg 1982; 64A:319–337.

22. Neer CS II, McCann PD, Macfarlane EA, Padilla N. Earlier passive motion following shoulder arthroplasty and rotator cuff repair. A prospective study. Orthop Trans 1987;2:231.

23. Neer CS II, Morrison DS. Glenoid bone-grafting in total shoulder arthroplasty. J Bone Joint Surg 1988;70A: 1154–1162.

24. Neer CS II. Shoulder reconstruction. Philadelphia: WB Saunders, 1990;143–271.

25. Post M, Jablon M, Miller H, Singh M. Constrainted total shoulder replacement: a critical review. Clin Orthop 1979; 144:135–150.

26. Wallensten R. Constrained total shoulder arthroplasty. In: Watson MS, ed. Surgical disorders of the shoulder. Edinburgh: Churchill Livingstone, 1991;511–517.

27. Wilde AH, Borden LS, Brems JJ. Experience with the Neer total shoulder replacement. In: Bateman JE, Welsh RP, eds. Surgery of the shoulder. St. Louis: CV Mosby, 1984;224–228.

6
Glenoid Deficiency in Total Shoulder Arthroplasty

David S. Morrison

INTRODUCTION

Articular surface replacements of the humeral head for degenerative changes and proximal humeral fractures were introduced by Neer in 1951 (3). In 1974, a glenoid surfacing component was included in the procedure, and the total shoulder replacement was popularized. Since that time, indications for total shoulder arthroplasty have expanded to include not only degenerative and rheumatoid arthritis but also posttraumatic arthritis and the arthritis associated with recurrent dislocations, rotator cuff tear arthropathy, and other lesions about the shoulder that result in significant bone destruction or loss (2, 4, 5). As the scope of the pathologies addressed through a total shoulder replacement has expanded, the prosthesis and the surgical technique have been modified to address the specific problems encountered in specific pathologies.

One of the most difficult situations to handle in shoulder replacement arthroplasty is the abnormal glenoid architecture resulting from loss of bone. This lack of adequate glenoid bone stock has led some to recommend the use of constrained prostheses. However, such prostheses have very poor long-term results due to almost universal loosening, which causes further destruction of the glenoid with significant pain and functional deficits (7, 8). Others have attempted humeral head replacement alone, but the results with regard to pain relief have not been satisfactory when compared to those obtained with a total shoulder. To address the problem, autologous bone grafting of the glenoid has been advocated by Neer, and has been shown to give excellent results in a long-term study published in 1988 (6). In a series of 463 consecutive total shoulder replacement procedures performed between 1973 and 1985, there were only two cases in which lack of bone made the implantation of a glenoid component impossible. In these patients, the glenoid was so severely damaged that there was insufficient stock to allow for adequate fixation of a bone graft. Of the remaining 65 cases with this problem, 20 were successfully treated with large internally fixed bone grafts, and 45 were treated with smaller cancellous and corticocancellous bone grafts that did not require internal fixation. The follow-up was 4.4 years, and the clinical results were judged to be excellent in 16, satisfactory in one, and two patients with rotator cuff tear arthropathy obtained their limited goals of pain relief and function at the side postoperatively. No clinical loosening or migration of the components occurred, and no patient required further surgery.

Only 4.3% of the 463 replacement surgeries required bone grafting to successfully complete a total shoulder arthroplasty. Although this is a relatively small number, an orthopaedic surgeon performing this procedure should be able to address this problem when it is encountered. If significant unexpected bone loss becomes apparent in the operating room, it must be corrected at that time if the surgery is expected to yield satisfactory results.

OPERATIVE PLANNING

A decision as to whether or not bone grafting of the glenoid will be necessary should be made prior to the time of surgery. The most useful tools in determining the degree of bone loss at the glenoid are an axillary radiograph and a CT scan. We have not found that the use of computer reconstructions add significantly to the information obtained through standard means, and the significant cost involved in this computer-generated data is probably not justified in most cases. The sole exception to this is in the case of a comminuted scapular fracture in which the alignment of the fragments cannot easily be appreciated on plain radiographs or routine CT.

Most patients requiring total shoulder arthroplasty have some amount of uneven wear of the glenoid. This minor asymmetry of the glenoid can easily be compensated for through slight changes in the version of the humeral component. Wear on the posterior aspect of the glenoid results in relative glenoid retroversion (Fig. 6.1A). This can then be compensated for by leveling off the high side of the glenoid (Fig. 6.2A) or by anteverting the humeral head to a degree equal to that of the retroversion of the glenoid. Anteversion of the glenoid component can be accommodated with a slight increase in the retroversion of the humeral component beyond the normal 35–40°. Occasionally, there is such severe destruction of the glenoid that simply altering the glenoid version not only fails to compensate for the degree of glenoid bone loss but results in glenohumeral instability. (Fig. 6.1B) In these cases, large cortical cancellous bone grafts are needed to support the glenoid prosthesis in proper version (Fig. 6.3). Such techniques as the use of an uneven glenoid component or reconstructing the normal architecture of the glenoid with excess methylmethacrolate have proved to be biomechanically unsound and lacking in the longevity of an adequately bone-grafted glenoid (Fig. 6.2B). These latter two techniques are prone to early glenoid loosening due to deformation of the polyethylene or a breakout of the excess cement.

SURGICAL TECHNIQUE

The surgical technique of the total shoulder arthroplasty is demanding and requires an intimate knowledge of the pathologic process of each diagnostic category as well as experience in major reconstructive surgery of the shoulder. With the

Figure 6.1. **A**, In degenerative arthritis and the arthritis of dislocations, wear is most often seen on the posterior aspect of the glenoid. **B**, If the glenoid component is inserted without correcting the abnormal version caused by posterior glenoid wear, the prosthesis will be unstable posteriorly.

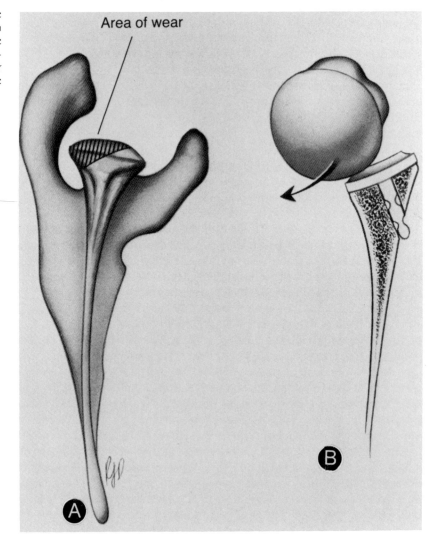

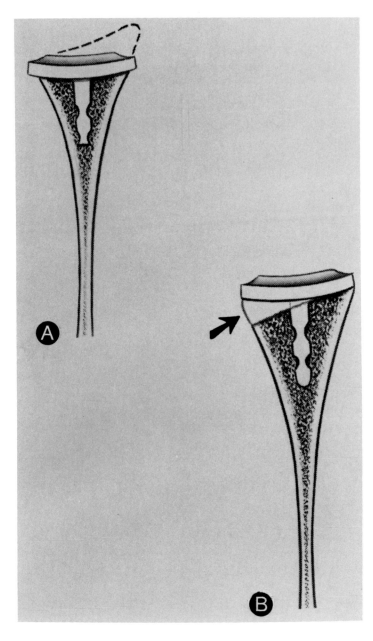

Figure 6.2. **A**, Minor problems with glenoid version can be corrected by lowering the high side of the glenoid and using a thicker humeral prosthesis. It is sometimes necessary to contour the keel of the prosthesis to fit within the shallow medullary canal often seen with centralization of the glenoid. **B**, Building up the high side of the glenoid using bone cement is contraindicated since this cement will fracture and become displaced, causing toggling and loosening of the glenoid component .

unique role played by the ligamentous and muscular stabilizer of the glenohumeral joint, meticulous soft tissue technique is essential. In addition, because of the tendency of the shoulder to form adhesions postoperatively, a well-planned and physician-supervised rehabilitation program is necessary. Input and active participation by the surgeon in the rehabilitation program is needed in every case, both complicated and simple, if optimum results are to be achieved.

The glenoid surface must be shaped to the contour of the glenoid component. In preparation of the severely worn glenoid, it is advisable to do this mostly by hand, using small curettes. When a power

burr is utilized, a blunt-tipped Swanson burr significantly reduces the chance of perforation of the glenoid cortex during preparation. However, if a minor perforation does occur, the cortical hole can be packed with cancellous bone fragments obtained from the humeral head, thereby decreasing extrusion of cement during final fixation.

A standard metal-backed prosthesis, or more recently, the screw-stabilized metal-backed prosthesis, is the device of choice in most cases. Eighty percent or more of the bearing surface of the metal prosthesis should be in contact with glenoid bone. If this cannot be achieved through contouring, the use

Figure 6.3. **A**, A large corticocancellous bone graft fashioned from the humeral articular surface is used to reestablish the normal contour and version of the glenoid. **B**, This graft is usually held in place with two lag screws that are countersunk into the articular surface to avoid contact with the glenoid component. The component is then cemented in place.

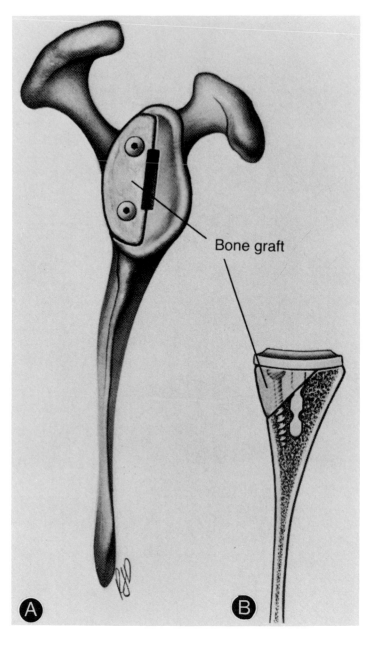

Bone graft

of a smaller glenoid component or glenoid bone grafting becomes necessary. If the medullary canal is too narrow or too shallow to allow implantation of the metal-backed prosthesis, then a polyethylene prosthesis may be used. The use of polyethylene enables the surgeon to contour the keel of the prosthesis to fit the anatomy of the scapular canal. When the medullary canal is too shallow to allow use of even the standard polyethylene component or if bone wear is so uneven that the glenoid component cannot adequately be supported, a large internally fixed bone graft should be considered. It is possible to contour the surface of the glenoid using a reamer, as sup-

plied by several manufacturers. It must be remembered, however, that the best support the glenoid prosthesis can have is subchondral bone, and not cancellous bone. With that in mind, only the minimal amount of reaming necessary to achieve adequate bone support should be attempted.

When bone grafting is necessary, large cortical cancellous grafts are obtained from a portion of the humeral head removed during the first part of the surgical procedure. The worn area of the glenoid is debrided down to bleeding bone, and the bone graft is shaped to fit the defect, thus reconstructing the normal anatomy of the glenoid. Whenever possible, the graft is secured to the glenoid with cancellous screws that are countersunk into the bone graft so that the screw heads are not in contact with the glenoid component. (Fig. 6.3) The screws should be long enough to obtain a solid cortical grip and lag the bone graft into place. If the shape or location of the defect makes it impossible to use screw fixation, or if the screws would interfere with the placement of the glenoid component, the bone graft may be wedged into the defect like a keystone and held in place with large nonabsorbable sutures passed through the graft and the remaining glenoid bone. The graft is then further stabilized by the cemented glenoid component. In rare cases, the use of stainless steel mesh may be needed to control cement extravasation from the scapula during implantation of the component.

Good cement technique is paramount for satisfactory fixation. The vast majority of lucent lines around the glenoid component are the result of poor technique, and can be seen on the immediate postoperative radiographs (1). We have found that these lucent lines can be minimized through the use of a double-cementing technique.

After satisfactory preparation of the glenoid fossa, the trough in the medullary bone of the glenoid neck is irrigated with antibiotic solution and packed with a dry gauze. The packing is then removed and the methylmethacrolate is injected into the canal with a catheter-tipped syringe while still in a liquid state. Gauze is then packed into the canal, pressurizing the cement and forcing the methylmethacrolate into the trabeculae of the medullary bone. This enhances fixation, and also provides hemostasis by tamponade. The sponge is then removed, and the now dry canal is immediately refilled with the semisoft methylmethacrolate, which is pressurized manually. All of the excess cement on the articular surface is removed, and the glenoid component is inserted, impacted into place, and held manually until the cement has hardened. It is important to realize that the cement acts simply as a grout and is meant to only hold the keel of the prosthesis within the medullary canal of the glenoid. The cement is not meant to form a bond between the back of the prosthesis and the subchondral bone of the glenoid. The goal is to obtain metal on bone contact over the glenoid surface, and to restrict the cement to the medullary canal as much as possible. Use of the screw-stabilized metal-backed glenoid component allows for maximum pressurization of the cement and immediate stability of the bone cement construct. In cases where a bone graft is necessary, it is possible to use the screws that stabilize the glenoid component to also stabilize the glenoid bone graft. At present, we prefer the use of the screw-stabilized metal-backed glenoid, which is cemented in place.

The postoperative regimen and duration of immobilization are determined by the stability of the bone graft and the quality of the soft tissues. Except when a massive bone graft is used or where the soft tissue is extremely deficient, the extremity is placed in a sling and a surgeon-directed in-hospital physical therapy program is begun in the first or second postoperative day. The program is a passive and passive-assisted range of motion program. The patient must be cautioned against any active attempts at elevation or impact loading on the shoulder over the first 8 weeks postoperatively. This rehabilitation program is begun early since the stability of the prosthesis and the bone graft depend upon the integrity and function of the active and passive stabilizers of the glenohumeral joint: the ligaments and the rotator cuff muscles.

PATTERNS OF GLENOID BONE LOSS

There are two major categories of glenoid destruction. The most common pattern is seen in conjunction with degenerative arthritis or the arthritis of recurrent dislocations where there is anterior or posterior sloping of the glenoid secondary to asymmetric wear.

The second type of bony destruction is gross loss of bone due to etiologies such as fractures, penetrating trauma, tumors, and rheumatoid arthritis. In these cases, the portion of glenoid that remains intact maintains a normal version, but the lack of bone stock makes the implantation of a glenoid component impossible due to lack of positive support.

Each of the different diagnostic categories presents with specific pathologic features and patterns of joint destruction that distinguish it from the others. Because of this, details of the surgical procedure vary with each group.

RHEUMATOID ARTHRITIS

In rheumatoid arthritis, granulation tissue causes massive erosion of the articular surfaces of both the humerus and the glenoid. The pattern of bone loss is usually a centralization of the glenoid, that is, there is equal bone loss along the entire surface of the glenoid fossa rather than asymmetrical anterior or posterior wear. These patients will also have large cysts within the glenoid, which may perforate the glenoid cortex. Most patients with rheumatoid arthritis and simple centralization of the glenoid can be treated with a standard glenoid component and a larger humeral head to maintain the tension on the myofascial sleeve of the shoulder. In some patients where the centralization has progressed beyond the base of the coracoid, there will be an insufficient medullary canal in the scapula to allow implantation of a standard glenoid component. In these cases, a polyethylene component may be necessary. The standard prosthesis keel is contoured in such a way as to allow its implantation into this very shallow medullary canal. When destruction has progressed to the point where even a modified polyethylene component will not fit within the medullary canal, then a glenoid bone graft is used. With severe centralization of the glenoid, a circular graft of the articular surface is necessary. A new articular surface of normal size and contour is fashioned out of a fragment of the removed humeral head and fastened to the remaining glenoid with screws. The thickness of this graft will usually be greater than 5 mm but not more than 10 mm. Adequate fixation is obtained by directing the screws up into the base of the coracoid and down the lateral border of the scapular body. In rare cases, the centralization has progressed beyond the base of the coracoid so that there is essentially no glenoid fossa remaining and the head is articulating with the body and spine of the scapula. In these cases, the coracoid will often be free-floating, since its attachment to the scapula has been worn away. These patients have inadequate scapular bone stock to allow for fixation of large bone grafts and should, therefore, be treated with a humeral head replacement alone. The goal in this case is pain relief rather than significant improvement in function. As mentioned, large glenoid cysts are frequently encountered in rheumatoid arthritis, and these must be curetted down to good quality bone and then packed with corticocancellous bone grafts prior to implantation of the glenoid component. These large glenoid cysts seen in rheumatoid arthritis comprise the majority of the patients who required smaller noninternally fixed bone grafts.

ARTHRITIS OF DISLOCATIONS AND OSTEOARTHRITIS

Osteoarthritis and the arthritis of recurrent dislocations are associated with uneven wear of the glenoid cavity. In the patient with osteoarthritis, the humeral head tends to sublux posteriorly, resulting in uneven wear along the posterior aspect of the glenoid. It is quite common to see 15–20° of posterior

glenoid version secondary to the normal posterior wear seen in osteoarthritis. Most of these patients have very good bone stock and have retained adequate height of the glenoid to allow implantation of a standard metal-backed component. In patients with only 5–15° of abnormal version, it is possible to insert the glenoid component in that amount of retroversion and correct for this by changing the anteversion of the humeral head by an equal amount. This will maintain the relationship between the humerus and the glenoid, and maintain normal stability and range of motion postoperatively. In patients where the degree of wear is greater, it is usually possible to level off the high side to bring the glenoid back to a more normal version (Fig. 6.2). In patients where the posterior wear is so severe that leveling off the high side of the glenoid would result in a very shallow glenoid medullary canal and therefore interfere with the insertion of a standard component, it is necessary to perform a posterior bone graft. The goal is to return the surface of the glenoid to normal version, and to maintain the depth of the medullary canal to such an extent that the keel of the metal-backed component can be completely implanted. This correction of abnormal wear on the glenoid must be performed with bony contouring and not through the use of extra cement. We have found that when cement is used to support a glenoid component and correct for abnormal glenoid version, the cement will eventually break out, causing toggling of the prosthesis and failure.

In patients with recurrent dislocations, the glenoid wear has two etiologies. In patients who have not had previous surgery for anterior instability, the wear takes place on the anterior inferior glenoid. This wear is due in part to abrasion secondary to subluxation and in part to bone loss secondary to fractures along the anterior inferior rim of the glenoid. When the wear is simply due to abrasion, the glenoid takes on the characteristic appearance of an osteoarthritic glenoid with the wear being anterior rather than posterior. These patients can be treated in a similar fashion to that described above. In those patients with gross bone loss of the anterior rim of the glenoid secondary to fractures, the remaining glenoid usually has a normal version. In these individuals, the bone graft is used to augment the existing glenoid and support the portion of the prosthesis overlying the area of wear. This is usually held in place with two or three screws passed into the remaining glenoid.

The second type of wear seen in patients with recurrent dislocation is caused by a too-tight anterior repair. This squeezes the head out the back of the glenoid and produces the characteristic changes of osteoarthritis. These patients will be treated in the same way as the patients with osteoarthritis, but in addition, they require a release of their tight anterior structures to allow for adequate external rotation postoperatively. If release is not performed, the posteriorly directed joint reaction force will cause posterior subluxation and loosening of the glenoid as well as limitation in postoperative motion.

CHRONIC UNREDUCED DISLOCATIONS

In these patients, the humeral head is locked outside of the glenoid fossa either anteriorly or posteriorly and articulates with the glenoid neck. The amount of bone destruction seen will be proportional to the amount of time that the humeral head has been locked in a dislocated position and how much physical therapy or attempted use has taken place. If the destruction is too extensive to consider an open reduction and transfer of the tuberosity to correct the instability, a nonconstrained total shoulder arthroplasty should be considered. In most cases, this requires loss of more than 50% of the humeral head or 50% of the glenoid fossa. The glenoid bone grafting is handled in a similar manner as discussed with the arthritis of recurrent dislocation, but in addition, the soft tissue balance must be addressed. In a patient who has had a chronically unreduced shoulder, either the posterior or the anterior structures will be quite tight secondary to scarring and lack of the normal excursion seen in an active shoulder. A posterior release is necessary in a fixed anterior dislocation, and an anterior release is necessary in a fixed posterior dislocation. When a bone graft alone is done without a soft tissue release, the range of motion postoperatively will be compromised. There is also the distinct possibility that a dislocation of the prosthesis will result. The stability and range of motion of the shoulder must be tested before the wound is closed to assure that there is no tendency towards redislocation.

GLENOID DYSPLASIA

Abnormal glenoid architecture may be due to a defect at birth, or a defect in development subsequent to birth. Here the glenoid is intrinsically deficient due to muscular paralysis or imbalance. The most common etiology of developmental glenoid dysplasia is brachial plexus palsy. The lack of a normal joint reaction force across the glenohumeral joint prevents the glenoid from developing normally. This often results in instability and chronic subluxation of the humeral head. The glenoid becomes further misshapen due to the abnormal wear caused by this painfully unstable situation. Because of the lack of any normal glenoid articulation, these patients usually require very large circumferential grafts similar to those used in patients with massive destruction due to rheumatoid arthritis. Sometimes the remaining glenoid may be used as a post for the attachment of the large bone graft, while in other patients a circular graft with fixation to the scapula is necessary. It must be remembered that in these patients the muscles are abnormal and the postoperative rehabilitation program should be geared towards stability and functional use at the side and not full active use of the shoulder.

LOSS OF BONE FROM TRAUMA OR PREVIOUS SURGERY

Another class of glenoid destruction is that seen in patients with penetrating trauma or previous surgery. Injuries such as gunshot wounds or severe scapular fractures result in loss of bone stock and severe distortion of the glenoid architecture. In failed surgery, the bone loss is of two varieties. With a failed glenoid osteotomy for instability, there can be avascular necrosis of the articular surface of the glenoid or failure of the articular surface to unite to the remaining glenoid. With a failed prosthesis, there is significant bone loss caused either intentionally at the time of the original procedure or subsequently due to the destruction caused by component malpositioning, loosening, or failure. In most constrained total shoulder prostheses, the glenoid component is anchored with multiple screws or a single massive one. In others, a significant portion of the glenoid is removed for placement of the glenoid component. When these fixed prostheses loosen or pull out, extensive destruction of the glenoid occurs. Both traumatic and revision surgery are further complicated by deficiencies in the muscles and nerves about the shoulder. For this reason, the bone grafting procedure is only a portion of the total reconstruction that is required to reestablish normal bony and soft tissue relationships. In the reconstruction of the severely traumatized shoulder, it must be remembered that the main goal is to return all bone, structures, and soft tissue to as near normal anatomy as possible. Only if this cannot be accomplished are procedures such as bone grafting and muscle transfer considered.

CUFF TEAR ARTHROPATHY

The diagnosis of cuff tear arthropathy implies a longstanding massive rotator cuff tear with resultant glenohumeral instability and superior migration of the humeral head. Often, this diagnosis is misused or is applied erroneously to a patient with degenerative arthritis of the glenohumeral joint and a concomitant rotator cuff tear. In the vast majority of these patients, a total shoulder replacement can be satisfactorily performed, and the rotator cuff repaired at the time of surgery. Even very large rotator cuff tears can usually be repaired in this situation because it is possible to decrease the volume of the glenohumeral joint by selecting a smaller head prosthesis. The recommended procedure includes osteotomy of the articular surface of the humeral head back to the articular margin followed by repair of the rotator cuff. In the case of very large rotator cuff tears, this often results in significant shortening of the rotator cuff and a decrease in the volume of the glenohumeral joint. This can be compensated for through the use of a smaller humeral head. In this way both the degenerative arthritis and the rotator cuff tear can be addressed at the same time.

The problem arises in patients who have true rotator cuff tear arthropathy, that is, a massive irreparable rotator cuff tear, with instability and absorption of the humeral head. This results in an incongruent humeral head that erodes into the acromion, the coracoid process, and the glenoid. Radiographic examination often gives the appearance of a Chargot joint. In the absence of a satisfactory rotator cuff or one that cannot be repaired in such a manner as to allow the implantation of a smaller humeral head prosthesis, we recommend humeral head replacement alone without the use of a glenoid component. The implantation of a glenoid component in a shoulder in which the rotator cuff cannot be repaired runs the risk of rapid glenoid loosening and failure. In these cases, the use of judicious glenoid reaming is probably beneficial both for enhanced stability and decrease in postoperative pain. An acetabler reamer is selected that has a radius of curvature the same or slightly larger than that of the selected humeral head. Reaming is very gentle, and minimal bone is removed. The goal is to contour the scapular articulation and enhance stability. In many of these patients, the remnant of the humeral head is articulating with the undersurface of the acromion, the base of the coracoid, and the spine of the scapula. The reaming, therefore, acts as a debridement of the glenoid and enhances containment of the humeral head.

Postoperative rehabilitation is directed toward limited goals of painless use at the side for activities of daily living.

References

1. Brems JJ, Wilde AH, Borden LS, Boumphrey FRS. Glenoid lucent lines. Orthop Trans 1986;10:231.
2. Neer CS II. Indications for replacement of the proximal humeral articulation. Am J Surg 1955;89:901–907.
3. Neer CS II. Articular replacement for the humeral head. J Bone Joint Surg 1955;37A:215–228.
4. Neer CS II, Watson KC, Stanton FJ. Recent experience in total shoulder replacement. J Bone Joint Surg 1982;64A: 319–337.
5. Neer CS II, Craig EV, Fukuda H. Cuff-tear arthropathy. J Bone Joint Surg 1983;65A:1232–1244.
6. Neer CW II, Morrison DS. Glenoid bone-grafting in total shoulder arthroplasty. J Bone Joint Surg 1988;70A:1154–1162.
7. Post M, Jablon J, Miller H, Singh MD. Constrained total shoulder joint replacement: a critical review. Clin Orthop 1979;144–145.
8. Post M. Constrained total shoulder arthroplasty: long term results. Orthop Trans 1987;11:238.

7
Complications of Humeral Head Replacement

Gregory W. Soghikian and Robert J. Neviaser

INTRODUCTION

Hemiarthroplasty of the shoulder has become an accepted treatment for certain proximal humerus fractures and fracture dislocations, as well as some cases of osteonecrosis, osteoarthritis, and rheumatoid arthritis. Unfortunately, as this procedure gains popularity, the number of associated complications has increased. This chapter outlines the more commonly encountered complications, makes some suggestions on how to avoid them, and discusses treatment options for dealing with those complications when they do occur.

PROSTHESIS MALPOSITION

Functional success and lower complication rates depend greatly on proper prosthesis position. The two most important components of humeral position are height and rotation.

Improper Height

The prosthesis should sit so that the superior point on the curvature of the head is above the tuberosities. If the prosthetic head is below the top of the greater tuberosity, the tuberosity will impinge against the acromion and block elevation (Fig. 7.1). A lower position or shorter prosthetic length will decrease the resting tension of the deltoid and cause weakness in elevation. It can also contribute to laxity of the rotator cuff and capsule with subsequent subluxation or dislocation.

Positioning the prosthesis too superiorly may also result in problems. There may be increased soft tissue tension, making cuff closure more difficult. It may also lead to improper tuberosity placement and nonunion.

Prevention of these problems begins with preoperative templating. Care should be taken to not make the neck osteotomy too inferior or too oblique. In general, preservation of as much of the neck and head as possible is recommended. Ideally, the calcar and some of the head are preserved for seating of the prosthesis, helping to prevent excessive shortening of the humerus or subsidence of the prosthesis (Fig. 7.2). If a preoperative fracture extends below the

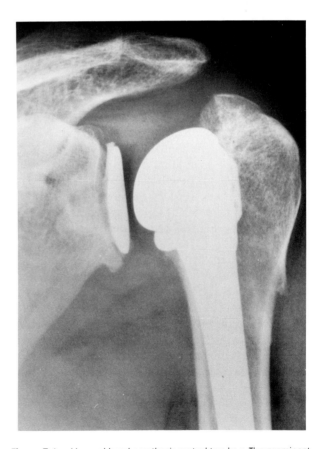

Figure 7.1. Humeral head prosthesis seated too low. The prominent tuberosity will impinge and block full elevation.

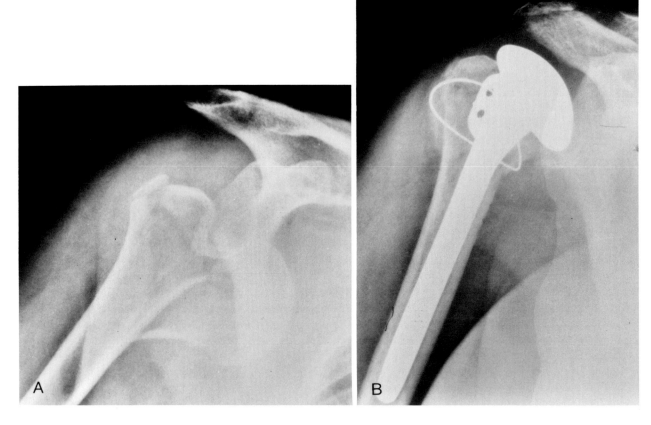

Figure 7.2. **A,** Fracture/dislocation of the humeral head. Note the piece of the medial metaphysis (calcar) attached to the head. **B,** The metaphyseal fragment has been retained and used to support the head, which is seated in the proper position.

level of the tuberosities, such that maintaining the length leaves the prosthesis unsupported, a prosthesis with a longer shaft and augmentation of the shaft with bone graft should be considered (2) (Fig. 7.3). This will also help achieve union of the reapproximated tuberosities. If there is any doubt concerning final stem length and height, intraoperative x-rays may be helpful prior to closure in selected cases.

If a patient has poor elevation after hemiarthroplasty, and radiographs show evidence of improper prosthesis height, then physical therapy is unlikely to be of benefit. The remaining options for improvement are subacromial decompression or revision. Revision is biomechanically advantageous but obviously technically more difficult. It may require reconstruction of length with an iliac crest bone graft to restore adequate height (Fig. 7.4).

Malrotation

Placing the prosthesis in 30–40° of retroversion along with cuff repair is one of the most important factors in preventing postoperative instability. If a prosthesis is not retroverted sufficiently, it will tend to subluxate anteriorly, while one that is excessively retroverted will subluxate posteriorly and limit external rotation.

In choosing rotational position the best points of reference are the tuberosities. The fin of the stem is placed just behind the bicipital groove. If, however, they are not intact, as is often the situation in displaced fractures, the surgeon should use the distal humeral epicondyles. With the elbow flexed and the hand pointing forward, the prosthesis should point directly at the glenoid.

One exception to the usual choice of retroversion is in the case of prosthetic replacement for the treatment of a chronic posterior dislocation. In that case, a position of less retroversion or even neutral rotation may provide improved stability. If the glenoid is eroded or deficient anteriorly or posteriorly, rotation is adjusted accordingly to assist stability.

If a patient presents postoperatively with subluxation or dislocation and radiographs show improper rotational positioning, reoperation may be

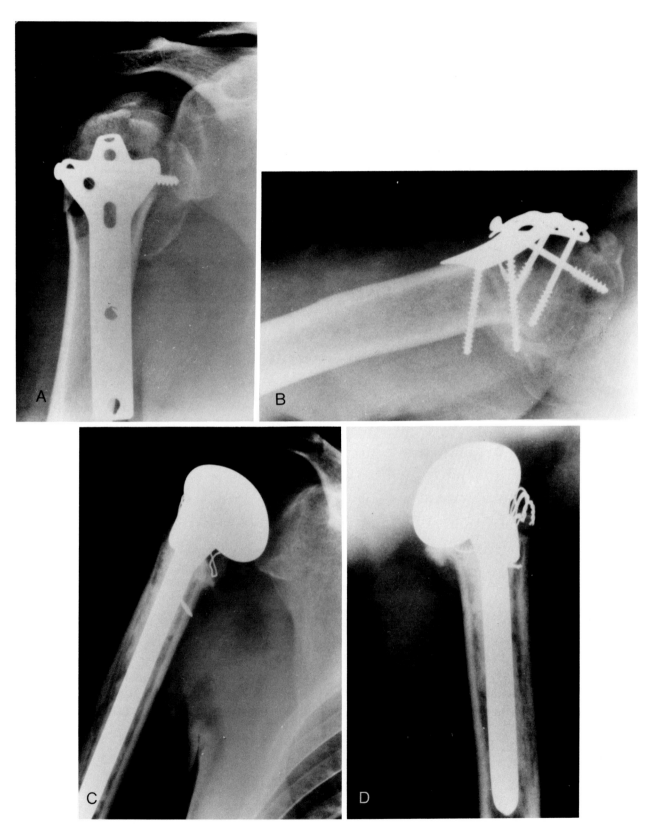

Figure 7.3. **A**, Proximal humeral fracture with inadequate internal fixation (AP). **B**, Axillary of the same fracture. **C**, Reconstructed with prosthetic replacement using an iliac crest bone graft to recreate a calcar for proper support and positioning of the prosthesis. **D**, Axillary of the same patient.

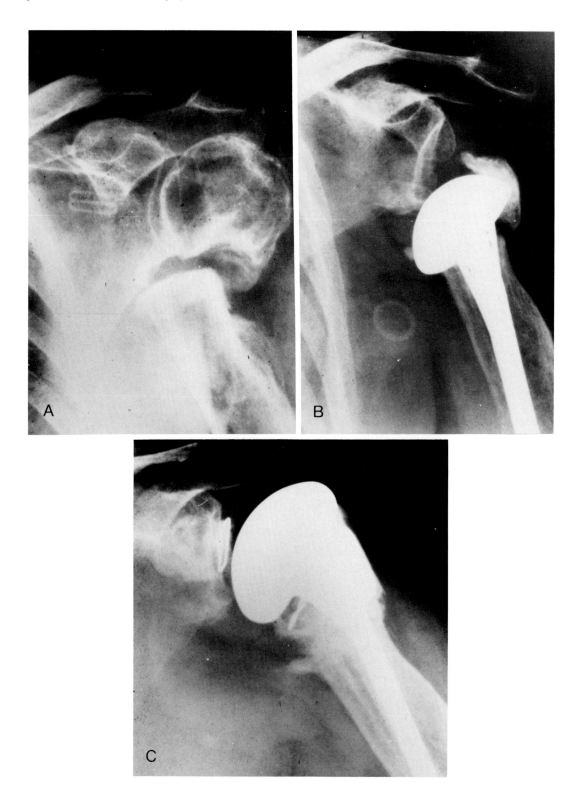

Figure 7.4.   A, Nonunion of a surgical neck fracture. **B**, Improperly used prosthesis seated on the shaft so that the tuberosities cannot be secured under the implant. **C**, Reconstructed using an iliac crest bone graft to raise the prosthesis to the proper height and allow the tuberosities to be seated under the head.

considered, but the surgeon should then pay particular attention to the condition of the soft tissues and not just the rotation of the prosthesis. At the time of revision, the stem will most likely need to be cemented to maintain the desired position of rotation (Fig. 7.5).

HUMERAL SHAFT FRACTURE

Humeral shaft fracture occurs most commonly during reaming, but can also occur while implanting the prosthesis or even when simply manipulating the arm. Since most of the patients requiring hemiarthroplasty are older, they may have disuse or senile osteoporosis and are at higher risk for fracture.

Careful hand reaming and attention to alignment of the reamer relative to the shaft to avoid excessive levering or torque can help prevent shaft injury. Overreaming will cause thinning of the cortex and increase the fracture risk. Attempting to implant an oversized or tight "press-fit" stem can also result in a fracture and is an unnecessary risk if cementing the prosthesis.

Choice of stem size can be approximated by preoperative radiographic templating, but the final determination should be made intraoperatively. If a press-fit is chosen, care must be taken when implanting the prosthesis. If the prosthesis is cemented, a smaller shaft can be used with less danger of fracture. Cement should be considered in patients with a wide medullary canal.

Spiral fractures are caused by torquing forces that occur during reaming or in attempting to change the rotational position of the prosthesis after it has been partially seated. Oblique or longitudinal fracture can be caused by attempting to seat an oversized stem. These fractures can frequently be treated by circlage wiring, especially if they are nondisplaced and do not extend beyond the prosthesis length.

Transverse fractures result from cortical penetration during reaming or by levering of the prosthesis or reamer within the shaft. These can be treated by using a long-stemmed prosthesis that extends beyond the cortical penetration or fracture by a minimum of two shaft widths (Fig. 7.6). For rotational control, the prosthesis should then be cemented into position unless the patient is young and the fit is snug or the fracture interdigitates well.

If repair of the fracture is felt to be at all tenuous, then longer postoperative protection, delayed rehabilitation, and an external brace should all be considered.

TUBEROSITY MALPOSITION

Malposition of the tuberosities can contribute to impingement symptoms, weak abductor function, and postoperative migration or subluxation. Choosing the correct position is particularly difficult in hemiarthroplasty for four-part fractures.

Understanding the configuration of the fracture pattern and tuberosity fragments begins preoperatively. A variety of radiographic views are helpful and should include AP views in neutral, internal and external rotation, as well as an axillary view and a lateral view in the scapular plane (10). If care is taken to position the shoulder gently, these can be obtained without causing great discomfort to the patient. A variety of radiographic views are helpful and should include AP views in neutral, internal and external rotation, as well as an axillary view and a lateral view in the scapular plane (10). If care is taken to position the shoulder gently, these can be obtained without causing great discomfort to the patient. Radiographs of the unaffected shoulder may also help in determining the premorbid position of the tuberosities. Computerized tomography may also be helpful.

Correct tuberosity placement will aid in the recreation of the appropriate amount of tension on the muscular attachments. Failure to restore correct tension can lead to a lax rotator cuff, which may in turn cause subluxation (Fig. 7.7).

A study by Rietveld showed that restoration of the "humeral offset" (the distance from the geometric center of the head to the lateral side of the greater tuberosity) is one of the most important factors in achieving good abductor function by maintaining the correct lever arm for the deltoid (8). If the greater tuberosity is reduced in size or malpositioned, it reduces the abductor power of the deltoid and increases its superior pull, raising the chances of postoperative superior migration, subluxation, and abductor weakness (3, 8). If the greater tuberosity is placed proximal to the prosthetic head, it may cause impingement problems.

Correction of postoperative problems secondary to tuberosity malposition can be difficult. It may also be difficult to assess which problem associated with malposition is the most symptomatic: impingement, subluxation, or weakness. If therapy to strengthen the shoulder muscles fails, reoperation is the only option. This may require decompression, retensioning of the soft tissues, or complete revision.

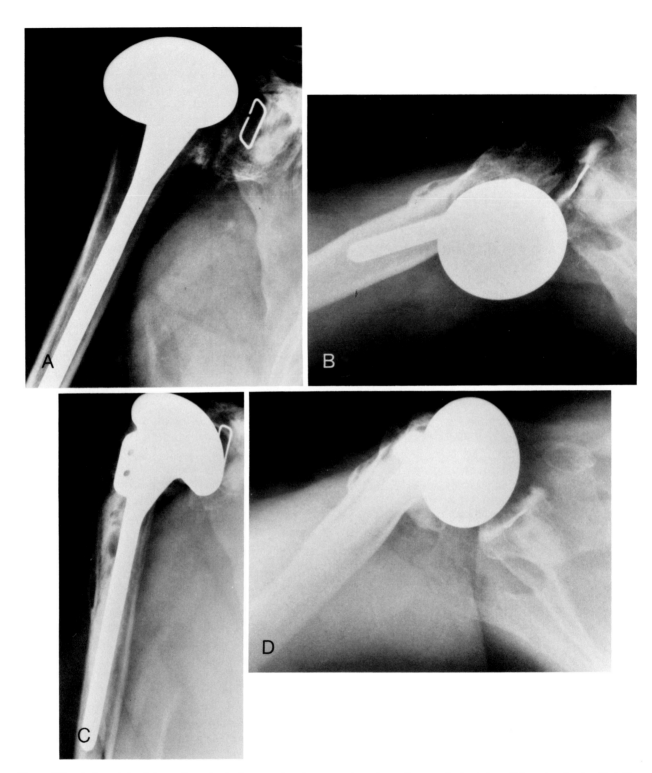

Figure 7.5. **A**, Posteriorly dislocated prosthesis due to malrotation and severe internal rotation contracture of the shoulder. **B**, Axillary view confirming the posterior dislocation. **C**, Prosthesis revised with more anteversion and concomitant anterior soft tissue lengthening. **D**, Axillary shows the reduced position.

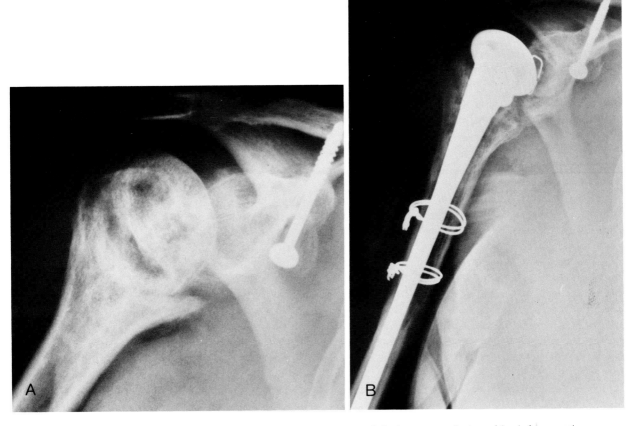

Figure 7.6.   **A**, Nonunion of the proximal humerus prior to replacement. **B**, During surgery, a fracture of the shaft occurred and was treated with circlage wiring and a bypass with a long-stemmed prosthesis.

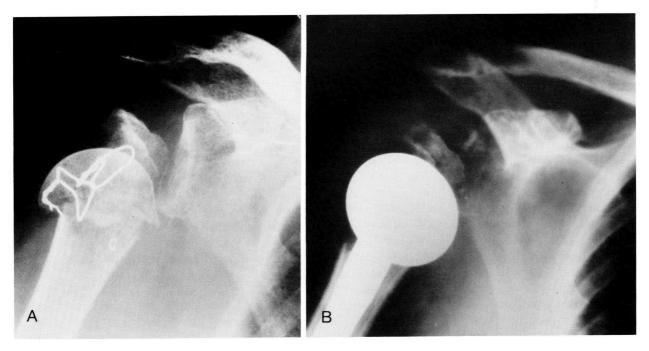

Figure 7.7.   **A**, Fractured treated by in situ wiring with neither reducing the head to its correct position nor reducing the tuberosities. **B**, Attempt at salvage with a prosthesis, but the tuberosities have not been seated under the lip of the prosthesis and secured to the bone of the shaft.

SUBLUXATION/PROXIMAL MIGRATION

Since good shoulder function involves a great deal of motion in several planes, the natural joint is necessarily minimally constrained. Because of this, the shoulder is highly dependent on the soft tissues to prevent subluxation. The main contributors to shoulder stability are the glenohumeral ligaments and capsule and the rotator cuff. In hemiarthroplasty the glenohumeral ligaments and the capsule are usually damaged. For this reason, the rotator cuff becomes the only major stabilizing force for the (prosthetic) humeral head. In patients requiring hemiarthroplasty for trauma or rheumatoid changes, the rotator cuff is frequently injured or abnormal preoperatively, making reconstruction that much more difficult and important.

During the initial approach, assessment of the condition of the cuff should be made. Mobilization of the rotator cuff will make both the initial exposure and later repair easier. In cases of massive rotator cuff defects, biceps tendon or freeze-dried rotator cuff grafts may be necessary (7). Contracture and shortening of the subscapularis in a chronic injury may require z-plasty lengthening (5). The availability of modular prostheses now allows smaller or larger heads to be used to help to overcome shortened or lax rotator cuff tendons.

Late rotator cuff dehiscence or reinjury can be associated with postoperative impingement. For this reason, the amount of clearance between the subacromial arch and the prosthesis and greater tuberosity should be assessed intraoperatively. If it is deemed to be inadequate, repositioning of the prosthesis or decompression of the arch should be considered.

Postoperative protection is important to preserve any rotator cuff repair, to allow for soft tissue healing, and to help prevent dislocation. Most authors use some variation of a sling and swathe. The schedule and aggressiveness of physical rehabilitation should be guided by the individual case and intraoperative assessment of stability of the prosthesis and strength of repair. Early mobilization (1–2 days postoperatively) may help gain better functional outcome, especially if the operation was for treatment of a chronic injury. However, in the case of acute fracture, Tanner and Cofield found that waiting for 2 weeks postoperatively before initiating motion increased the chances of proper tuberosity and rotator cuff healing and resulted in better eventual function (10), especially when fixation is of concern.

Dislocation of the prosthesis is most likely to occur in the early postoperative period before the soft tissues have healed. Most can be treated with closed reduction, under general anesthesia if necessary, and immobilization with postponement of physical rehabilitation. Subluxation and proximal migration occur more frequently later and can become a progressive problem. Although some patients will be asymptomatic, others will develop poor abduction and may have increased pain. Proximal migration is often secondary to a poor rotator cuff repair, stretching out of the repair, or dehiscence of the cuff. Prolonged protection or targeted strengthening of the cuff may help, but if the problem is persistent, painful, or progressive, it may require reoperation and repair.

EARLY INFECTION

As in any major joint surgery, infections do occur and can be devastating. Both early and late wound infections have been reported (4, 6, 9). Perioperative antibiotics should be used immediately prior to surgery and continued for 24–48 hours postoperatively. Careful preoperative scrubbing is essential, and some advocate putting an antibiotic-soaked pad in the axilla the night prior to surgery.

In cases of prior failed open reduction and internal fixation, intraoperative cultures, frozen section, Gram's stain, and tissue samples should be considered to rule out the presence of a preoperative infection.

Throughout a proximal humerus replacement, as in any operation, careful attention should be paid to hemostasis. Hematoma formation increases the risk of infection and can also increase postoperative scarring and adhesions. Closed-system drains may be placed deep to the rotator cuff and between the cuff and deltoid to help prevent hematoma collection in wounds that are not sufficiently dry intraoperatively.

In the event of a large postoperative hematoma or superficial infection, some authors advocate early return to the operating room to decompress the hematoma and debride most of the superficial infection. More minor superficial infections can be treated by appropriate intravenous antibiotics.

HETEROTOPIC OSSIFICATION

Heterotopic bone formation, in particular periscapular bony deposits, has been reported by several authors (1, 10), but is rarely a significant problem. Irrigation and debridement to remove all fracture fragments or bone debris from the soft tissues at the time of operation should help to reduce the incidence of problems. Any periscapular bone already formed preoperatively should also be debrided. In patients with a history of heterotopic bone formation or severe closed-head injury, prophylactic treatment with indomethacin or radiation therapy can be considered. If significant amounts have formed, they can be excised when mature if they inhibit adequate motion or cause pain (10).

MALUNION/NONUNION

Nonunion of the tuberosities is an infrequent problem, but in cases of injured vascular supply to the proximal humerus or loss of bone stock because of trauma, nonunion can be more common.

Prevention of nonunion begins with adequate intraoperative fixation. Most surgeons advocate the use of a heavy nonabsorbable suture or # 20 gauge wire (5, 10). Late breakage and possible migration of wire can occur in delayed or nonunion cases. Fixation of the tuberosities is most secure if taken through holes in both the prosthesis and proximal humeral shaft. The goal is not only to seat the tuberosities under the prosthesis but also to achieve union between them and the shaft, since bone will not heal to metal (Fig. 7.8). If fixation is tenuous, postoperative motion should be delayed.

Preservation of the bulk of the tuberosities will increase the area of cancellous bone available for union and will also allow for correct tensioning of the attached musculature. In cases where significant bone stock is missing from the proximal shaft, primary bone grafting may be prudent. This will help with union of the tuberosities as well as fixation of the shaft.

If nonunion or malunion of the tuberosities occurs and causes significant loss of function or pain, refixation and bone grafting may be necessary.

LOOSENING/SETTLING

The incidence of prosthetic loosening in shoulder hemiarthroplasty is low. However, loosening can occur, especially in more active patients. Settling of the prosthesis has also been reported but is more common in uncemented hemiarthroplasty.

By cementing the prosthesis with good technique, the risk of significant loosening is reduced.

This begins with adequate retraction and complete exposure of the proximal end of the humeral shaft. Use of a cement restrictor and a cement gun will reduce the volume of cement used distally and ensure adequate filling of the shaft.

When an uncemented prosthesis is used, a true "press-fit" must be achieved. If using a prosthesis with proximal flutes, the flutes should be well seated in bone to prevent rotation. If the bone stock is questionable (but cement is not used), then primary bone grafting should be considered (Fig. 7.9).

If loosening or settling occurs and becomes clinically significant, treatment should be based on the symptoms. Settling can cause weakening of the deltoid lever arm, impingement, and pain. If the only symptom is weakness, physical therapy with deltoid and cuff strengthening may alleviate the problem. If there is radiographic and clinical evidence of impingement, reoperation to decompress the subacromial space or to revise the prosthesis may be necessary. If revision is performed, a cemented prosthesis should be considered, augmented by bone grafting the calcar.

LATE INFECTION

As with any joint replacement, hemiarthroplasty of the shoulder can be complicated by late infection—either from an indolent contaminant at the time of surgery or by seeding from another site. Prophylactic antibiotic coverage during dental or urologic procedures is recommended and should be considered.

If a late, deep infection does occur, it is much more troublesome than early infection. Reoperation is necessary with removal of all hardware and cement, as is a minimum of 6 weeks of appropriate intravenous antibiotics. After that time, if there is no evidence of recurrence, a new prosthesis can be considered for implantation with antibiotic-impregnated cement.

References

1. Aliabadi P, Weissman B, Thornhill T, et al. Evaluation of a nonconstrained total shoulder prosthesis. AJR 1988;151: 1169–1172.
2. Gristina AG, Romano RL, Kammire GC, Webb LX. Total shoulder replacement. Orthop Clin North Amer 1987;18: 445–453.

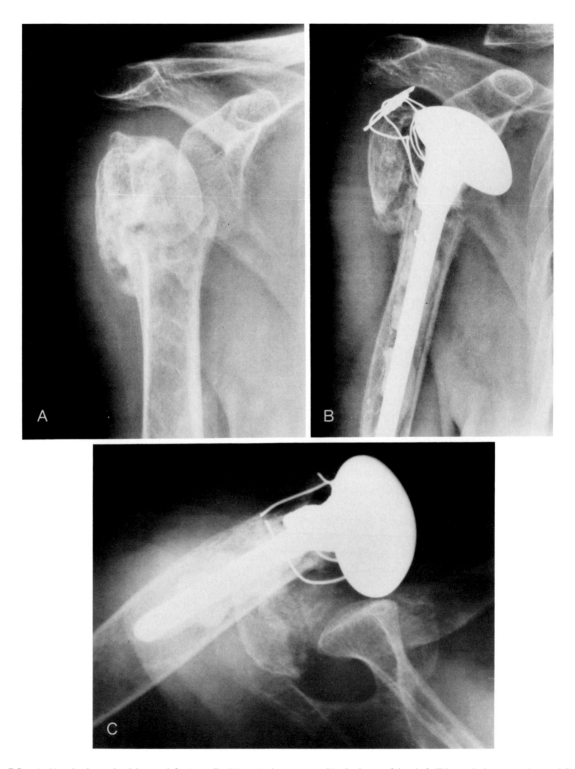

Figure 7.8. **A**, Ununited proximal humeral fracture. **B**, Attempted reconstruction with a prosthesis, but the tuberosities have not been secured to the bone of the shaft. This results in a nonunion and **C**, Dislocation of the prosthesis and posteriorly displaced greater tuberosity.

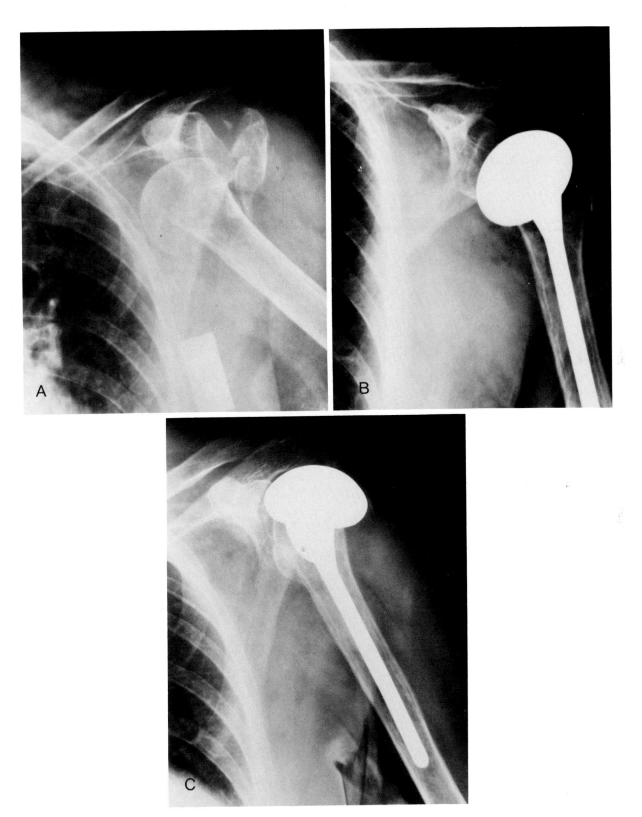

Figure 7.9.   **A**, Fracture/dislocation of the shoulder. **B**, Treated by a prosthesis, but the stem is too small for the wide medullary canal, and cement was not used. **C**, This resulted in the prosthesis rotating within the shaft.

3. Kay SP, Amstutz HC. Shoulder hemiarthroplasty at UCLA. CORR 1988;228:42–48.

4. Kraulis J, Hunter G. The results of prosthetic replacement in fracture-dislocations of the upper end of the humerus. Injury 1976;8:129–131.

5. Neer CS, Watson KC, Stanton FJ. Recent experience in total shoulder replacement. JBJS 1982;64A:319–337.

6. Neer CS. Displaced proximal humeral fractures. JBJS 1970;52A:1090–1103.

7. Neviaser JS, Neviaser RJ, Neviaser TJ. The repair of chronic massive ruptures of the rotator cuff by use of a freeze-dried rotator cuff. JBJS 1978;60A:681–684.

8. Rietveld AB, Daanen HA, Rozing PM, Obermann WR. The lever arm in glenohumeral abduction after hemiarthroplasty. JBJS 1988;70B:561–565.

9. Stableforth PG. Four-part fractures of the neck of the humerus. JBJS 1984;66B:104–108.

10. Tanner MW, Cofield RH. Prosthetic arthroplasty for fractures and fracture-dislocations of the proximal humerus. Clin Orthop Rel Res 1983;179:116–128.

8
Complications of Shoulder Fusion

John J. Brems

INTRODUCTION

Fortunately, the indications for shoulder fusion are becoming less and less common. In the last 40 years, the evolution of shoulder joint replacement has eliminated the need for fusion in the treatment of painful arthritis. Whereas treatment of septic joints by fusion was once common, new generation antibiotics have made septic destruction of joints distinctly uncommon in Western societies. Furthermore, the advent of the polio vaccine in 1955 has had a dramatic effect on diminishing the paralytic states that at one time were best managed, in the case of the shoulder, with an arthrodesis. As we read of the reappearance of the polio virus, especially in Third World countries, however, we are reminded that things can go wrong at any time. Even though as orthopaedic surgeons we will find less occasion to perform shoulder fusions, we must be aware of the complications that may occur.

Clearly, any operative procedure has risks and complications independent of the procedure itself. There are the inherent risks of the anesthesia, blood loss and its replacement, nerve injuries, and wound infections. Postoperative complications of fluid imbalance, deep vein thrombosis, pulmonary emboli, and the sequelae of prolonged immobilization often attendant with orthopaedic procedures are not uncommon even with the most observant care. As surgeons, we must be keen not only to the specific complications of our specific procedures; we must also be fully aware that we are operating on a whole person—not just a joint.

SPECIFIC COMPLICATIONS OF SHOULDER FUSION

Complications of Position

The most common complication related to shoulder fusion is malposition of the fused components, i.e., the humerus and scapula. The important requisites following shoulder fusion are that the hand should reach the face, head, and midline of the body anteriorly and posteriorly; that the arm should be in a position of maximum strength for lifting, pushing, and pulling; that the shoulder should be comfortable when the arm is at the side of the body, and that the scapula should not be prominent while in this position (19). Numerous articles have been written describing the optimal positioning in terms of arm abduction, forward flexion, and internal rotation. The surgeon must recall that probably the most important *functional* requirement of the shoulder is external rotation. Without it, the largest functional impairment of the fused shoulder results. In 1942, the Research Committee of the American Orthopaedic Association reported on the results of shoulder fusion (1):

Early in the course of the investigation, certain facts became apparent. We have felt that, in all of the 102 shoulders on which an arthrodesis had been attempted, some benefit had been received through increased stability, regardless of the position and whether or not fusion had occurred. However, less than 10% of the cases met all the criteria necessary to be classed as excellent. The results in the large majority of the arthrodesed shoulders were below the possible optimum, because of some relatively minor defect in management, the most frequent of which was some error in postoperative position. It would seem that too little attention was paid by the surgeon to the relative position of humerus and scapula. The majority of us have been placing the humerus in relation to the trunk and neglecting its relationship to the scapula. Too much emphasis has been placed, also, on securing abduction but not enough on the degree of rotation of the arm.

In the more contemporary reports, disagreement remains regarding the role of glenohumeral positioning at the time of arthrodesis. Cofield and Briggs studied 71 shoulders in 70 patients and concluded that the position of fusion had little effect on the functional results, but no patient had abduction greater than 58° (2, 6, 18). However, in 1983, Rowe published the findings with a series of shoulder fusions, and noted that excessive abduction or forward flexion and especially external rotation, must be avoided (17). With the literature promoting a variety of "optimal" positions that are ideal for shoulder arthrodesis, how is one to know? To complicate matters, it is very difficult to perform intraoperative angular measurements and to identify the bony landmarks from which one can make the measurements. It has been my experience to position the patient in a true lateral decubitus position on the operating table with the back straight and perpendicular to the floor and the arm draped free. At the time of glenohumeral positioning, the hand is placed at the mouth and the elbow abducted from the side approximately 45° relative to the floor. With the arm held in this position, the hardware of choice is placed. This assures the physician that at the very least the patient can reach his mouth. With this technique of positioning, patients can usually reach their mouths as well as the anal region for hygiene, and this amount of abduction usually permits patients to reach their opposite axilla. Radiologic analysis of this position demonstrates true abduction (medial scapular border to humerus) of approximately 40°. Forward flexion (humerus to coronal plane of body) is approximately 20°, and internal rotation also approximates 20°.

Of all the joints for which fusion is common, shoulder arthrodesis has the highest incidence of continued pain. Malposition, especially excessive abduction, can result in increased back pain and interscapular pain. With fusion in excessive abduction, as the arm comes down to the side the scapula is rotated on the thorax, placing an abnormal increased tension on scapular stabilizing muscles including the trapezius, rhomboids, levator scapulae, and serratus anterior. The patients complain of muscle ache and

fatigue symptoms in addition to pain. Similarly, increased forward flexion can result in increased forces of retraction on the scapula and result in chronic interscapular pain and neck pain. With the increased lever arm provided by the fusion, rotational moments on the scapula are dramatically increased.

Another complication of malposition (excessive abduction) is weakness. With increasing abduction, the hand becomes farther away from the fulcrum of the shoulder and therefore diminishes the lifting and functional strength (17). Barton recommended a trial of immobilization in a cast prior to arthrodesis in the anticipated position of fusion to assess relief of pain. However, two of his patients who had complete relief of their symptoms while in their spica casts were among those who continued to complain of pain following their shoulder fusions (2).

In children, fusion of the shoulder in excessive abduction may result in bowing of the arm and growth arrest. Some authors have recommended diminished abduction and that fusion be delayed until skeletal maturity (11).

Complications due to malposition do not only relate to excessive abduction. Rotational malposition can be equally disabling, not so much from pain, but more for function. Hawkins and Neer wrote that the position of humeral rotation was the most critical factor in approaching optimal function. Fusions with excessive internal rotation have diminished ability to comb hair, wash the face, or perform other activities near the head and neck. With excessive external rotation, reaching the opposite axilla and reaching the behind to pass a belt become very difficult (8). The ideal range of humeral rotation is 25–35° relative to the frontal plane of the body.

Complications of Healing

The glenohumeral joint has a very small surface area for the fusion to occur. Consequently, nonunion and pseudarthrosis are not rare. In 1942, the American Orthopaedic Association reported nonunion rates approaching 22% with internal fixation techniques. Cofield summarized the literature and found an overall pseudarthrosis rate of 10% in nearly 500 reported cases (7). Because of the high failure rates, various fixation techniques have been described in the literature (3, 7, 9, 12, 15, 18, 20). Barton reviewed his series of arthrodeses for degenerative conditions and found that all four patients who had cuff tears prior to surgery eventually complained of pain after their arthrodesis. He theorized that when the rotator cuff is intact, the weight of the abducted arm tends to force and hold the humeral head in the glenoid cavity. When there is a large tear in the supraspinatus, this leverage is lost and cannot be compensated by the already atrophic deltoid (2). This diminished force may result in a higher rate of nonunion.

Regardless of the method of fixation, one must remember that the area of bone contact is minimal in nearly all contemporary techniques for shoulder arthrodesis by intra-articular and extra-articular fixation methods. Autograft and allograft are often important adjuncts to local measures of fusion. Published series with both glenohumeral and acromiohumeral fixation have been advocated. Tension wires, bone plugs, plates, and internal fixators all have their proponents, but each technique carries its own complications.

Complications of fixation also may occur secondary to inadequate immobilization. Prolonged immobilization and continuance of fixation are critical. Polo and Monterrubio reported a 42% incidence of nonunion if the external fixation was discarded at 10 weeks or less from the time of surgery (14).

Complications of Fixation

Improved technology and modern metallurgy have provided today's orthopaedic surgeon with super alloys, ultra-high tensile-strength materials, and metals of indefinite fatigue life. Consequently, primary failure of these devices used as an initial fixation device is rare.

However, whereas the chain is only as strong as its weakest link, the device is only as strong as the bone into which it is placed. The polio, paralytic, and postinfectious shoulder usually has remarkably osteoporotic bone. The glenoid and humeral head, in particular, are osteopenic and incapable of supporting screws and have a high potential for loosening and pull-out. Screws and plates are prominent on the scapular spine and may cause pain and erode through the skin (16, 20). Cofield and Briggs published a series where 17 of 66 patients (24%) required a second operation because of painful and prominent internal fixation devices (6).

Occasionally, smooth and threaded pins are used as an adjunct in the fixation techniques for shoulder fusion. However, there is a high incidence of complications related to pin migration. At the American Shoulder and Elbow Surgeons Meeting in 1990,

Lyons and Rockwood presented a paper describing the perils of pins in shoulder surgery (10). Not only can pins break and migrate, infection may occur when these devices are used transcutaneously. Johnson and his coworkers published the results of shoulder fusion with the Hoffman external fixator on only four patients, one of whom developed a significant pin tract infection that ultimately responded to antibiotics (9). Charnley also reported a 10% incidence of pin tract infection with his external compression device when used for shoulder fusion (5).

MISCELLANEOUS COMPLICATIONS OF SHOULDER FUSION

Complications Related to Bone

Several other potential complications must be considered. With a successful glenohumeral fusion, significant bending stresses arise in the proximal humerus. This has resulted in an unexpectedly high rate of humeral fractures. Cofield reported on 10 fractures in 70 patients, eight in the humerus, one in the ulna, and one in the radius. Half of these fractures occurred in patients with a paralytic condition (6).

The acromion, clavicle, and AC joint may present complications and require consideration in a shoulder fusion. The acromion provides another bone surface to incorporate during arthrodesis. There is debate over whether or not to osteotomize the acromion and bring it "down" to the humerus or whether to bring the humerus "up" to meet the acromion process. There is little doubt that the addition of the acromion in the fusion mass significantly adds to the union rate. When the acromion is osteotomized and brought distally, it significantly alters the cosmetic appearance and symmetry of the shoulders. On the other hand, if the arm is brought cephalad and up under the acromion, the shoulder contour and cosmesis are maintained, but the elbow flexors and coracoid muscles are shortened with subsequent weakness of elbow flexion and supination.

Although most authors recommend preservation of the clavicle for cosmesis and stability, the increase in scapular motion that results from the arthrodesis may cause late acromioclavicular joint pain. If this pain becomes severe enough, lateral clavicular resection may be indicated. Pipkin studied patients who had partial (lateral) and total claviculectomy. He noted that there was a significant improvement in motion and thus function with claviculectomy, but that there was a concomitant increase in cosmetic deformity. He further concluded that resection of the lateral clavicle provided as much benefit as total claviculectomy with improved cosmesis. However, he cautioned against this procedure in patients who are crutch ambulators or who otherwise had weakened muscles and needed the entire clavicle for muscular support (13).

Complications of Soft Tissues

MUSCLE

The complications of persistent pain following shoulder fusion have already been mentioned. The most common cause seems to be related to malposition and its secondary effects on soft tissues, especially muscle. Whereas many fusions are performed for paralytic conditions, one must carefully assess all scapular muscles prior to the arthrodesis. Ideally, the trapezius, rhomboid, and serratus anterior must be of good quality. At the very least, the trapezius should have moderate strength to support the limb. May reviewed 14 cases of shoulder fusion and determined that only those patients who had a strong trapezius and serratus were able to elevate and rotate their shoulders against resistance (12).

NERVE

Another complication of shoulder arthrodesis is traction neuritis. The neuritis may involve the suprascapular nerve, which is more commonly seen with the arm fixed in excessive abduction. Humeral osteotomy or lateral clavicle resection may relieve these symptoms. Ulnar neuritis may develop at the elbow as a patient "subconsciously" seeks chairs with arms and other supports for their arms while at work. The constant external pressure over the elbow may result in ulnar symptoms enough to necessitate nerve transposition. Cases have been reported of reflex sympathetic dystrophy of the extremity following shoulder fusion. Whereas prevention is the best treatment, sympathetic ganglion blocks have usually proven beneficial in the established condition.

INFECTION

Recognizing that the indication for shoulder fusion many times is active or remote infection, it is not surprising that this may be a postoperative complication. Virtually all publications in the literature that discuss shoulder fusion remark about infection as a postoperative complication. Cofield found that although primary infections occur during shoulder arthrodesis, they are no more common than in other orthopaedic procedures (7). Carnesale and Stewart stated that wound infections exclusive of a pin tract infection probably occur in 3–5% of the patients undergoing arthrodesis of the shoulder. (4) In all cases, the basic prophylactic measures must be followed. Keep in mind that viable tissue rarely becomes infected. One must debride devitalized tissue, prevent desiccation of tissue during prolonged procedures, use judicial perioperative antibiotics, respect normal tissue planes, and avoid dead space formation.

SUMMARY

Table 8.1 is a generalized listing of complications to consider when attempting shoulder fusion. The development and techniques of shoulder arthroplasty, the polio vaccine, and modern antibiotics have dramatically lessened the indications and frequency for shoulder fusion. With fewer procedures performed, it becomes easy to recall the benefits of the procedure, but rather difficult to remember other risks and complications. Before performing a shoulder fusion, one should again be reminded of the

Table 8.1.   Complications of Shoulder Arthrodesis

Malposition
    Excessive abduction
    Excessive external rotation
Persistent Pain
Pseudarthrosis
    Nonunion
Failure of Fixation
    Plates
    Screws
    Pins
Fracture
Acromion
    AC joint arthritis
    Limited motion
    Cosmesis
Muscle
    Chronic pain/strain
    Weakness
Nerve
    Neuritis
    Reflex sympathetic dystrophy
Infection
Growth Arrest/Bowing
    Skeletally immature bone

work of the Research Committee of the American Orthopaedic Association (1): "The results in a large majority of the arthrodesed shoulders were below the possible optimum because of some relatively minor defect in management."

With the proper indications and with attention to the details of position, fixation techniques and proper postoperative management, shoulder fusion can be a useful reconstructive procedure that will decrease pain and improve function.

References

1. Barr JS, Freiberg JA, Colonna PC, Pemberton PA. A survey of the end results on stabilization of the paralytic shoulder: report of the Research Committee of the American Orthopaedic Association. J Bone Joint Surg 1942;24:699–707.
2. Barton NJ. Arthrodesis of the shoulder for degenerative conditions. J Bone Joint Surg 1972;54A:1759–1764.
3. Beltran JE, Trilla JC, Barjou RA. A simplified compression arthrodesis of the shoulder. J Bone Joint Surg 1975; 57A:538–541.
4. Carnesale PG, Stewart MJ. Complications of arthrodesis surgery. In: Epps CH, ed. Complications in orthopaedic surgery. Philadelphia: JB Lippincott, 1978;1123–1129.
5. Charnley J, Houston JK. Compression arthrodesis of the shoulder. J Bone Joint Surg 1964;46B:614–620.
6. Cofield RH, Briggs BT. Glenohumeral arthrodesis. J Bone Joint Surg 1979;61A:668–677.
7. Cofield RH. Shoulder arthrodesis and resection arthroplasty. In: Instructional Course Lectures, AAOS. St. Louis: CV Mosby, 1985:268–277.
8. Hawkins RJ, Neer CS. A functional analysis of shoulder fusions. Clin Orthop 1987;223:65–76.
9. Johnson CA, Healy WL, Brooker AF, Krackow KA. External fixation shoulder arthrodesis. Clin Orthop 1986;211:219–223.
10. Lyons FR, Rockwood CA. Perils of pins: migration of pins used in shoulder surgery. Presented at The American Shoulder and Elbow Surgeons Society Open Meeting 1990; New Orleans, La.
11. Makin M. Early arthrodesis for a flail shoulder in young children. J Bone Joint Surg 1977;59A:317–321.
12. May VR. Shoulder fusion. J Bone Joint Surg 1962;44A:65–76.
13. Pipkin G. Claviculectomy as an adjunct to shoulder arthrodesis. Clin Orthop 1967;54:145–159.
14. Polo G, Monterrubio AC. Arthrodesis of the shoulder. Clin Orthop 1973;90:178–182.
15. Ralston EL. Arthrodesis of the shoulder. Orthop Clin North Amer 1975;6:585–591.
16. Richards RR, Sherman RM, Hudson AR, Waddell JP. Shoulder arthrodesis using a pelvic-reconstruction plate. J Bone Joint Surg 1988;70A:416–421.
17. Rowe CR. Arthrodesis of the shoulder used in treating painful conditions. Clin Orthop 1983;173:92–96.
18. Schroeder HA, Frandsen PA. External compression arthrodesis of the shoulder joint. Acta Orthop Scand 1983;54: 592–595.
19. Vastamaki M. Shoulder arthrodesis for paralysis and arthrosis. Acta Orthop Scand 1987;58:549–553.
20. Wilde AH, Brems JJ, Boumphrey FRS. Arthrodesis of the shoulder: current indications and operative technique. Orth Clin North Amer 1987;18:463–472.

9
Complications Following Anterior Instability Repairs

Tom R. Norris

INTRODUCTION

Diagnosis and treatment of the unstable shoulder is one of the more difficult problems in orthopaedic surgery. There is confusion between the normal laxity with translation and subluxation of the humeral head relative to the glenoid and an abnormal amount of laxity, leading to pain and dysfunction (33, 36, 55). Increasingly, shoulder instability is being recognized as a pathological entity in the absence of a fixed dislocation documentable by x-ray. This enhanced appreciation of subtle shoulder subluxation as a pathological entity, however, brings with it increased risk of error in both the diagnosis and treatment.

Unfortunately, there is no single treatment that applies to all lesions. It is imperative, therefore, that an accurate diagnosis be made, including the directions and degree of shoulder instability as well as any coexisting problems. Anatomical defects must be defined. The psychological motivation of the individual may also require exploration, since patient understanding and cooperation are critical to successful treatment.

In this review, common factors that could most readily compromise instability repairs are examined. These include techniques for making an accurate diagnosis with identification of the precise anatomical pathology, and the rationale for appropriate surgical treatment with the avoidance of technical complications such as unnecessary hardware or exposures that might lead to residual instability, arthritis, and nerve or vascular injuries. Additional injuries may be prevented by careful rehabilitation postoperatively to restore shoulder stability, flexibility, and endurance prior to an individual's return to stressful sports or work (45).

ANATOMY AND BIOMECHANIC CONSIDERATIONS

The normal laxity of the humeral head relative to the glenoid allows translation in anterior and posterior planes of up to 50% of the humeral head diameter. When tightened, the capsule and ligaments serve as a barrier against instability, as well as a restraint against displacement to the opposite side. However, the positions of elevation and rotation are significant factors that must be taken into account. Each can alter exam findings when the patient is either awake or under anaesthesia (20, 55). Thus, ligamentous detachment on one side of the joint will permit increased instability in the direction of the detachment as well as in the opposite direction. This explains why a shoulder with a large anterior labral detachment can be translated a greater distance posteriorly either clinically or with the patient under anaesthesia, without posterior instability being the primary problem. However, stabilization of the inferior capsular pouch by repair of the anterior ligamentous detachment will stop the abnormal posterior laxity, without requiring a posterior repair as well.

Another important anatomical consideration is that overly tight instability repairs will cause an obligate translation of the humeral head in the opposite direction. Hence, an overly tight anterior repair will cause a shift of the humeral head posteriorly. If the underlying anterior ligaments have been left unrepaired, this shift posteriorly will increase. Overly tight repairs may also lead to early arthritic degeneration of the humeral head and glenoid, even in young individuals (37).

The rotator interval or seam, between the subscapularis and supraspinatus distal to the base of the coracoid, may extend to the biceps groove. Imbrication of this interval lessens posterior and inferior instability (34).

The ligamentous structures are thought to be the prime restraint against shoulder instability (51, 83, 84). Anteriorly, there is a superior, middle, and inferior glenohumeral ligament (32). The inferior glenohumeral ligament normally attaches to the anterior labrum at the rim of the glenoid (23). It is the prime restraint against anterior and inferior instability (60, 84). This inferior glenohumeral ligament has an anterior and posterior band (63). Between the two bands is the inferior pouch (61), to which much attention is directed in the treatment of multidirectional instability (53) or when treating failed instability repair when there is a residual inferior component with an unidirectional anterior or posterior repair (56).

The posterior ligaments and tendons are less substantial than their counterparts on the anterior side. This relative tissue deficiency leads to many operative procedures directed at bony reconstruction to obtain posterior stability. However, even with this relative deficiency, bone blocks and osteotomies have been less effective than capsular procedures (31, 35, 79).

Neurovascular Anatomy

A key issue in any approach to the shoulder has been how to handle techniques involving the deltoid muscle and the various nerves about the shoulder. From Erb's point, the brachial plexus passes just medial to the coracoid muscles (Fig. 9.1A). With detachment of the coracoid muscles, the brachial plexus can be put on stretch more easily. In addition, the musculocutaneous nerve passes between 1.7 and 8 cm below the coracoid tip (30) (Fig. 9.1B). This nerve is at risk with any anterior procedure, especially if the coracoid is detached and transposed. Revision surgery is typically more difficult secondary to scarring. However, it is especially difficult if the coracoid muscles have been transposed, with corresponding loss of the normal anatomical landmarks.

The branches of the suprascapular nerve (Fig. 9.1C) are at risk in direct posterior approaches, since these elevate tissues medial to the glenoid (i.e., Boyd-Sisk and posterior Putti-Platt), and in anterior approaches that involve transscapular drilling (Fig. 9.2), (i.e., Bristow and arthroscopic screw or suture placement through the scapula). The safe distance medial to the posterior margin is only 1.5–2.0

cm (30, 85). Hence, the nerve can easily be injured if this safe distance is not observed.

The axillary nerve is at risk in anterior or posterior inferior capsular procedures, or in any deltoid detaching or splitting techniques (Fig. 9.1) (17). It is also at risk with anterior dislocation of the shoulder (4). Sensory testing in the axillary distribution does not correlate predictably with the status of the motor function (14).

PATTERNS OF FAILURE

In general, failed instability repairs can be classified as those resulting from errors in diagnosis, failure to repair the detached labrum, excessive capsular laxity, iatrogenic or technical complications, incomplete rehabilitation, or severe reinjury.

If the error in diagnosis was one in which impingement was not recognized as being secondary to glenohumeral instability, treatment of the impingement lesion alone will not suffice. The primary lesion is that of the glenohumeral instability, and should be repaired to eliminate recurrence of secondary rotator cuff impingement. This is particularly common in the younger, athletic population and is most often the result of an overhand throwing motion like that used by pitchers or swimmers. Another error in diagnosis would occur if the wrong side of the shoulder were tightened, thereby displacing the humeral head in the direction of the original instability and forcing it out of the center of the glenoid cavity. This is a variation of Rockwood's contention that the most common cause of failed instability repair is missed multidirectional instability, with repair of only one side (73).

Displacement of the humeral head to the opposite side can be caused by repairing the wrong side, or by overtightening the proper side, particularly in a loose-jointed shoulder. It can also be caused by shortening the rotator cuff on the appropriate side. Failure to repair an underlying capsule or labral detachment facilitates humeral head displacement to the opposite side. Failure to appreciate excessive inferior capsular laxity, or to repair a widened rotator interval superiorly, leaves the potential for inferior subluxation of the humeral head, even with a tight anterior-posterior repair.

A third iatrogenic cause of failed repairs involves the use of metal, which can break, pull loose, or migrate within the joint or to nearby neurovascular structures (5, 43, 59, 87). The nerves most fre-

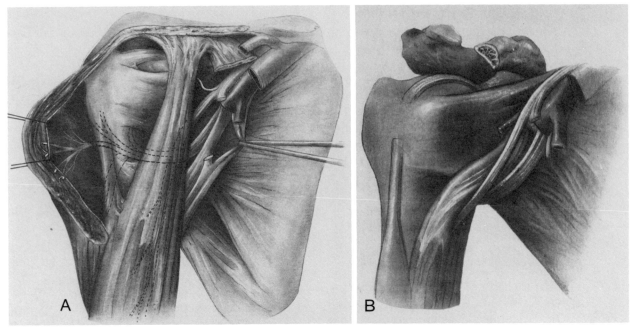

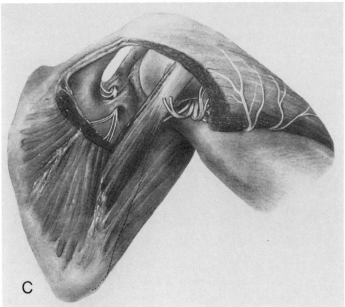

Figure 9.1.   Relevant neuroanatomy about the shoulder. **A**, The coracoid muscles serve to protect the underlying brachial plexus during traction of shoulder reconstructive procedures. The plexus passes just medial to the coracoid muscles with the musculocutaneous nerve entering the coracoid muscles between 1.8–8 cm from the coracoid tip (30). The axillary nerve passes over the subscapularis muscle around the posterior humeral neck and enters the deltoid approximally 5 cm from the acromion. **B**, The musculocutaneous and axillary nerves are at greatest risk with anterior shoulder procedures. They are better visualized with the removal of the coracoid tip. From either the anterior or posterior approach, the axillary nerve is at risk with any procedure involving the dissection of the inferior capsule. **C**, The suprascapular and axillary nerves are at risk with any posterior procedures. The suprascapular nerve is at risk with any dissection greater than 1.5 cm medial to the glenoid rim. The axillary nerve is at risk with inferior capsule dissections, particularly at the inferior edge of the teres minor or if the deltoid is split greater than 5 cm.

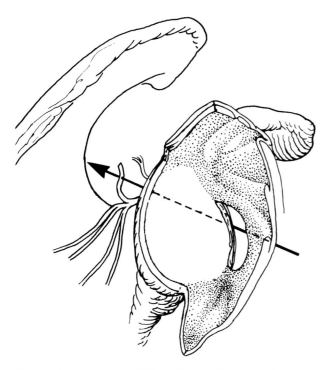

Figure 9.2. Transscapular drilling with open Bristow or arthroscopic suture or screw fixation, injuring the suprascapular nerve.

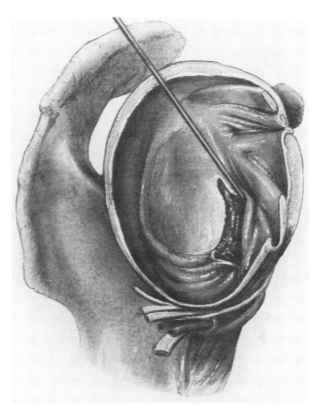

Figure 9.3. Anterior labral detachment. The detachment of the anterior-inferior glenoid labrum appears to be the most common traumatic cause for anterior shoulder instability. Failure to repair this ligament has been the most common finding in failed instability surgery.

quently at risk include the axillary, musculocutaneous, suprascapular, and, to a lesser extent, the entire brachial plexus. The plexus is at greater risk with coracoid detachment procedures because traction can be placed on an unprotected plexus.

FAILURE DUE TO DIRECTION OF REPAIR

Failed Anterior Repairs

The most frequent cause of failed anterior repair is a detached anterior inferior glenoid labrum (Fig. 9.3) (56, 65, 75). This was found to be the case in 84% of Rowe's review (75). With a large labral detachment, the examination may resemble multidirectional or posterior instability with increased laxity in these other directions.

FAILED PUTTI-PLATT AND MAGNUSON-STACK PROCEDURES

By different methods, these two techniques achieve the shortening of the subscapularis. In the Magnuson-Stack procedure, the subscapularis is moved from its insertion on the lesser tuberosity to the lateral side of the biceps groove, and is fixed in a bony trough by either sutures or a staple. In the Putti-Platt, the subscapularis is opened with a more

medial incision. The lateral subscapularis is sutured to the anterior glenoid rim. Variations have included overlapping the subscapularis without suture of the lateral portion to the glenoid. Technical problems associated with shortening of the subscapularis include failure to repair the detached glenoid labrum. The humeral head subsequently undergoes an obligate translation posteriorly (33, 37). Not only is valuable external rotation lost, but the fixed posterior displacement of the humeral head causes more pressure on the posterior glenoid, resulting in arthritic degeneration and eccentric glenoid wear (Fig. 9.4). In a review of failed Magnuson-Stack and Putti-Platt procedures, 43% of these patients developed degenerative arthritis by the time of revision (56). Instability directly inferior is still present in individuals with unrepaired labral detachments, or in those who had multidirectional instability for which only the anterior side was tightened.

The main principles in revising these procedures are to regain subscapularis length, repair any labral detachments, and then assess the capsular laxity to determine if any additional capsular

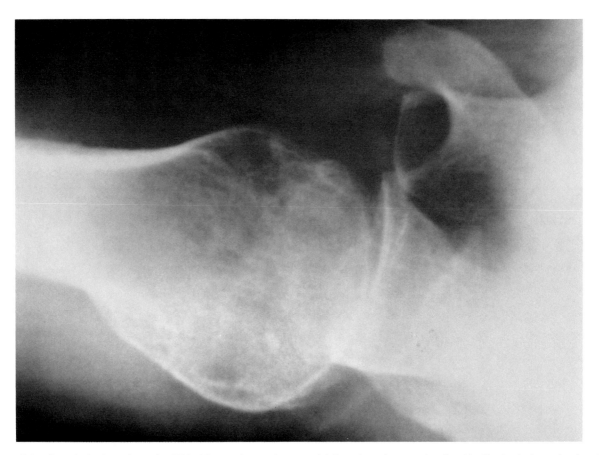

Figure 9.4. Capsulorrhaphy arthropathy. With tight anterior repairs, there's an obligate posterior translation of the humeral head on the glenoid. Over time, the posterior glenoid will selectively erode, changing the version of the glenoid, as the secondary osteoarthritis develops.

shifting is needed. Usually, if the labrum has been detached, repair of the labrum alone should be sufficient. However, if the labrum was initially intact, then this procedure may have been done for a patient with multidirectional shoulder instability. Attention will then need to be directed to the capsule and with an inferior capsular shift performed. Fixed displacement of the humeral head in these situations is more appropriately treated by regaining length in the anterior structures, than by opening the opposite side and attempting to push the head back into the glenoid cavity with an overly tight posterior repair.

FAILED BRISTOW

The Bristow procedure has undergone numerous modifications following Helfet's original description (3, 9, 16, 38, 41, 48). However, the essential features of the procedure include coracoid detachment with transfer of the coracobrachialis and short head of the biceps tendon through the subscapularis muscle to the anterior scapular neck. The coracoid is then secured to the scapula with a screw. Some au-

thors perform the procedure without opening the joint capsule, thereby missing any articular pathology. The procedure gained wide popularity among sports enthusiasts with the hope that the "minimal distortion of anatomy" from the repair would allow a throwing pitcher to return to his preinjury status. In Hill and Lombardo's study, this was true for only 6 of 42 pitchers (39). The muscle-sling effect of the coracoid muscle transfer has been shown to be obsolete and ineffective (78). Transfer of the coracoid muscle through the subscapularis serves to limit external rotation, a step deemed unnecessary if the Bankart labral detachment is repaired (16, 74). The bone block itself may obliterate the pseudopouch medial to the labral detachment, but does not control subluxation (78). Repair of the labral detachment alone would have sufficed. More reports have noted the significant potential complications and disadvantages of the procedure (86). In Albrektsson et al.'s study, there were 27 complications in 31 patients including recurrent dislocation, nerve injury, marked stiffness, and pain (1).

Complications that have plagued the procedure include: coracoid nonunion; coracoid malunion with humeral head impingement upon the coracoid or its screw fixation; subscapularis tethering; coracoid malposition superiorly, inferiorly, medially, or laterally (1, 40); neurovascular injuries (1, 5, 6, 43, 71, 86, 87); and recurrence of instability in the same or in a different direction (59). Placement of the coracoid and its muscles through the subscapularis tendon either too medial or too inferior allows continued instability in the same direction. When it is placed too superior, the humeral head subluxes or dislocates below the transfer (41). As a result, the coracoid fixation bypass fails to obliterate the labral detachment pathology. If it is placed too lateral, then the humeral head may be damaged by subluxing onto or impinging on the bony block or the screw, with resultant cavitation of the humeral head and eventual capsulorrhaphy arthropathy (Fig. 9.5).

Tethering of the subscapularis has also resulted in loss of external rotation and elevation (16, 78). Each of these losses compromises overhead throwing and potentially produces glenohumeral arthritis from an overly tight repair (56, 59, 86).

Hardware complications include migration of the screw into the nearby neurovascular plexus with rupture of the axillary artery (87) and pseudoaneurysms of the axillary artery with permanent paralysis of the upper extremity (5, 43). With transcorporal drilling of the scapula, the screw may be too short, leading to inadequate fixation (Fig. 9.6A). If the screw is too long, it can cause suprascapular nerve paresis or infraspinatus irritation (41) (Fig. 9.6B, C). Other neurovascular injuries associated with Bristow and Putti-Platt procedures include suture ligation of the musculocutaneous, axillary, median and ulnar nerves, and laceration of the axillary artery (71).

Rockwood (72) has often stated that the Bristow is the worst operation in orthopaedic surgery because of the great difficulty in revising it. The distorted anatomy no longer has intact coracoid muscles attached to the coracoid to protect the brachial plexus from the retractors used for expo-

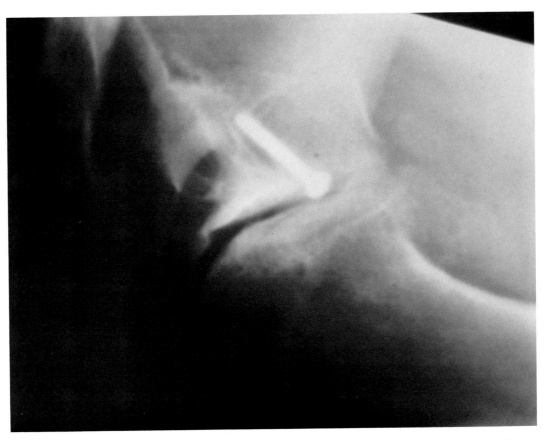

Figure 9.5. Capsulorrhaphy arthropathy—failed Bristow. Multiple factors contribute to this joint destruction including hardware and coracoid impingement, an unrepaired labrum, and a scarred tight subscapularis.

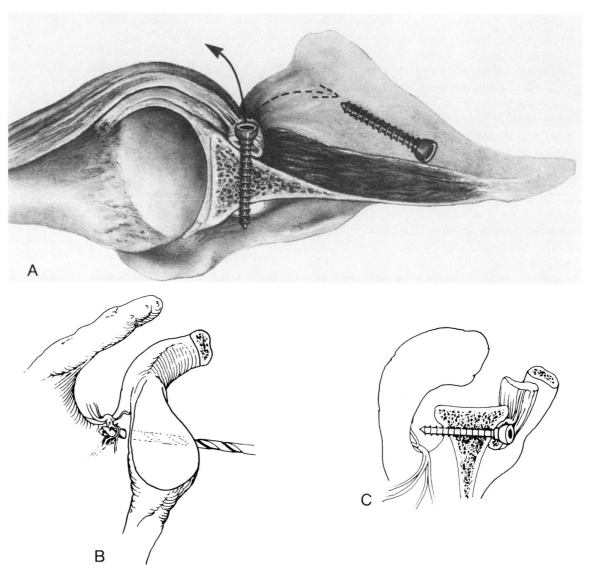

Figure 9.6. **A**, Transfer of the coracoid muscles with a portion of the coracoid has been plagued with hardware problems. If the screw is too short, it may easily loosen, leading to a coracoid nonunion with recurrent instability. **B**, Transscapular drilling risks wrapping up the suprascapular nerve and significant injury. **C**, Long screw fixation risk suprascapular nerve injury as well as tethering of the infraspinatus.

sure. The subscapularis, coracoid muscles, deltoid, pectoralis, axillary nerve, and musculocutaneous nerves form one mass of scar. This is a serious challenge to the reconstructive surgeon's efforts to recreate more normal anatomy, with a freed subscapularis and anterior capsule suitable for revision. The subscapularis may be shortened and the anterior capsule may be deficient. The contracted anterior scar may push the humeral head posteriorly, resulting in capsulorrhaphy arthropathy both from coracoid impingement and from an overly tight anterior repair. This is compounded if the detached labrum has not been repaired.

Factors to consider at the time of revision include: freeing the tethered subscapularis; reestablishing the normal length of the subscapularis; neurolysis and protection of the brachial plexus, most specifically, the musculocutaneous and axillary nerves; repair of any labral detachment; closure of the rotator interval; reassessment; and, if necessary, shifting of the inferior capsule to rebalance all three sides, paying careful attention not to overly tighten the anterior structures. By not dissecting medial to the transplanted coracoid, the musculocutaneous nerve can be protected. If there is a bony deficit in the anterior glenoid, repair of the anterior capsule to the remaining glenoid rim will suffice in lieu of adding the coracoid as a bone block or bone graft.

If the joint is arthritic, the considerations for a joint replacement are applicable. In an arthritic shoulder, regaining motion is a more difficult problem than recurrent instability in the same direction.

Identification of the axillary nerve is crucial to any inferior capsular procedure (49). When the nerve is bound in concrete-like scar, an alternative to direct identification is to find the posterior cord and then proceed from proximal to distal. This is accomplished by removing the upper half of the pectoralis insertion on the humerus. Just deep to this and medial to the long head of the biceps, the latissimus dorsi and teres major insert on the medial aspect of this combined tendon, the radial nerve can be identified. Follow it proximally to its junction with the axillary nerve at the posterior cord, and then proceed distally along the axillary nerve to free it from the scar and inferior capsule. The nerve can thus be identified and protected during any capsular reconstruction.

FAILURE OF PROCEDURES INVOLVING REATTACHMENT OF THE ANTERIOR GLENOID LABRUM

The Bankart is the most common procedure performed to repair a detached anterior glenoid labrum (7, 8). In the method described by Rowe (74, 77), the subscapularis is elevated as a separate layer, the arm is fully externally rotated, and the capsule is incised vertically at the level of the glenoid. This is sutured down to the rim of the glenoid in a double-layered reinforced repair, with sutures placed horizontally through the glenoid and then tied in a vertical manner outside of the joint. The subscapularis is then returned to its normal position. Rowe prefers taking off the coracoid for better visualization. There are potential difficulties with this method. It can be a technically difficult problem to separate the capsule from the subscapularis without leaving one thin or deficient. If the arm is not fully externally rotated or if the incision is placed more laterally in the capsule, a shortened capsule is sutured to the glenoid rim. This creates a fixed internal rotation contracture. Revision of this procedure is easier if the coracoid muscles have not been detached. The subscapularis can be dissected off of the anterior capsule.

If the capsule is shortened, it can be incised at its most lateral point closest the lesser tuberosity insertion. The arm is externally rotated, and the joint is inspected to ensure that adequate healing has occurred at the medial aspect. The most lateral edge of the capsule can be sutured through the middle of the subscapularis tendon as a means of lengthening the capsule. When sutured through the subscapularis, the lateral half of the capsule will be the undersurface of the subscapularis, and the medial half will be the previously shortened capsule which was left attached to the glenoid.

Matsen's preferred technique of performing the Bankart repair involves a more laterally placed arthrotomy without separation of the capsule and subscapularis (10, 81). An inside-out repair is performed, and the sutures attaching the capsule to the glenoid are tied within the joint. The potential disadvantage of the sutures knots catching the joint cavity has not been a problem, as these sutures are well covered with synovium by 3 weeks.

The author's preferred technique is to open the joint with a longitudinal incision through the subscapularis and capsule, 1 cm medial to the attachment on the lesser tuberosity (Fig. 9.7A). This gives adequate tissue for repair laterally at the time of closure. Four sutures tag the capsule and subscapularis superiorly and inferiorly on both the capsular and subscapularis sides. Starting medially and from below, a scalpel is used to separate these two tissues in the soft muscular area, bringing the scalpel from medial to lateral (Fig. 9.7B). One-half of the thickness is left with the capsule to thicken and strengthen—the primary restraint against recurrent instability. The axillary nerve is adequately protected throughout this maneuver. Exposure is improved if a "T" is made in the capsule (Fig. 9.7C). If the labrum is detached, it is repaired with sutures passed through drill holes in the rim of the glenoid (Fig. 9.7D). The detached capsule can be brought back directly to the glenoid rim. The shoulder is then assessed for inferior or posterior capsular laxity (Fig. 9.7E). If there is no significant inferior laxity, the capsule and subscapularis are repaired anatomically. If there is an abundant recess, it is obliterated by transferring the inferior limb superiorly (Fig. 9.7F). The rotator interval between the supraspinatus and subscapularis is closed. The superior limb is then transferred inferiorly to overlap the inferior limb (Fig. 9.7G). The subscapularis is closed anatomically without shortening it.

An iatrogenic form of posterior instability, namely, that of an overly tight anterior repair, can be corrected by lengthening the anterior structures. A second type of posterior instability associated with

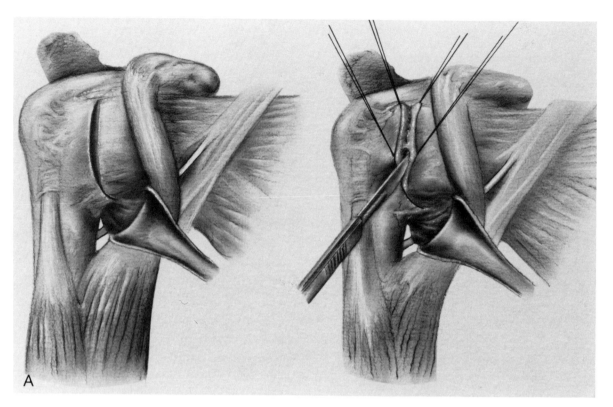

Figure 9.7. Operative approach for anterior and multidirectional instability. **A**, The subscapularis and capsule are divided 1 cm lateral to their insertion on the lesser tuberosity. **B**, With sutures attached to the superior and inferior aspects of both the capsule and subscapularis, a scalpel is brought from medial to lateral. This begins in the muscular portion of the subscapularis at the level of the glenoid, separating the capsule from the subscapularis with an equal thickness on each side. **C**, A "T" is made in the underlying capsule. **D**, Any detachment of the labrum is repaired back to the rim of the glenoid with drill holes in bone facilitated with the Rowe glenoid punches and tenaculum. **E**, The inferior capsular laxity can be assessed clinically. It is likely to play less of a role once any labral detachments have been repaired. **F**, The inferior limb is brought superiorly to obliterate any excess capsular recess if multidirectional instability is present. **G**, The superior limb is brought inferiorly to overlap the inferior limb once the rotator interval has been closed.

multidirectional instability can be corrected by an anterior-inferior capsular shift through an anterior approach after detaching the humeral origin at the anterior band of the inferior glenohumeral ligament complex. Caution is appropriate when combining a labrum reattachment and an anterior-inferior shift. The two may overly tighten the anterior structures, and thus limit postoperative external rotation and elevation.

An alternative method of opening the capsule is through a "T" with the top of the "T" on the glenoid side rather than on the humeral side (2). The repair is essentially the same as the above-described repair with the exception that the capsulotomy begins on the glenoid side rather than on the humeral side.

The Dutoit staple repair was another means of reconnecting a detached labrum back to the anterior glenoid (27). However, its shortcomings included the use of hardware, which has the potential for tearing through the capsular repair and thus allowing for recurring instability (75, 76), abrading the humeral head by joint penetration or because of being a hard unyielding structure, eroding the humeral head, and resulting in further anterior subluxations. With an average of 19 years follow-up, the Dutoit procedure was found to have an unacceptable failure rate (64).

The Eden-Hybbinette procedure for glenoid rim fractures or glenoid erosion has been seldom encountered in the last 15 years (28, 42). These bone-block procedures and their variations are associated with an increased arthrosis and higher complication rate, both from hardware loosening and from erosion of the humeral head due to direct contact of the humeral head on the bone block. Recommendations for repair include an open reduction and internal fixation of the rim fracture, assuming the ligaments are still attached to the anterior glenoid rim. If not, the ligaments should be transferred to the edge of the rim fracture. Bone blocks should not be placed in an

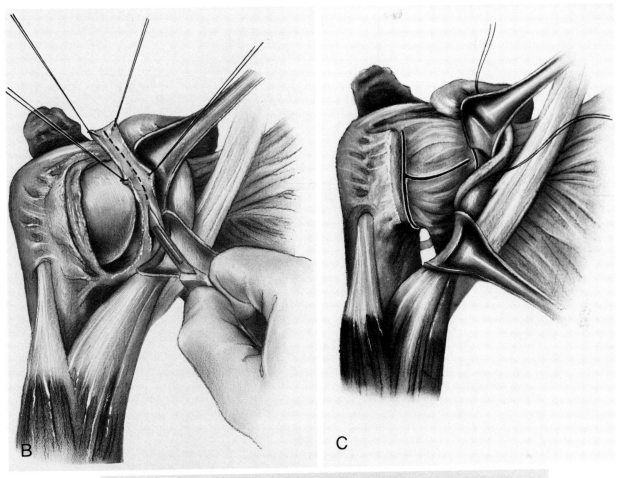

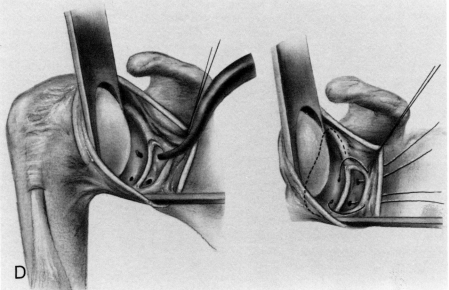

Figure 9.7.   **B–D.**

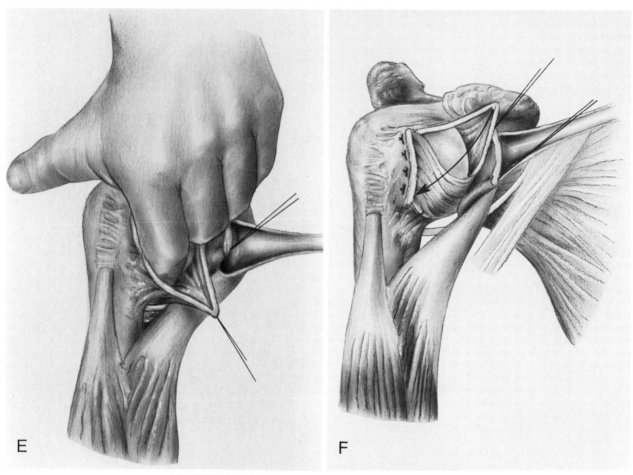

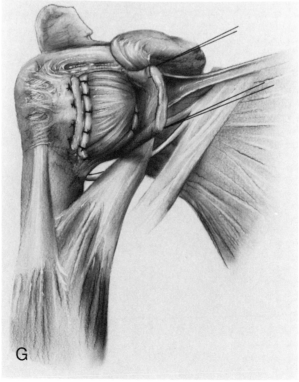

Figure 9.7. E–G.

intra-articular position, where the cartilage of the humeral head will articulate with the bone block, nor should they be placed higher than the joint surface outside the capsule.

Failed Multidirectional Instability Repairs

The mechanisms of failure in a patient treated for multidirectional instability arise from use of anterior or posterior repairs alone, in which the inferior capsular component has not be addressed. An overly tight tendon or tendon and capsular repair will displace the humeral head to the opposite side if all sides are not balanced. Not only should the inferior capsular pouch be obliterated with the arm in near neutral rotation, but the superior rotator interval should be closed to assist in controlling the posterior and inferior instability. Postoperative support should avoid inferior subluxation. The axillary nerve is at risk from either the anterior or posterior approaches (49). It is advisable to isolate this nerve at any time the inferior capsule is dissected from either the humerus or glenoid and shifted to a new position. Five to 6 weeks' immobilization has been recom-

mended to permit early healing for these presumed collagen-deficient individuals who are more likely to stretch out the repair. Postoperative roentgenographs assure that the joint is reduced without evidence of inferior subluxation. If inferior subluxation is found, the cast is modified to push the humerus upward (Fig. 9.8).

IMAGING STUDIES

Combined with the history and physical examination, imaging studies assist in confirming the suspected diagnosis. Beyond this, the goal is to determine the presence of articular defects, labral or cuff detachments, or gross arthritis, which would alter the operative reconstruction.

Plain roentgenographs begin with five screening views, including a true AP of the glenohumeral joint in the scapular plane, a lateral scapula, an axillary view, and anterior-posterior (AP) rotational views in internal and external rotation (62). With these five views, it is possible to assess articular cartilage thickness, whether or not there is a humeral head impression fracture, and if there is gross

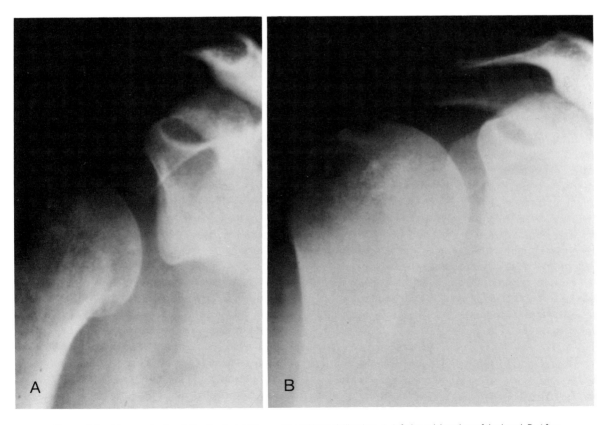

Figure 9.8. X-ray evaluation following instability repair and immobilization. **A**, Inferior subluxation of the head. **B**, After cast modification and with reduction of the humeral head.

displacement of the humeral head from a fixed subluxation or dislocation. More obvious displacement from an anterior dislocation can be identified on the plain AP view. A locked posterior fracture dislocation is most clearly seen on the axillary view, while the internal rotation view allows visualization of a Hill-Sachs defect (57). Additional plain films to evaluate an anterior labral detachment include the West Point axillary view, as well as an axillary view in full external rotation. These projections attempt to image the anterior inferior glenoid rim without other overlapping bony structures, so that a rim fracture or ectopic calcification adjacent to the rim can be seen. Additional views for evaluation of posterior-lateral humeral head defects include the Stryker notch view and Didee view. The Bloom-Obata view is an alternative to the axillary view for the diagnosis of a posterior fracture/dislocation (15). However, in the author's radiology department, it is difficult to position an elderly patient for this view, so other radiologists have not been eager to use it.

More sophisticated methods of diagnosing labral detachments include CT scans (26), CT with double contrast (114), and MRI scans with or without the use of gadolinium contrast. Each of these techniques has achieved a high degree of accuracy, approaching 95% (69). The advantage of MRI is that it provides more information about the rotator cuff and status of the humeral head, in addition to the labral pathology (66). The advantage of a CT scan in more advanced arthritic cases is the ability to see, in one view, the entire scapula in the axial plane. This is very useful in determining eccentric glenoid erosion in planning for total shoulder arthroplasty (58). CT arthrography better delineates the shoulder capsule, and MRI provides superior imaging of the glenoid labrum and intraarticular structures (44, 66).

Under anaesthesia, the degree and direction(s) of instability can be confirmed with C-arm fluoroscopy (55). This is most useful in the axial plane. More direct imaging under anaesthesia, such as arthroscopy or open visualization, are seldom necessary to make a diagnosis of the direction(s) and degree of instability. However, these direct methods of visualization are the most accurate in determining labral detachment (66).

SPECIFIC TECHNIQUES OF REPAIR

Failed Anterior Procedures

There is a systematic approach for each of the types of failed anterior instability repairs. The pa-

tient is placed on the operative table in a modified semi-Fowler's position on a Gelfoam mattress pad. The opposite arm is placed at the side with a Gelfoam pad placed around the elbow and padding around the wrist. It is tucked at the side to prevent abduction of the arm in an effort to avoid a brachial plexus injury to the nonoperative side (22). The cervical spine is protected with a padded headrest that frees up the neck area for surgery on the involved shoulder. The patient is tilted slightly to the opposite side with a gel pad under the scapula, then draped in a manner to expose all sides of the shoulder, arm, and upper chest. The previous scar is reopened, if at all possible, in an effort to avoid creating additional flaps with loss of blood supply to the skin. A deltopectoral approach is preferred to one with deltoid detachment. The intact deltoid is freed from the underlying humerus and rotator cuff. If the coracoid muscles are in their normal position, they are left intact to the coracoid to protect the brachial plexus during medial retraction. The subscapularis is freed from the overlying coracoid and its tendons. As much thickness of the subscapularis as possible is preserved. All extra-articular adhesions between the acromion, the deltoid, and the coracoid muscles are freed prior to opening the joint. The subscapularis is incised 1 cm from its lesser tuberosity insertion, providing good tissue for closure without the necessity of drilling holes in the lesser tuberosity. The most common reason for failed anterior repairs is a persistent detachment of the labrum from the glenoid rim (56, 75, 76). In these cases, a repair and reattachment of the labrum are necessary. This is facilitated by decortication of the anterior scapular neck, creation of drill holes in the glenoid, and suture repair of the detached labrum (10, 81).

To obtain more complete visualization for repair of multidirectional instability, or to lengthen the subscapularis, the subscapularis and capsule must be separated. The standard technique for separating the subscapularis and capsule involves a direct arthrotomy 1 cm medial to the subscapularis insertion. This tissue is elevated en bloc and then, beginning at the inferior margin just inside the preserved anterior circumflex humeral vessels, the subscapularis and capsule are divided, leaving an equal thickness of tissue with each. The subscapularis is retracted medially with the intact coracoid muscles (Fig. 9.7). A "T" is made down to, but not through, the inferior glenohumeral ligament in the capsule. The capsular "T" facilitates evaluation of any labral detachment. If the labrum is detached, the anterior glenoid neck is decorticated with an osteotome, curette, or burr.

Then, using curved Rowe awls and tenaculums, a series of drill holes is made, entering just inside the rim on the articular surface of the glenoid and exiting through the anterior scapular neck. The repair is augmented if two sutures are placed through each drill hole. The side that exits on the articular surface is passed through the detached labrum and capsule to secure it back to the *rim* of the anterior glenoid. The sutures are tied outside of the joint between the level of the capsule and the subscapularis.

If there is still excessive capsular laxity after reattachment of the glenoid, consideration is given to an anterior-inferior capsular shift or cruciate capsule repair (24, 68). More capsule may need to be separated from the humerus to free up the anterior band of the inferior glenohumeral ligament, and to tighten the inferior pouch. With the arm in neutral to 10° of external rotation, superior traction on the inferior limb will obliterate the inferior pouch. The inferior limb is then sutured through the supraspinatus at the rotator interval or at least to the undersurface of the lateral subscapularis tag on the humerus. The rotator interval is closed prior to pulling the superior capsular limb inferiorly. This forms a cruciate capsular repair. The subscapularis is then repaired at its normal insertion.

Variations of this approach are needed when the anterior tendon and capsular structures have been overly tightened. In a Magnuson-Stack procedure, the subscapularis is elevated from the lateral side of the biceps tendon in order to return it to its normal length. If a Putti-Platt subscapularis shortening has been performed, then lengthening is more complicated. Often the anterior structures appear to be a thick, shortened mass of scar. The subscapularis must be separated from the underlying capsule without opening the capsule and removing it directly off the lesser tuberosity. The capsule is then opened in its midportion. If there is a labral detachment, the medial portion of the capsule is repaired by placing sutures at the rim of the capsule. Upon external rotation, the two edges of the capsule become widely separated. The subscapularis is lengthened by suturing it to the lateral capsular flap. The medial edge of the capsule has been reattached to the glenoid. Its most lateral border is sutured up through the subscapularis tendon. More lengthening than this is difficult while still preserving attachment of the capsule to the glenoid.

If there is a large Hill-Sachs defect, repairing the labrum to the rim of the glenoid is sufficient. The Connolly procedure (21), more recently advocated by Rowe (75), involves transfer of the infraspinatus into the posterior lateral humeral head defect. This has not been necessary in the author's experience. Once there is a 40–50% defect in the articular surface, a humeral head or total shoulder replacement is preferred.

In the revision of a failed Bristow procedure, any loose or bent screws should be removed. With extensive scar around the musculocutaneous nerve, it is safest not to dissect medial to the transplanted coracoid (59). If necessary, the coracoid muscles can be released from the superficial surface of the tethered subscapularis. Then the repair can be continued as determined by the pathology, such as a detached labrum, a scarred subscapularis that might need lengthening, or an arthritic joint that may require replacement.

For failed multidirectional instability procedures, it is important to ensure that the rotator interval is closed, the labrum is attached both anteriorly and posteriorly, and the capsular flaps being shifted are attached securely to the glenoid. If the capsular dissection traverses obliquely from the humeral side to the glenoid side inferiorly, traction on the inferior flap will pull only on the anterior tissue attached to the glenoid. The pull is lost on the remaining inferior and posterior pouch. The goal is to eliminate excessive capsular laxity on all three sides. If, in the process of performing a capsular shift, it is discovered that the capsule is detached from the glenoid on the opposite side, then that side needs to be opened and the capsule reattached. All three sides must then be balanced from both operative approaches. Rarely, however, are both anterior and posterior approaches needed to correct multidirectional instability. Postoperative immobilization for multidirectional instability, with either the anterior or posterior approach, is with the arm at the side in neutral–10° of external rotation, and supported with a light-weight fiberglass waistband and arm cast (Fig. 9.9). It is risky to use removable immobilization, for the patient may remove it prematurely. The return to overhead activities and sports with preserved stability has approached 90% in athletes (13).

THE ROLE OF ARTHROPLASTY

Indications for humeral head or total shoulder replacement include capsulorrhaphy arthropathy, anterior and posterior dislocations with greater than 40–50% humeral head impression fractures, and secondary osteoarthritis from recurrent shoulder instability. The most common form of capsulorrhaphy

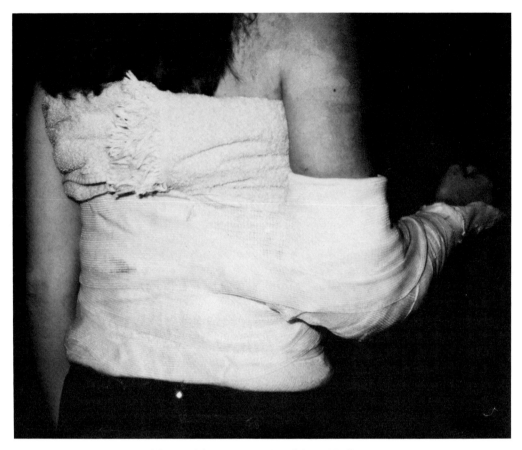

Figure 9.9.   Postoperative immobilization following MDI repair. A light-weight fiberglass cast supports the arm upward into the glenohumeral joint and in 10° of external rotation for 5 weeks.

arthropathy is an overly tight anterior shoulder repair, with capsule or tendon shortening. It can occur in an individual with multidirectional instability with an anterior tightening procedure, in whom no adjustments are made for the loose inferior and posterior capsule. An alternative mechanism occurs in individuals with traumatic anterior-inferior instability in whom the labrum is not repaired. This unrepaired labrum allows the humeral head to be easily displaced in the opposite direction when the subscapularis alone is shortened (Fig. 9.4). The next most common form of capsulorrhaphy arthropathy involves prominent or intra-articular hardware from a Dutoit staple capsulorrhaphy, an arthroscopic staple Bankart repair, or a Bristow procedure in which the bone block or screw is prominent and impinges on the humeral head as it subluxes (Fig. 9.10). A more rare cause is from a posterior glenoid osteotomy. All of these examples can lead to glenohumeral joint destruction.

In the assessment, adequate imaging studies of the glenoid will assist the surgeon in determining whether or not a glenoid replacement will be needed at surgery and, if so, whether or not there is still adequate bony stock in the glenoid to accept a prosthesis. With an overly tight anterior repair, the humeral head is displaced posteriorly. Attempted strengthening and stretching exercises increase the force on the posterior glenoid surface, resulting in eccentric wear of the glenoid as the humeral head flattens. Because of loss of rotation and elevation, abduction can be a problem in obtaining an adequate axillary view. A CT scan is the most reliable view for assessment of the glenoid.

Principles of surgery include those of arthroplasty, and also special techniques intended to restore the joint balance. If less than 10° of external rotation is present, then the operative approach should include subscapularis lengthening. Prior operative skin incisions may be incorporated into a long deltopectoral approach, with an attempt to preserve the cephalic vein either with the deltoid or pectoralis. The coracoid muscles are left intact. The subscapularis is dissected free from the overlying coracoid muscles, and the deltoid is elevated from the underlying humerus. The subacromial space is recreated. If the coracoid muscles have been transferred through the subscapularis, then greater care is needed in the dissection to avoid injuring the brachial plexus. The usual expectations of placement of the neurovascular bundle is not assured once the coracoid muscles have been transferred. In unusual cases, the coracoid muscles have been transferred under or through the brachial plexus. This requires extremely careful dissection to recreate near normal anatomy.

If the subscapularis is shortened, it needs to be opened laterally and separated from the underlying capsule. The underlying capsule is released from the glenoid margin, and the humerus is externally rotated. If the humerus is locked in a posteriorly displaced position, then a flat Darrach elevator can be placed posteriorly to pry the humeral head laterally. With enough soft tissue releases, a second instrument can be placed under the remaining articular surface, and the humeral head can be reduced into the joint using the flat elevator as a shoehorn. The patient is placed on the operative table so that the arm can be extended over the edge of the table. This extension, in conjunction with external rotation, will permit the humeral head to be brought up into the deltopectoral interval. The articular surface is removed, with consideration of whether or not an altered version would be beneficial.

If there is a large posterior pouch where the head has been dislocated posteriorly, then altering the version of the humeral component toward neutral, rather than the usual 35–40° retroversion, is one of several steps that will prevent recurrent posterior instability. With the head out, the posterior capsule itself can be incised and plicated from inside-out.

In instances with more posterior than anterior glenoid wear, the glenoid version can also be returned to normal by reaming to lower the high anterior side. This assumes that sufficient bone remains to place a glenoid component. Posterior glenoid bone grafting is an option when lowering the high anterior side would centralize the glenoid too far to accept a component (58, 58a).

In the most severe cases of glenoid bone loss, either both components can be reamed to match each other's version, or the high side can be lowered to correct version and restore some stability. If a component will not fit in the glenoid because of too much centralization with loss of bone stock in the glenoid neck, the glenoid is omitted and only the humeral head replaced. The soft tissue and rotator cuff is tensioned by the version of the humeral component, lengthening of the subscapularis and, if necessary, tightening of the posterior capsule.

Postoperatively, pendulum motion to prevent strong subacromial and subdeltoid adhesions, without stressing the repair, is recommended. The surgeon should assess the safe limits of motion prior to closure at surgery.

Hardware Complications

Many authors report complications with hardware used in shoulder instability repairs, whether done open or arthroscopically (18, 27, 29, 41, 56, 59, 71, 72, 86, 87). Also, many other authors have reported their successful use of hardware. It is important to note that cases in which hardware was used did not have a lower recurrence rate for instability. In addition, hardware with staples, screws, or pins are seldom needed to correct the anatomical pathology. There is also a higher complication rate with loosening, breakage, bending, nonunion, and migration to nearby neurovascular structures (5, 43). Intra-articular penetration of the joint will, in a short time, destroy the articular surface of the joint (64).

If hardware is used, means to ensure its proper placement include avoidance of placing hardware that will be prominent at the periphery of the joint. Neurovascular structures must be identified and protected on the same side of the surgery, and avoided during any transscapular approaches on the opposite side. Fixation must be secure, confirmed by x-ray, and followed at intervals forever. The hardware should be removed if it is displaced, broken, loose, or if there is any suggestion that it has penetrated the joint.

Rehabilitation

The most frequent complication in rehabilitation is recurrent instability due to inadequate healing time prior to resuming motion. This is either due to physician error or patient noncompliance. Three weeks are thought to be the minimum time necessary for early capsular reattachment; hence any stress should be avoided on this portion of the repair during that time. A second rehabilitation complication results from inadequate motion, strength, or endurance prior to return to activities. An otherwise satisfactory repair may be disrupted by premature return to sports or stressful activities beyond the capabilities of the tissue. For anterior repairs, early pendulum exercises would help avoid tension on the capsular repair, and is thought to be safe unless there is an indication that the patient is noncompliant. Then, consideration should be given to immobilization with a nonremovable fiberglass support.

For posterior and multidirectional instability repairs, a nonremovable fiberglass cast support in neutral rotation, with the arm at the side, has been reliable. The emphasis is on active stretching rather than on passive assisted stretching exercises in the first 3 months. The three groups of muscles for rehabilitation include the rotator cuff, the deltoid, and the scapular stabilizers. The rotator cuff muscles can be strengthened with light resistive exercises, concentrating on the internal and external rotators with the arm down at the side. The supraspinatus is strengthened with resistive abduction exercises between 0–80°, with the arm in internal rotation. All three divisions of the deltoid can be strengthened in the plane of their muscle fibers. The scapula stabilizers—namely, the serratus, the trapezius, and the rhomboid muscles—are additional key elements in support of the shoulder joint. The serratus is strengthened by push-ups on the wall with the patient upright; the trapezius and rhomboids are strengthened by resistive shoulder shrugs in the direction of their muscle fibers (50, 67).

CONCLUSION

In summary, complications from instability repairs can be avoided if an accurate diagnosis is established preoperatively, and then reconfirmed by an examination under anesthesia at the time of surgery. Operative approaches that protect the neurovascular structures, detach the least amount of deltoid and rotator cuff, allow for repair of any labral or capsular detachments, rebalance the joint with regard to capsular laxity on all three sides, and avoid shortening of the rotator cuff muscles permit the most anatomical repair without further injury. If at all possible, hardware should be avoided because it can eventually bend, break, or migrate. A carefully planned rehabilitation program that allows escalation of flexibility, endurance, and strength, while permitting stability prior to the return to sports or other combat activities, will go a long way in reducing the incidence of redislocation (50, 52). A psychological assessment of the patient's motivation and ability to understand these factors may benefit the patient and the surgeon immensely. The success rate of repeated surgical repairs intended to correct recurrent disloca-

tion of the shoulder after prior repairs, has been quite high when nonoperative means were tried and found unsuccessful. At times, however, either injury or iatrogenic causes has lead to the development of advanced arthritis, with the need for prosthetic replacement. The final result depends upon pain relief and the ability to regain motion and strength. Motion requires release of contractures and scar. Stability requires rebalancing the soft tissues. Strength depends upon the integrity of the rotator cuff, and the deltoid, on preservation of the neurovascular structures and release of scar for it to be clinically useful.

The treatment of shoulder instability is one of the more challenging endeavors in orthopaedic surgery, especially since there are so many pitfalls to consider. It also has become very rewarding as the techniques and understanding continue to advance.

References

1. Albrektsson BE, Herberts P, Korner L, et al. Technical aspects of the Bristow repair for recurrent anterior shoulder instability. In: Bayley I, Kessel L, eds. Shoulder surgery. New York: Springer-Verlag, 1982:87–92.
2. Altchek DW, Warren RF, Ortiz G, et al. T-Plasty: A technique for treating multidirectional instability in the athlete. Orthop Trans 1989;13:561.
3. Allman F. Symposium on sports injuries to the shoulder. Contemp Surg 1975;7:82.
4. Antal CS, Conforty B, Engelberg M, et al. Injuries to the axillary due to anterior dislocation of the shoulder. J Trauma 1973;13:564.
5. Artz T, Huffer JM. A major complication of the modified Bristow procedure for recurrent dislocation of the shoulder. J Bone Joint Surg 1972;54A:1293–1296.
6. Bach BR Jr, O'Brien SJ, Warren RF, et al. An unusual neurological complication of the Bristow procedure. J Bone Joint Surg 1988;70A:458–460.
7. Bankart ASB. Recurrent of habitual dislocation of the shoulder joint. Br Med J 1923;2:1132–1133.
8. Bankart ASB. The pathology and treatment of recurrent dislocation of the shoulder joint. Br J Surg 1938;26:23–29.
9. Barry TP, Lombardo SJ, Kerlan RK, et al. The coracoid transfer for recurrent anterior instability of the shoulder in adolescents. J Bone Joint Surg 1985;67A:383–387.
10. Berg EA, Ellison AE. The inside-out Bankart procedure. Am J Sports Med 1990;18:129–133.
11. Bigliani LU, Singson R, Feldman F, et al. Double contrast CT arthrography in shoulder instability. Proceedings of the Third International Conference on Surgery of the Shoulder, Professional Postgraduate Services, Tokyo, 1987;82–85.
12. Bigliani LU, Endrizzi DP, McIlveen SJ, et al. Operative management of posterior shoulder instability. Orthop Trans 1989;13:232.
13. Bigliani LU, Kurzweil PR, Schwartzbach CC, et al. Inferior capsular shift procedure for anterior-inferior shoulder instability in athletes. Orthop Trans 1989;13:560.
14. Blom S, Dahlback LO. Nerve injuries in dislocations of the

shoulder joint and fractures of the neck of the humerus. Acta Chir Scand 1970;136:461–466.

15. Bloom MH, Obata WG. Diagnosis of posterior dislocation of the shoulder with use of velpeau axillary and angle-up roentgenographic views. J Bone Joint Surg 1967;49A:943–949.

16. Braly WG, Tullos HS. A modification of the Bristow procedure for recurrent anterior shoulder dislocation and subluxation. Am J Sports Med 1985;13:81–86.

17. Bryan WJ, Schauder K, Tullos HS. The axillary nerve and its relationship to common sports medicine shoulder procedures. Am J Sports Med 1986;14:113–116.

18. Burkhead WZ, Richie MF. Revision of failed shoulder reconstruction. Contemp Orthop 1992;24:126–133.

19. Butters KP, Curtis RJ, Rockwood CA Jr. Posterior deltoid splitting shoulder approach. J Bone Joint Surg Transactions 1987;11:233.

20. Cofield RH, Irving JF. Evaluation and classification of shoulder instability. Clin Orthop 1987;223:32–43.

21. Connolly JF. Humeral head defects associated with shoulder dislocations—their diagnostic and surgical significance. In: Instructional Course Lectures, The American Academy of Orthopaedic Surgeons. St. Louis: CV Mosby, 1972;21:42–54.

22. Cooper DE, Jenkins RS, Bready L, et al. The prevention of injuries of the brachial plexus secondary to malposition of the patient during surgery. Clin Orthop 1988;228:33–41.

23. Cooper DE, Arnoczky SP, O'Brien SJ, et al. Anatomy, histology, and vascularity of the glenoid labrum. J Bone Joint Surg 1992;74A:46–52.

24. Craig EV. The posterior mechanism of acute anterior shoulder dislocations. Clin Orthop 1984;190:212–216.

25. Cyprien JM, Vasey HM, Burdet A, et al. Humeral retrotorsion and glenohumeral relationship in the normal shoulder and in recurrent anterior dislocation (scapulometry). Clin Orthop 1983;175:8–17.

26. Danzig L, Resnick D, Greenway G. Evaluation of unstable shoulders by computed tomography. Am J Sports Med 1982;10:138–141.

27. Du Toit GT, Roux D. Recurrent dislocation of the shoulder. J Bone Joint Surg 1956;38A:1–12.

28. Eden R. Zur operation der habituellen schulterluxation unter mitteilung eines neuen verfahrens bei abriss am innren pfannenrande. Dtsch Z Chir 1918;144:269–280.

29. Ferlic DC, DiGiovine NM. A long-term retrospective study of the modified Bristow procedure. Am J Sports Med 1988;16:469–474.

30. Flatow EL, Bigliani LU, April EW. An anatomical study of the coracoid muscles. Clin Orthop 1989;244:166–171.

31. Fronek J, Bowen M, Warren R. Posterior subluxation of the glenohumeral joint. J Bone Joint Surg 1989;71:205–216.

32. Grant JCB, Agar AMR, eds. Grant's atlas of anatomy. 9th ed. Baltimore, Williams & Wilkins, 1991:353–397.

33. Harryman DT, Sidles JA, Clark JM, et al. Translation of the humeral head on the glenoid with passive glenohumeral motion. J Bone Joint Surg 1990;72A:1334–1343.

34. Harryman DT, Sidles JA, Harris SL, et al. The role of the rotator interval capsule in passive motion and stability of the shoulder. J Bone Joint Surg 1992;74A:53–66.

35. Hawkins RH, Kopper G, Johnston G. Recurrent posterior instability (subluxation of the shoulder). J Bone Joint Surg 1984;66A:169.

36. Hawkins RJ, Schutte JP. The assessment of glenohumeral translation using manual and fluoroscopic techniques. [Abstract]. Fourth Annual Meeting, American Shoulder and Elbow Surgeons, 1988.

37. Hawkins RJ, Angelo RL. Glenohumeral arthritis. A late complication of the Putti-Platt repair. J Bone Joint Surg 1990;72:1193–1197.

38. Helfet AJ. Coracoid transplantation for recurring dislocation of the shoulder. J Bone Joint Surg 1958;40B:198–202.

39. Hill JA, Lombardo SJ, Kerlan RK. The modified Bristow-Helfet procedure for recurrent anterior shoulder subluxations and dislocations. Am J Sports Med 1981;9:283–287.

40. Hovelius L, Akermark C, Albrektsson B, et al. Bristow-Latarjet procedure for recurrent anterior dislocation of the shoulder. Acta Orthop Scand 1983;54:284–290.

41. Hovelius L, Korner GL, Lundberg B, et al. The coracoid transfer for recurrent dislocation of the shoulder. Technical aspects of the Bristow-Latarjet procedure. J Bone Joint Surg 1983;65A:926–934.

42. Hybbinette S. De la transpantation d'un fragment osseux pour remedier aux luxations recidivantes de l'epaule: constatations et resultats operatories. Acta Chir Scand 1932;71:411–445.

43. Iftikhar TB, Kaminski RS, Silva I. Neurovascular complication of the modified Bristow procedure. J Bone Joint Surg 1984;66A:951.

44. Jahnke AH, Petersen S, Neuman C, et al. A prospective comparison of computerized arthrotomography and magnetic resonance imaging of the shoulder. Am J Sports Med 1990;18:556.

45. Jobe FW, Moynes DR, Brewster CE. Rehabilitation of the shoulder joint instabilities. Orthop Clin North Am 1987;18:473–482.

46. Johnston GH, Hawkins RJ, Haddad R, Fowler PJ. A complication of posterior glenoid osteotomy for recurrent posterior shoulder instability. Clin Orthop 1984;187:147.

47. Kretzler JJ. Scapular osteotomy for posterior shoulder dislocation. J Bone Joint Surg 1980;62B:127.

48. Latarjet M. A propos du traitement des luxations recidivantes de l'epaule. Lyon Chir 1954;49:994–997.

49. Loomer R, Graham B. Anatomy of the axillary nerve and its relation to inferior capsular shift. Clin Orthop 1989;243:100–105.

50. Mendoza FX, Nicholas JA, Sands A. Principles of shoulder rehabilitation in the athlete. In: Nicholas JA, Hershman EB, eds. The upper extremity in sports medicine, St. Louis: CV Mosby 1990;251–264.

51. Moseley HF, Overgaard B. The anterior capsular mechanism in recurrent anterior dislocation of the shoulder. J Bone Joint Surg 1962;44B:913–927.

52. Moynes DR. Prevention of injury to the shoulder through exercise and therapy. Clin Sports Med 1983;2:413.

53. Neer CS II, Foster CR. Inferior capsular shift for involuntary inferior and multidirectional instability of the shoulder. J Bone Joint Surg 1980;62A:897–908.

54. Neer CS II. Involuntary inferior and multidirectional instability of the shoulder: etiology, recognition and treatment. Instructional Course Lecture 1985;34:232–238.

55. Norris TR. C-arm fluoroscopic evaluation under anesthesia for glenohumeral subluxations. In: Bateman JE, Welsh RP, eds. Surgery of the shoulder. Philadelphia: BC Decker, 1984:22–25.

56. Norris TR, Bigliani LU. Analysis of failed repair for shoulder instability—A preliminary report. In: Bateman JE, Welsh RP, eds. Surgery of the shoulder. Philadelphia: BC Decker, 1984:111–116.

57. Norris TR. Diagnostic technique for shoulder instability. In:

American Academy of Orthopaedic Surgeons, Instructional Course Lectures. St. Louis: CV Mosby, 1985.

58. Norris TR. Bone grafts for glenoid deficiency in total shoulder replacements. The shoulder. Proceedings of the Third International Conference on Surgery of the Shoulder, Professional Postgraduate Services, Tokyo, 1987;373–376.

58a. Norris TR. Unconstrained prosthetic shoulder replacement. In: Watson MS, ed. Surgical disorders of the shoulder. London: Churchill Livingstone, 1991.

59. Norris TR, Bigliani LU. Complications following the modified bristow procedure for shoulder instability. Orthop Trans 1987;11:232–233.

60. Norris TR. History and physical examination of the shoulder. In: Nicholas JA, Hershman EB, eds. The upper extremity in sports medicine. St. Louis: CV Mosby, 1990.

61. Norris TR. Recurrent posterior subluxations. Hosp Med 1990;26:45–63.

62. Norris TR. Fractures of the proximal humerus and dislocations of the shoulder. In: Browner BD, Jupiter JB, eds. Skeletal trauma. Philadelphia: WB Saunders 1991.

63. O'Brien SJ, Neves M, Rozbruck R, et al. Anatomy and histology of the inferior glenohumeral ligament complex. Orthop Trans 1989;13:231.

64. O'Driscoll SW, Evans DC. Long-term results of the staple capsulorrhaphy for recurrent anterior instability of the shoulder; Twenty years of experience in six Toronto hospitals. Orthop Trans 1988;12:674.

65. Perthes G. Uber Operationen bei Habitueller Schulterluxation. Deutsch Ztschr Chir 1906;85:199–227.

66. Petersen SA, Jahnke AH, Neumann CH. Diagnostic imaging of glenohumeral instability: a prospective comparison study of CT arthrography and MRI of the shoulder. Orthop Trans 1991;15:763.

67. Pink M, Jobe FW. Shoulder injuries in athletes. Orthopaedics 1991;11:40–47.

68. Protzman RR. Anterior instability of the shoulder. J Bone Joint Surgery 1980;62A:909–918.

69. Rafii M, Minkoff J, Bonamo J, et al. Computed tomography (CT) arthrography of shoulder instabilities in athletes. Am J Sports Med 1988;16:352–361.

70. Randelli M, Gambrioli PL. Glenohumeral osteotry by computed tomography in normal and unstable shoulders. Clin Orthop 1986;208:151.

71. Richards RR, Hudson AR, Bertoia JT, et al. Injury to the brachial plexus during Putti-Platt and Bristow procedures. Am J Sports Med 1987;15:374–380.

72. Rockwood CA, Gerber C. Failed shoulder reconstruction. Orthop Trans 1985;9:1.

73. Rockwood CA Jr. The shoulder: facts, confusions and myths. Internat Orthop 1991;15:401–405.

74. Rowe CR, Patel D, Southmayd WW. The Bankart procedure. J Bone Joint Surg 1978;60A:1–16.

75. Rowe CR, Zarins B, Ciullo JV. Recurrent anterior dislocation of the shoulder after surgical repair. J Bone Joint Surg 1984;66A:159–168.

76. Rowe CR. Failed surgery for recurrent dislocations of the shoulder. American Academy of Orthopaedic Surgeons Instructional Course Lectures 1985;34:264–267.

77. Rowe CR. The Bankart procedure: improvements and options. Surgical Rounds for Orthopaedics 1990;Feb:15–22.

78. Schauder KS, Tullos HS. Role of the coracoid bone block in the modified Bristow procedure. Am J Sports Med 1992;20:31–34.

79. Schwartz W, Warren RF, O'Brien SJ, et al. Posterior shoulder instability. Orthop Clin North Am 1987;18:409–419.

80. Scott DJ Jr. Treatment of recurrent posterior dislocations of the shoulder by glenoplasty. J Bone Joint Surg 1967;49A:471.

81. Thomas SC, Matsen FA III. An approach to the repair of avulsion of the glenohumeral ligaments in the management of traumatic anterior glenohumeral instability. J Bone Joint Surg 1989;71A:506–513.

82. Tibone JE, Prietto C, Jobe FW, et al. Staple capsulorrhaphy for recurrent posterior shoulder dislocation. Am J Sports Med 1981;9:135–139.

83. Townley CO. The capsular mechanism in recurrent dislocation of the shoulder. J Bone Joint Surg 1950;32A:370–380.

84. Turkel SJ, Panio MW, Marshall JL, Girgis FG. Stabilizing mechanisms preventing anterior dislocation of the glenohumeral joint. J Bone Joint Surg 1981;63A:1208–1217.

85. Warner JJP, Krushell RJ, Masquelet A, et al. Anatomy and relationships of the suprascapular nerve: anatomical constraints to mobilization of the supraspinatus and infraspinatus muscles in the management of massive rotator cuff tears. J Bone Joint Surg 1992;74A:36–45.

86. Young DC, Rockwood CA Jr. Complications of a failed Bristow procedure and their management. J Bone Joint Surg 1991;73A:969–981.

87. Zuckerman JD, Matsen FA. Complications about the glenohumeral joint related to the use of screws and staples. J Bone Joint Surg 1984;66A:175–180.

10
Complications of Posterior Instability Repairs

Richard J. Hawkins and James D. Cash

INTRODUCTION

Posterior instability of the shoulder can be difficult to diagnose, confusing to classify, and often frustrating to treat. The terminology used in much of the literature to describe this spectrum of disorders is often vague and ambiguous. Consequently, even orthopaedists who see a fair number of shoulder problems may hesitate to make this diagnosis, which we feel is poorly understood and often underdiagnosed.

The incidence of posterior dislocation has been reported to be between 1 and 4% of all shoulder dislocations. This is a reflection of the fact that acute posterior shoulder dislocations are very rare compared with anterior dislocations. Conversely, posterior shoulder subluxation is much more common than posterior dislocation and is probably greatly underdiagnosed. Many previous references to posterior dislocation in the literature may have in fact been posterior subluxations. If all shoulder instabilities were considered (both subluxations and dislocation), the incidence of posterior instability would be much higher than reported. In this chapter, we will discuss and attempt to clarify the classification, diagnosis, treatment, and complications involved with surgery for posterior instability of the shoulder. Since the most common complication is incorrect diagnosis, emphasis will be placed on classification, examination, diagnosis, and selection of appropriate treatment.

CLASSIFICATION

Understanding posterior instabilities begins with knowledge of the types of patients presenting with these problems. The classifications of these disorders (Table 10.1) allows a more definitive diagnosis and is imperative in determining the correct treatment and prognosis. The acute posterior dislocation in the absence of an impression defect in the humeral head, usually attributed to violent trauma, is extremely rare. The senior author has seen this only twice in 13 years of practice. If initially diagnosed, reduced, and immobilized in external rotation, acute posterior dislocation without an impression defect should not result in recurrent dislocation. The acute posterior dislocation with an impression defect can also be successfully managed, the treatment being dependent upon the size of the impression defect (8) (Table 10.2). If undiagnosed, this can result in a chronic locked (missed) posterior dislocation, as described by McLaughlin (Fig. 10.1) (14). Despite Sir Astley Cooper's observation in 1844 that "It is an accident which cannot be mistaken," (2) the majority of these cases continue to be misdiagnosed by the physician who initially sees the patient (7, 8, 14, 21). The term "missed," which is often associated with locked posterior dislocations, could be eliminated if appropriate x-ray views were instituted with significant trauma involving the shoulder. These injuries would then most commonly result from postictal or posttraumatic states where a previously semi-alert patient finally communicates his shoulder discomfort, prompting x-rays to be ordered.

The largest group of patients with posterior shoulder instabilities are those with recurrent subluxation. Past reports have referred to this entity as "dislocation" when in fact most cases represent a subluxation. Four subgroups of posterior subluxators have been suggested (Table 10.1), and most patients fit predominantly into one of these distinct groups with some overlap. A small but notorious group of these patients are those with a personality disorder who solely by selective muscle contraction can subluxate their shoulder. This phenomenon was investigated by Rowe et al. in an electromyographic study that demonstrated the selective suppression of

Table 10.1.   Classification of Posterior Shoulder Instability

Acute Posterior Dislocation
    Without impression defect
    With impression defect

Chronic Posterior Dislocation
    Locked (missed) with impression defect

Recurrent Posterior Subluxation
    Voluntary
        habitual (willful, personality disorder)
        muscular control (not willful)
    Involuntary
        positional (demonstrable by patient)
        not demonstrable by patient

Table 10.2.   Guidelines for Treatment of Locked Posterior Shoulder Dislocations

Time Since Dislocation		% Defect in Humeral Head	Treatment[a]
6 weeks	and	20%	1. Closed reduction[b] 2. If closed reduction unsuccessful, transfer lesser tuberosity (Neer)[b]
6 weeks–6 months	and	20–45%	Transfer lesser tuberosity[b]
6 months	and/or	45%	1. Hemiarthroplasty[c] 2. Total shoulder arthroplasty if glenoid destroyed[c]

[a] If patient is inactive, asymptomatic, or poor risk for surgery, no treatment is indicated.
[b] Postreduction immobilization for 6 weeks with the arm at the side and the shoulder in 20° of external rotation.
[c] Immediate rehabilitation as per Neer protocol.

half of the "force couple" (20). The patient with this psychiatric or habitual type of subluxation is often an adolescent girl with apparent psychiatric problems in whom surgery will not be helpful and is in fact contraindicated (19, 20). These patients have a subconscious desire to frustrate any attempts at treatment and will succeed in causing any reconstruction to fail. Although it is important to recognize this subset of patients, in our experience it is not common.

The voluntary muscular posterior subluxator (not willful) should not be confused with the previously discussed habitual (willful) subluxator. It is inaccurate to suggest that simply because patients can demonstrate the instability, they have psychiatric problems and therefore should be denied surgical

treatment when indicated. In the senior author's experience, most patients with posterior shoulder instability can demonstrate the instability in their shoulders but do not have a willful desire to do so, nor a psychiatric or personality disorder (6). These patients are most often normal, active people who have a component of involuntary instability with certain movements or activities that may or may not be painful and functionally disabling. They happen to also be able to subluxate their shoulder by muscular contraction, therefore are categorized as voluntary (not willful) posterior subluxators.

The third group of recurrent posterior subluxators is involuntary—the patient cannot demonstrate the instability with pure muscular contraction. The positional posterior subluxator may be able by himself or with examiner assistance to position his arm such that with motion (usually from the forward flexed position) toward the coronal plane, the humerus will audibly and visually relocate.

The final group of recurrent posterior subluxators cannot demonstrate the instability by arm positioning or muscular contraction, yet they have a complaint of instability with or without pain. This condition offers a considerable diagnostic challenge. In the past, examination under anesthesia has been used to confirm the diagnosis. However, examination under anesthesia may demonstrate up to 50% posterior translation of the humeral head within the glenoid in normal patients (15). "Symptomatic translation" can be used as an aid in establishing the diagnosis. When the proximal humerus is pushed posteriorly in the glenoid socket, the patient may appreciate reproduction of symptoms leading to the diagnosis.

DIAGNOSIS

Posterior Dislocations with Impression Defect (Locked or Missed)

McLaughlin has warned that "posterior dislocators of the shoulder . . . (create) a diagnostic trap for the unwary surgeon" (14). Hawkins, Neer, et al. found in 41 locked posterior dislocations that the average interval from injury to diagnosis was 1 year (7).

Patients with posterior dislocation of the shoulder present with a history of indirect force in which there is a fall on the outstretched hand, causing sudden internal rotation, adduction, and flexion of the arm. Other precipitating events are multiple trauma, seizures, or an alcohol related event. Occasionally a patient may be referred fol-

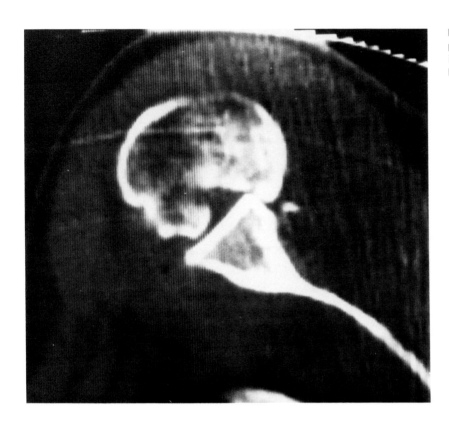

Figure 10.1.   CT scan of chronic locked posterior shoulder dislocation. Note large impression defect on anterior aspect of humeral head.

lowing a failed course of physiotherapy with a diagnosis of "frozen shoulder." The chief complaint at late presentation is a functional disability with difficulty in combing hair, washing, shaving, and even eating (Fig. 10.2). Although pain is frequently present, it is usually only mild and not a factor precipitating referral (7).

Physical examination reveals a marked internal rotation deformity, often as much as 60°. This internal rotation deformity is the key physical sign in establishing the diagnosis. On inspection, the humeral head is prominent posteriorly, and the acromion is squared off anteriorly. The coracoid is likewise prominent anteriorly. When visualizing the shoulder from the lateral side, there is malalignment of the humeral shaft under the acromion, in that it is a more posterior position. Forward elevation and internal rotation, although limited to varying degrees, are often surprisingly functional (7). Rowe and Zarins have described the presence of limitation of supination of the palm when the arm is extended, due to the shoulder being locked in internal rotation (21).

Routine AP and lateral x-rays may be insufficient to make the diagnosis and are often interpreted as normal. A true AP x-ray with the beam directed at right angles to the scapula may fail to clearly demonstrate the posterior dislocation, although many signs are described that suggest the diagnosis. These signs include internal rotation of the humerus, upward displacement of the humerus, disappearance of the normal half-moon overlap of the glenoid fossa, a "trough line" from impaction of the humeral head, and a positive "rim" sign (Fig. 10.3). (When the humerus is internally rotated in posterior dislocation, an increased space may be visible between the anterior glenoid rim and the medial portion of the humeral head.) The lateral scapular view is often difficult to interpret since due to the impression defect, only part of the humeral head is out of the glenoid fossa. An interruption has been noted in the normal scapulohumeral arch (sometimes known as Moloney's line) (3) formed by the axillary border of the scapula and the inferior border of the neck and shaft of the humerus.

The axillary view not only demonstrates very clearly the posterior subluxation, but also delineates the size of the impression defect, characteristically at the level of the lesser tuberosity. This "key investigation" will establish the diagnosis, direct treatment, and will be a guide to prognosis. So valuable is the axillary view that it should be part of the routine trauma series for shoulder injuries along with the AP and lateral views relative to the scapular plane (16, 18). In the injured patient with a painful shoulder, where the x-ray technician is reluctant to move the patient's arm, the physician should aid the techni-

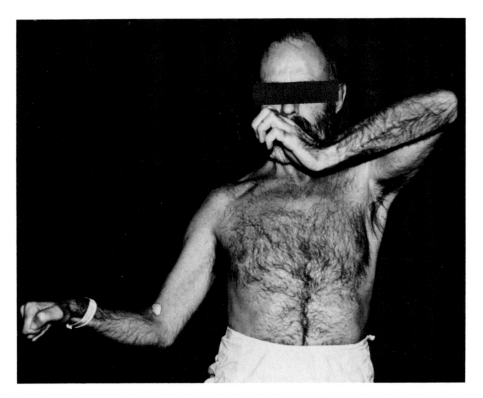

Figure 10.2.   Patient with locked posterior dislocation showing typical difficulty in raising left hand to head due to lack of external rotation.

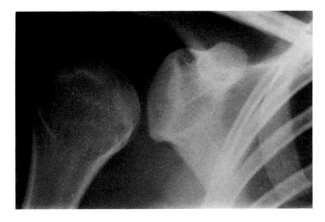

Figure 10.3.   AP x-ray of posterior shoulder dislocation showing typical internal rotation of humeral head and positive "rim sign" (increased space between the anterior glenoid rim and medial portion of the humeral head).

cian by simply abducting the shoulder 20–30° to allow the axillary view to be obtained. If this rule is followed, the diagnosis of missed posterior dislocation of the shoulder should be eliminated, assuming an early x-ray is obtained. Tomograms or CT scans can aid in defining the impression defect and any other abnormalities of the articular surfaces (8) (Fig. 10.1).

Recurrent Posterior Subluxation

The presentation and physical findings of patients with recurrent posterior subluxation are much more subtle and varied than those of locked posterior dislocation. The usual complaint is that of pain often accompanied by a feeling that the shoulder is "coming out." Hawkins et al. found only 11 of 50 shoulders to have a history of trauma initiating the instability (6), and usually it was minor. As the years progressed, the affected shoulder would come out with increasing frequency. Eighty percent of the patients in this series were able to subluxate the shoulder themselves by using certain maneuvers. Often this voluntary motion was not painful, but the unintentional subluxation that occurred daily in 70% of the patients in the series was sometimes painful and was responsible for the patients' concern, leading them to seek medical attention (6).

The most common maneuver used by the patient is forward elevation of the internally rotated and adducted arm. When the arm is elevated between 30 and 100°, the humeral head subluxates posteriorly. As forward elevation continues above 100° and the arm approaches the coronal plane of the body, the subluxation is reduced with a visible, audible, and palpable "clunk." It is the reduction that should be obvious to the examiner. Posterior subluxation rarely if ever occurs when the shaft of the humerus is posterior to the coronal plane of the body. This is the description of the positional subluxator. The voluntary subluxator can with muscular control subluxate the shoulder posteriorly, usually with the arm next to the thorax. If there is suspicion that the voluntary subluxator has a psychological disorder, a psychiatric evaluation should be obtained, as an habitual (willful) subluxator will fail with surgical reconstruction.

Physical examination should include attempts to translate the humeral head posteriorly on the glenoid fossa in the sitting and supine position while noting the patient's response to such testing (Fig. 10.4). As was previously noted, up to 50% translation of the humeral head on the glenoid may be normal (15). Thus, the examiner must compare this translation with the nonaffected shoulder and appreciate an episode of "symptomatic translation," which may reproduce the symptoms.

The differentiation between unidirectional posterior instability and multidirectional instability with a posterior component is often difficult but cru-

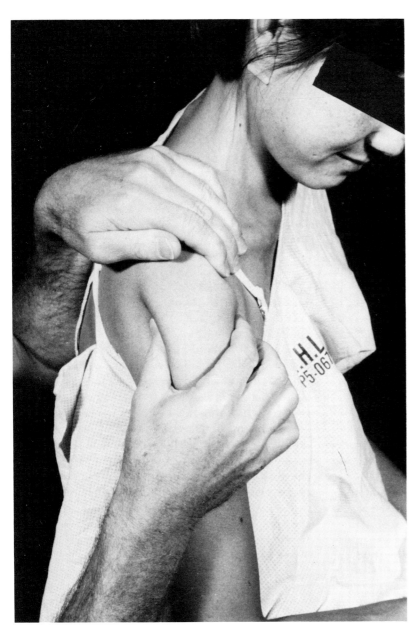

Figure 10.4. Examiner demonstrating position to best examine posterior translation of the humeral head.

cial to treatment. The condition most commonly confused with posterior subluxation is multidirectional instability (MDI). The presentation of these two conditions may be very similar in that both are atraumatic in origin, subluxations, and not true dislocations, often associated with a generalized hyperlaxity or collagen disorder and often have minimal symptoms. The examiner should test for inferior subluxation with distal traction on the affected arm, checking for the "sulcus sign" (a hollow between the humeral head and lateral edge of the acromion). It is our impression that there are patients who truly have unidirectional posterior subluxation without a significant component of inferior instability. Still, care must be taken to differentiate between the two. A major cause of failure after procedures for anterior and posterior instabilities has been incorrect diagnosis and failure to eliminate a redundancy of the inferior part of the capsule if multidirectional instability is present (17).

TREATMENT

Posterior Dislocations (Locked)

The extremely rare acute posterior dislocation can be reduced by traction and external rotation with gentle direct forward pressure over the displaced head. Reduction might be blocked by a large impression defect on the humeral head, muscular contraction by an apprehensive patient, or interference of the long head of the biceps tendon (3).

Treatment of a chronic locked posterior dislocation depends upon the duration of the dislocation, the size of the impression defect, the condition of the glenoid fossa, and the general health of the patient. Hawkins and Neer have recommended the following treatment plan (Table 10.2). If the patient is inactive, a poor risk for surgery, and cannot cooperate in a rehabilitation program, no treatment should be administered. If the dislocation is less than 6 weeks old and the defect involves less than 20% of the articular surface as seen on the axillary x-ray, closed reduction should be attempted. If this is successful (three of 12 patients in a previous series) (7), immobilization is necessary for 6 weeks with the arm at the side and the shoulder in 20° of external rotation. If closed reduction is unsuccessful, transfer of the lesser tuberosity into the impression defect as described by Neer (18) should be performed. Transfer of the lesser tuberosity into the defect provides more secure fixation than the subscapularis tendon transfer, as described by McLaughlin (13). If the dislocation is 6 weeks to 6 months old and the defect involves 20–45% of the articular surface as seen on the axillary view, transfer of the lesser tuberosity may be followed by immobilization, as previously described. Possible complications with these transfer procedures would be recurrence of dislocation (seen in five of nine patients) (7), loosening of hardware, or intraarticular placement of hardware, leading to articular cartilage damage.

If the glenoid is normal and the dislocation is more than 45% of the articular surface as seen on the axilary x-ray, a hemiarthroplasty may be required, allowing immediate rehabilitation. If the glenoid has been destroyed, total shoulder replacement may be indicated, followed by immediate rehabilitation (7).

Complications involved with shoulder arthroplasty have been well documented (4, 9). Intraoperative complications can involve glenoid or humeral shaft fractures. Late complications can include symptomatic loosening of glenoid or humeral components, dislocation of the components, or infections. In the previously mentioned series of locked posterior shoulder dislocations (7), nine patients were treated with hemiarthroplasty and 10 treated with total shoulder arthroplasty. Three of the nine hemiarthroplasties had a failed result with moderate pain, narrowing of the cartilage space between the humeral component and the glenoid, and sclerosis of the glenoid. These three patients were revised to total shoulder arthroplasty and all had good relief of pain.

One of the 10 patients in this series treated by total shoulder arthroplasty had the shoulder dislocate during the immediate postoperative period, and the patient refused additional treatment. The humeral component in this patient had been inserted in 20° of retroversion. The usual amount of retroversion of the humeral component must be reduced in these lesions to lessen the tendency of the head to subluxate posteriorly. The longer the dislocation has been present, the more the retroversion must be reduced. The correct amount of version can be determined by inserting the trial components and testing the stability of the shoulder at the time of surgery, making adjustments as required. If necessary, the posterior part of the capsule can be plicated through the anterior approach after the humeral head is osteotomized and before the components are inserted. When the trial components are in place and the amount of version has been adjusted, any persistent tendency toward posterior subluxation or redundancy of the posterior capsule can be ascertained and corrected by plication of the capsule (7).

Recurrent Posterior Subluxation

Once a diagnosis of recurrent posterior subluxation of the shoulder has been made and a personality disorder has been ruled out, the degree of disability must be determined. Many of these patients have minimal pain and disability with their instability. There is no evidence that a future disability will develop due to either wear on the articular cartilage or increasing instability, and this group of asymptomatic or minimally symptomatic patients can be reassured that no treatment is necessary. The posterior subluxators who are symptomatic can benefit from a rotational and scapular strengthening program (18). This can be achieved with the use of a resistant rubber exerciser with the emphasis on external rotator strengthening combined with balanced internal rotator strengthening. Scapular strengthening can be achieved by push-ups, with the arms in the adducted position. Recent reports suggest that in patients with posterior instability there is an excellent chance of success in diminishing symptoms of pain and instability with a rehabilitation program (4, 18).

The indications for surgical treatment of the patient with recurrent posterior subluxation are: (a) significant pain and disability; (b) failure of physiotherapy; and (c) psychologically normal. The ideal patient is one who has had an acute traumatic subluxation or dislocation, goes on to a recurrent symptomatic instability, and has failed a supervised course of physiotherapy. We rarely see this type of ideal surgical candidate.

The different types of surgical procedures that have been described to correct recurrent posterior shoulder subluxation can be separated into soft tissue, bony, and combination procedures (Table 10.3). Posterior glenoid osteotomy was first described by Scott in 1967 (22), who described its advantages as: (a) forming a stable buttress; (b) alleviating prolonged immobilization due to rapid graft incorporation; (c) only one surgical exposure is necessary to perform the procedure and obtain the graft; and (d) capsulorrhaphy or bone-block procedure can be performed at the same time if necessary. Of three patients reported, there was one complication of an anterior dislocation in the immediate postoperative period. In fact, most authors who report using this procedure add a soft tissue reconstruction to the bony procedure, making it difficult to determine which procedure is truly contributing to the stated results. Bell (ASES, Fall 1988, Santa Fe) and Hurley et al. (10) found excessive glenoid retroversion in

Table 10.3. Procedures for Posterior Instability (Symptomatic)

Irreducible Locked Posterior Dislocation
  Benign neglect
  Subscapularis transfer (McLaughlin)
  Lesser tuberosity transfer (Neer)
  Arthroplasty
  Arthrodesis

Recurrent Posterior Subluxation
  Bone
    scapular osteotomy
    posterior bone block
  Soft Tissue
    reverse Putti-Platt
    biceps tendon transfer
    inferior capsular shift
    infraspinatus tendon transfer
    posterior capsulorrhaphy
  Combinations

their patients with posterior shoulder subluxation. With combined glenoid osteotomy and posterior Bankart repair, Bell reported only one failure, in a patient found to have multidirectional instability. Kretzler (12) reported four recurrences out of 28 patients (14%) with various posterior instabilities treated with scapular osteotomy. Norwood and Terry (19) performed posterior glenoid osteotomies on 11 patients with unidirectional posterior instability and had recurrences of "mild instability" in only two. Hawkins and Koppert reported that capsular plication and infraspinatus tendon overlap in conjunction with posterior glenoid osteotomy in 17 shoulders resulted in a 41% recurrence rate and a 29% complication rate (6). Two patients developed significant degenerative glenohumeral osteoarthritis, one due to penetration of the joint during the osteotomy cut, leading to avascular necrosis in this segment of the glenoid (Fig. 10.5). The related severe disability necessitated a total shoulder arthroplasty (11). The other patient was a 23-year-old female physical education student who had undergone posterior glenoplasty with capsular plication and whose shoulder had been immobilized in maximum external rotation. When a severe external rotation contracture developed, a posterior release was performed and the deformity recurred. Subsequent fluoroscopy suggested both anterior and inferior subluxation as well as some glenohumeral osteoarthritis. A combined posterior release and anterior stabilization was then performed. Two years later, the patient continued to have significant limitation of shoulder movement, with pain. She chose to defer any other operative

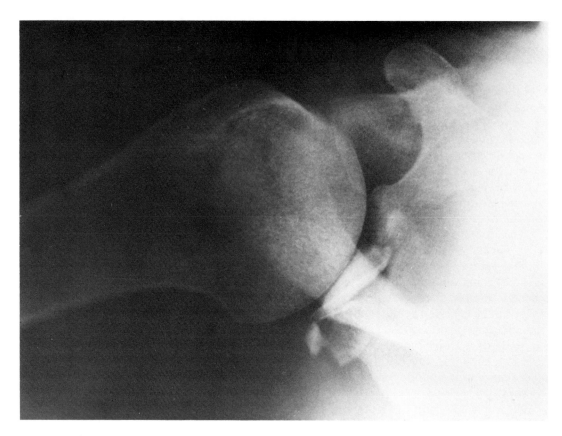

Figure 10.5. Axillary x-ray of glenoid fracture after osteotomy for recurrent posterior subluxation.

treatment (6). The remaining three complications consisted of an ulnar nerve neuropraxia that resolved over 3 months in one patient; prolonged stiffness for a period of 12 months for unknown reasons in one patient; and unremitting shoulder pain for which no cause was determined in another patient (6).

The other type of stabilizing procedure that attempts to alter the bony anatomy of the glenohumeral articulation is the posterior bone block to provide a buttress to prevent posterior subluxation, as described by Fevre and Mialaret (5). Reports of results of this technique are sporadic. Certainly, one would be concerned with hardware near the glenohumeral joint, the possibility of nonunion of the graft to the glenoid, and humeral head destruction with a noncartilagenous surface.

Soft tissue procedures to prevent recurrent posterior shoulder subluxation are designed either to eliminate the enlarged retroglenoid space (reverse Putti-Platt, capsular shift, infraspinatus tendon transfer) or form a sling around the back of the shoulder (biceps tendon transfer). Hurley and associates (10) in 1987 reported on a group of 22 patients undergoing 29 soft tissue procedures with a recur-

rence rate of 72% at an average of 5 years follow-up. Two patients in the surgical group also showed mild degenerative changes on x-ray, while none of the 25 nonoperated patients showed these changes. Boyd and Sisk reported their preliminary results on eight patients who underwent posterior capsulorrhaphies combined with posterior transfer of the long head of the biceps tendon. With an average follow-up of 28.6 months, there were no recurrences or complications (1). Hawkins et al. performed a biceps transfer in the manner of Boyd and Sisk on three patients with one recurrence (6). Of their six patients that had a reverse Putti-Platt-type operation (consisting primarily of a capsular plication with infraspinatus tendon overlapping), all but one (83%) had posterior instability at follow-up. The recurrences appeared at an average of 18 months postoperatively.

Bigliani and associates in 1988 (ASES Fall 1988, Santa Fe) reported on a group of 25 patients having failed conservative treatment who underwent posterior inferior capsular shift procedures. He did not, however, separate these patients into unidirectional, posterior subluxators, and those with multidirectional instabilities. He did say that posterior was the primary direction of instability, but a majority also had inferior subluxation. These patients therefore may not represent unidirectional posterior instability. Nevertheless, with an average follow-up of 3.3 years, 88% were rated as good or excellent. Three patients had poor ratings due to persistent pain; one developed degenerative arthritis, and another coracoid impingement. Recurrent instability was not a problem.

Possible surgical complications (Table 10.4) other than those already mentioned include infection and neurovascular injury. Certainly the proximity of the axillary nerve to the inferior border of the subscapularis, inferior capsule, and teres minor could subject it to injury during an episode of posterior dislocation or surgical reconstruction for this problem. Neer's report of one axillary nerve neuropraxia that resolved in 6 weeks after a posterior approach for inferior capsular shift is the only report of axillary nerve injury in our review.

Failed Surgical Reconstruction

After surgical reconstruction for posterior instability, if the patient follows the postoperative protocol and still ends up with a painful, stiff, or unstable shoulder, the complex world of posterior shoulder instability becomes even more so. One should exercise extreme caution in dealing with this most difficult problem. It is important to focus on the source of the problem and specifically to determine if the diagnosis was initially incorrect. The patient may demonstrate an instability not previously diagnosed. Inferior and/or anterior components of multidirectional instabilities are often present with

Table 10.4. Possible Surgical Complications Associated with Posterior Instability Surgery

Early
  Incorrect diagnosis
  Glenoid fracture
  Humerus fracture
  Neurovascular injury
  Infection
  Recurrence of instability

Late
  Incorrect diagnosis
  Recurrence of instability
  Pain
  Stiffness
  Hardware in joint
  Osteoarthritis
  Infection
  Avascular necrosis

posterior instabilities, and if present, should be detected. Repeat radiographs should be taken to check for avascular necrosis associated with glenoid osteotomy, degenerative osteoarthritis associated with bony and soft tissue procedures, loose hardware, and redislocations. If significant degenerative changes are present, hemiarthroplasty, total shoulder arthroplasty, or arthrodesis may be the patient's only hope for resolution of the problem. With recurrence of the same posterior instability, one should pursue all avenues of nonoperative therapy including scapular and rotational strengthening and modification of lifestyle and activities prior to considering another surgical reconstruction.

SUMMARY

Posterior instability of the shoulder is a broad spectrum of disorders whose diagnosis can be subtle, classification confusing, and treatment difficult. The most frequent complication involved with treatment of posterior instability is incorrect diagnosis. We have tried to clarify these problems by reviewing the keys to diagnosis that will allow classification of the disorders according to clinical presentation (Table 10.1).

The treatment of the rare posterior dislocation with an impression defect depends upon the duration of the dislocation, the size of the impression defect, the condition of the glenoid fossa, and the general health of the patient (Table 10.2). Recurrent posterior subluxation, on the other hand, is much more common than previously recognized. Fortunately, many of these patients are asymptomatic and most of the rest can be treated conservatively with a rotational and scapular strengthening program. If surgery becomes necessary, the probability of success will be maximized by careful attention to patient selection, exclusion of those with personality disorders, accurate diagnosis of unidirectional posterior instability, confidence that significant pain and functional limitations are present, and utilization of the best tissues of the posterior aspect of the shoulder for reconstruction (8).

The authors' preferred surgical treatment has evolved after reporting suboptimal results with a variety of procedures (6). Worse than a chance for recurrence is the prospect of degenerative osteoarthritis after a procedure, which has now happened in three patients who have undergone glenoid osteotomy in our experience. We have therefore abandoned this procedure as routine treatment of recurrent posterior shoulder subluxation. Many of the recurrences of instability after soft tissue procedures have been due to inadequate strength of tissues (thin posterior capsule and muscular portion of infraspinatus). We currently use a technique utilizing a tenodesis of the capsule and the thick tendinous portion of the infraspinatus tendon into the glenoid labrum. The postoperative regimen includes 6 weeks of immobilization with the arm at the side in 20° of external rotation, then a physiotherapy program progressing slowly from passive to active motion, followed by resistance exercises. The preliminary results with this procedure with recurrent posterior unidirectional subluxation have been encouraging with no recurrences to date.

Complications, other than incorrect diagnosis, associated with surgery for posterior shoulder instability (Table 10.4) are similar to those encountered with other surgical reconstructions about the shoulder. Hopefully, familiarity with others' complications encountered and more frequent recognition and treatment of these disorders will allow surgeons to deal with posterior instabilities more safely and effectively in the future.

References

1. Boyd HB, Sisk TD. Recurrent posterior dislocation of the shoulder. J Bone Joint Surg 1972;54A:779-786.
2. Cooper A. A treatise on dislocations and fractures of the joints. In: BB Cooper, ed. Philadelphia: Lea & Blanchard, 1844.
3. Dorgan JA. Posterior dislocation of the shoulder. Am J Surg 1955;89:890-900.
4. Farek J, Pavlov BH, Warren R. Posterior subluxation of the glenohumeral joint—nonsurgical and surgical treatment. Orthop Trans 1986;10:220.
5. Fevre MM, Mialaret J. Indications et technique des butees retroglenoidiennes dans les luxations posterieures de l'epaule. J de Chir 1938;52:156-167.
6. Hawkins RJ, Koppert G, Johnston G. Recurrent posterior instability (subluxation) of the shoulder. J Bone Joint Surg 1984;66A:169-174.
7. Hawkins RJ, Neer CS, Pianta RM, Mendoza FY. Locked posterior dislocation of the shoulder. J Bone Joint Surg 1987;69A:9-18.
8. Hawkins RJ, McCormack RG. Posterior shoulder instability. Orthopaedics 1988;11:101-107.
9. Hawkins RJ, Bell RH, Jallay B. Total shoulder arthroplasty. Clin Orthop 1989;242:188-194.
10. Hurley JA, Anderson TE, Dear W, Andvish JT, Bergfeld JA, Weiker GG. Posterior shoulder instability: surgical vs. nonsurgical results. Orthop Trans 1987;11:458.
11. Johnston GH, Hawkins RJ, Haddad R, Fowler PJ. A complication of posterior glenoid osteotomy for recurrent posterior shoulder instability. Clin Orthop 1984;187:147-149.
12. Kretzler HH. Scapular osteotomy for posterior shoulder dislocation. J Bone Joint Surg 1974;56A:197.
13. McLaughlin HL. Posterior dislocation of the shoulder. J Bone Joint Surg 1952;34A:584-590.
14. McLaughlin HL. Locked posterior subluxation of the shoulder: Diagnosis and treatment. Surg Clin North Am 1963;43:1621-1628.
15. Morton KS. The unstable shoulder: recurring subluxation. Injury 1978;10:304-306.
16. Neer CS. Displaced proximal humeral fractures. Part I. Classification and evaluation. J Bone Joint Surg 1970;52A:1077-1089.
17. Neer CS, Foster CR. Inferior capsular shift for involuntary and multidirectional instability of the shoulder. A preliminary report. J Bone Joint Surg 1980;62A:897-908.
18. Neer CS, Rockwood CA. Fractures and dislocations of the shoulder. In: Rockwood CA, Green DP, eds. Fractures in adults. Philadelphia: JB Lippincott, 1984:833-856.
19. Norwood LA, Terry GC. Shoulder posterior subluxation. Am J Sports Med 1984;12:25-30.
20. Rowe CR, Pierce DS, Clark JG. Voluntary dislocation of the shoulder. A preliminary report on a clinical, electromyographic and psychiatric study of twenty-six patients. J Bone Joint Surg 1973;55A:445-460.
21. Rowe CR, Zarins B. Chronic unreduced dislocations of the shoulder. J Bone Joint Surg 1982;64A:494-504.
22. Scott DJ. Treatment of recurrent posterior dislocations of the shoulder by glenoplasty. J Bone Joint Surg 1967;49A:471-476.

11
Chronic Unreduced Shoulder Dislocations

Efrain D. Deliz and Evan L. Flatow

INTRODUCTION

Chronic, unreduced shoulder dislocations are difficult to treat, and may be the source of significant disability. Although some may occur in patients who did not seek medical evaluation after their initial injury, for many, the dislocation is missed on the initial evaluation, and only diagnosed after extended therapy for a "frozen shoulder." By this time, secondary pathology such as contracture of the soft tissues, articular degeneration, and bone loss have created a far more complex situation. Minimally displaced proximal humerus fractures may often coexist with unreduced dislocations. This chapter will not consider dislocations with displaced fractures.

A thorough understanding of the historical, physical, and radiographic findings in shoulder dislocations will help the orthopaedist to make the correct diagnosis on the initial evaluation. Furthermore, the orthopaedist embarking on the treatment of a chronic, unreduced shoulder dislocation must keep in mind the special anatomic distortions generally present if a successful result is to be achieved.

CHRONIC ANTERIOR DISLOCATIONS

Anterior shoulder dislocations are sufficiently common that most orthopaedists are familiar with the usual physical and radiographic findings, which are generally obvious enough that these injuries are rarely missed if the shoulder is evaluated for acute trauma. However, if dramatic injuries elsewhere have diverted attention from the shoulder (e.g., in a patient with multiple trauma), if the history is obscured (e.g., by coma), or if medical attention has not been sought acutely (e.g., as in an alcoholic patient), an anterior dislocation may not be recognized until the patient's functional complaints trigger an evaluation. This can occur some time after the onset of the dislocation, as once the initial pain and swelling subside, the clinical findings are less evident (6).

Clinical Findings

While a history of an injury is helpful if present, a patient with an altered mental status or an unrecognized seizure disorder may be unclear as to the timing of the onset of shoulder impairment. Nocturnal hypoglycemia has been reported as an etiology of anterior shoulder dislocation (15).

Even if the initial dislocation is diagnosed and reduced, redislocation may occur unrecognized. This is especially possible in older, osteoporotic patients, if a large anterior fracture of the glenoid produces a "ski-jump" effect, so that the humerus can slide out the front (14) (Fig. 11.1).

Although patients with longstanding unreduced anterior dislocations can often be remarkably pain-free (10, 23), many are painful, especially when there is late arthritic degeneration. Most have significant functional deficits, with reduced elevation and rotation.

Plain radiographs, once obtained, will generally demonstrate the dislocation. The posterolateral head defect can be quite large in longstanding dislocations (9) (Fig. 11.2). Glenoid fractures are best demonstrated on axillary views and on axial CT-scan cuts. With time, a "false glenoid" develops on the anterior scapula where it is in contact with the dislocated head (5, 6, 13). Such chronic changes can be helpful in establishing that a dislocation is not acute, in a patient presenting after the most recent of many falls on the arm. If this is not recognized, an attempt at manipulative reduction may result in fracture, or an open reduction may be undertaken in a patient not prepared, consented, or appropriate for the complex reconstruction that may be necessary. Nerve injuries are frequently present, and should be carefully evaluated.

Figure 11.1. This patient had her anterior dislocation reduced, but was later noted to have redislocated with her arm in a sling. The axillary view demonstrates that her humeral head has slid anteriorly to rest in a large glenoid compression fracture.

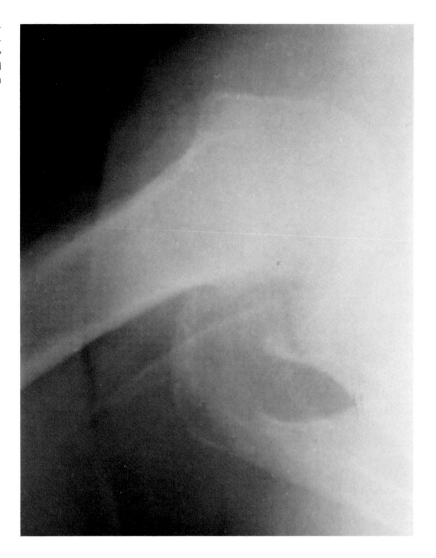

Treatment

Patients with little pain who can accept their functional deficit may decline intervention (23, 24) (Fig. 11.3). Active patients, however, are generally unhappy with the limitations. If the dislocation is of less than 2–3 weeks' duration, a gentle closed reduction may be tried. Regional or general anesthesia reduces the risk of further injury, and excessive force should be avoided. If closed reduction is successful, the patient should be initially protected in a sling, and then gradual motion and strengthening employed. If a patient over the age of 40 is persistently weak or in pain after a closed reduction, consideration should be given to imaging the rotator cuff to look for a concomitant rotator cuff tear (8).

Dislocations of longer duration should not be manipulated, but an open reduction with reconstruction planned. If the posterolateral head defect involves less than 40% of the articular surface, and if the dislocation is of fewer than 6 months' duration, the articular surfaces may generally be preserved. Open reduction is performed through an anterior, deltopectoral approach. An extensive release of the contracted capsule and other soft tissue distortions must be performed to allow reduction of the humerus from its dislocated position (2, 8, 11, 18, 26). The empty glenoid is frequently obliterated with scar tissue, and must be cleared to accept the humeral head (8, 18).

Various stabilization procedures have been combined with open reduction, including screws or pins transfixing the glenohumeral or acromiohumeral articulation (17, 25), fascial suspensions (7), bone block procedures (4, 20), and capsular procedures (1). However, it is important to remember that an inadequate soft tissue release cannot be compensated for by a pin holding the humerus in joint—the head will spring out again when the fixation fails or is removed. Rowe emphasized that if an adequate release and open reduction are followed by keeping the arm anterior to the coronal plane of the body with a sling, stability will generally be assured (23). Metallic transfixation of the joint might only damage the articular surfaces and restrict the possible beneficial effects of joint motion on the articular cartilage (23, 24).

Large rotator cuff defects may be encountered, and should be reconstructed as best as possible. If the humeral head defect comprises greater than 40% of the articular surface, or if the joint surfaces are damaged, replacement arthroplasty should be considered (16) (Table 11.1). If the dislocation has ex-

isted for more than 6–12 months, the part of the head out of contact with the scapula becomes soft, and the articular surface can be indented like a ping-pong ball (23) (Fig. 11.4). The soft head will flatten if reduced into the glenoid.

Mild anterior glenoid bone deficiency can usually be managed by lowering the posterior glenoid and by accepting some altered component version. However, large defects, especially those resulting from compression fractures in elderly patients with osteoporosis, may require bone grafting (16, 27) (Fig. 11.5). Rotator cuff defects can generally be repaired through the same anterior deltopectoral approach. Rehabilitation is progressed as healing allows, with passive movement within the forward range.

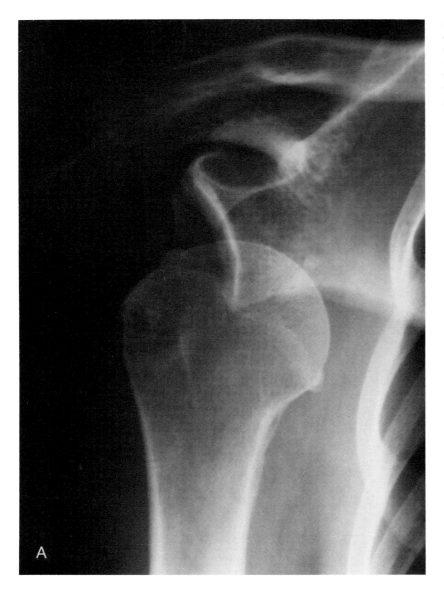

Figure 11.2. **A**, Chronic anterior dislocation of 1 year's duration. **B**, The patient had significant pain and little use. **C**, A large humeral head defect was seen at surgery. **D**, A total shoulder replacement with extensive soft tissue realignment was performed. **E**, Active elevation at 2 years' follow-up.

A

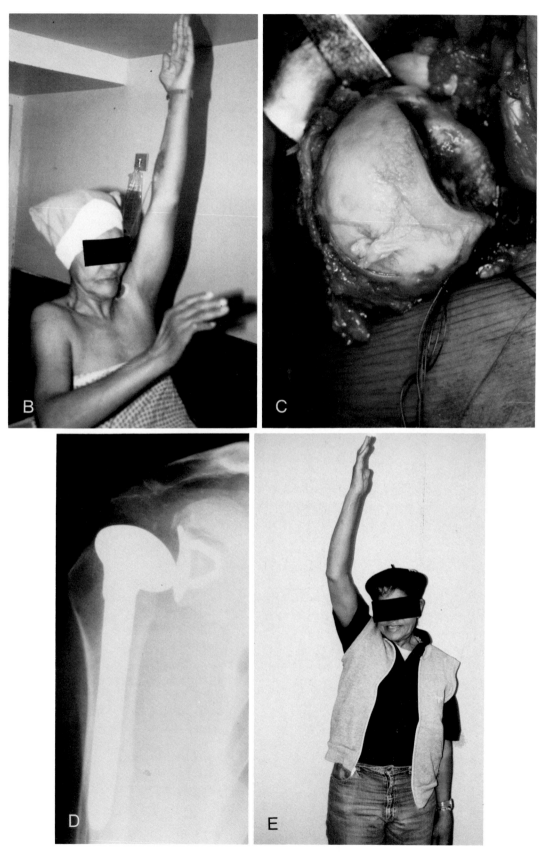

Figure 11.2.   B–E.

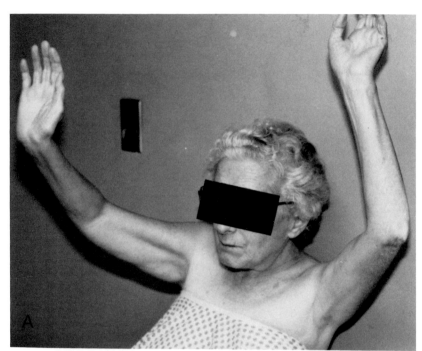

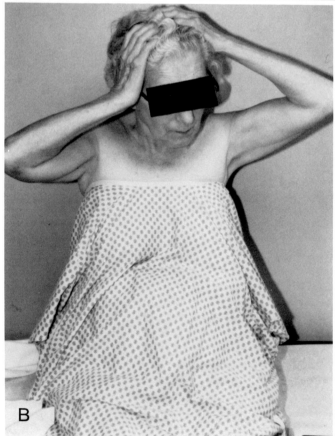

Figure 11.3. **A**, This elderly patient has a chronic unreduced anterior dislocation of her right shoulder. **B**, The patient was brought in by her daughter for evaluation. She had no pain, and felt that her shoulder was "fine" and not in need of treatment.

Results

The literature on chronic, unreduced anterior shoulder dislocations is very limited, and often gives a pessimistic outlook. Many series were collected before the arthroplasty era, when resection of the humeral head was all that was available for destroyed articular surfaces. Reports frequently combine chronic unreduced posterior as well as anterior dislocations, and fail to separate those with displaced proximal humerus fractures. Additionally, only small numbers of chronic anterior dislocations treated operatively have been reported (Table 11.2).

Table 11.1. Treatment of Chronic Anterior Shoulder Dislocations

< 3 weeks old + head defect < 40% → Closed reduction
3 weeks to 1 year old + articular surfaces viable → Open reduction
> 1 year old or head defect > 40% → HHR or TSR

Technical Issues
   Glenoid bone deficiency → Bone graft
   Cuff tear → Repair
   Increase HHR retroversion for stability

At our center, we have reviewed a series of 17 chronic, unreduced anterior shoulder dislocations treated in the arthroplasty era (16). Patients with displaced proximal humerus fractures, cuff-tear arthropathy, or neuromuscular deficits (e.g., stroke) had been excluded. There were 11 women and six men, with an average age of 67 years (range 36–88). There were 13 right and four left shoulders. The duration of dislocation averaged 2.3 years (8 weeks to 8 years).

Seven patients were treated nonoperatively despite functional deficits, for reasons of health or motivation. Ten were treated surgically. Those with preserved joint surfaces dislocated less than 1 year underwent open reduction. A liberal release including the pectoralis major and subscapularis was performed, with cleanout of scar from the glenoid. Those with destroyed articular surfaces underwent unconstrained replacement arthroplasty. Humeral retroversion was increased for stability. The soft tissues were reattached and rehabilitation modified as with a repair of recurrent dislocations. Anterior glenoid erosion was often present, and required grafting in four shoulders. Two chronic rotator cuff tears re-

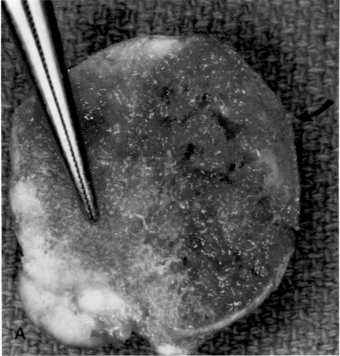
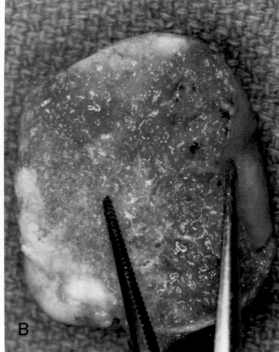

Figure 11.4. A, The excised humeral head from a shoulder that has been dislocated for over a year. The portion of the head that was in contact with the scapula (clamp) is sclerotic and eburnated, while the portion out of contact has softened, and the subchondral bone has resorbed (*arrow*). **B,** The soft portion of the head can be indented like a ping-pong ball, and will collapse if reduced into the glenoid. A total shoulder replacement was performed.

quired repair. Follow-up ranged from 1 to 7 years, with an average of 3.0 years. There were seven excellent, two good, and one satisfactory result. Although the reconstruction is complex, the surgical results were clearly superior to those of the nonoperative group.

CHRONIC UNREDUCED POSTERIOR DISLOCATIONS

The diagnosis and treatment of locked posterior dislocations are reviewed in depth in Chapter 10. Several points merit repetition for emphasis. Any patient with a shoulder locked in internal rotation should be carefully evaluated to rule out a posterior dislocation, which can occur without a history of trauma or known seizures. We have seen several patients in whom our diagnosis of a locked posterior shoulder dislocation initiated an evaluation that uncovered a hitherto unknown seizure disorder, or an improper insulin schedule leading to nocturnal hypoglycemic seizures (Fig. 11.6).

The axillary view is the key investigation. If a standard supine, abducted view is not possible, a modified view such as the velpeau axillary view (3) can almost always be obtained. This is especially important if other injuries, such as fractures, divert attention (Fig. 11.7).

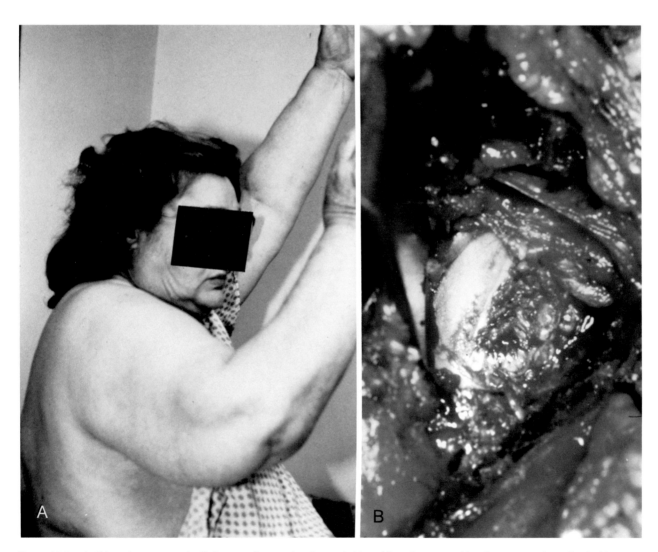

Figure 11.5.   A, This patient presented with longstanding anterior dislocation and significant pain and functional limitations. **B,** An anterior glenoid compression fracture, seen at the time of total shoulder replacement, shows loss of the anterior 60% of the glenoid. **C,** A bone graft was fashioned from the removed head segment and was fixed with screws to the glenoid in the damaged areas before the glenoid component was cemented. **D,** Three-year follow-up, AP radiograph. **E,** Three-year follow-up, axillary radiograph. **F,** Active elevation at 3-years' follow-up.

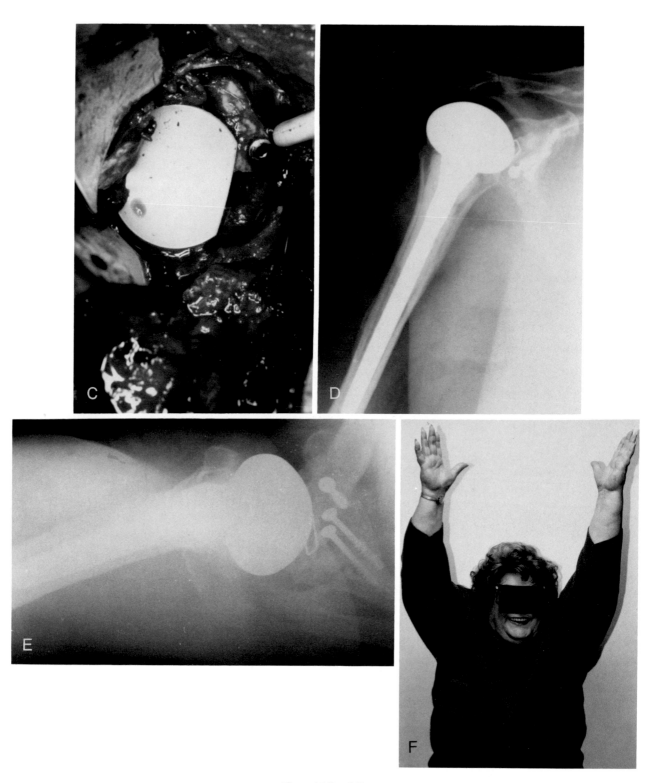

Figure 11.5.   C–F

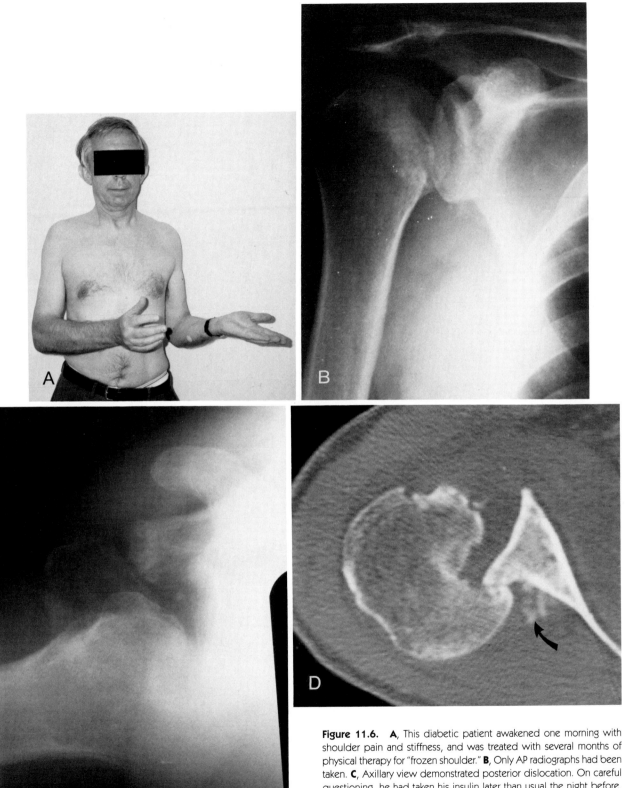

Figure 11.6. **A,** This diabetic patient awakened one morning with shoulder pain and stiffness, and was treated with several months of physical therapy for "frozen shoulder." **B,** Only AP radiographs had been taken. **C,** Axillary view demonstrated posterior dislocation. On careful questioning, he had taken his insulin later than usual the night before, and omitted his before-bed snack. **D,** CT scan shows size of head defect and demonstrated postglenoid periosteal changes (*arrow*) indicative of a longstanding dislocation.

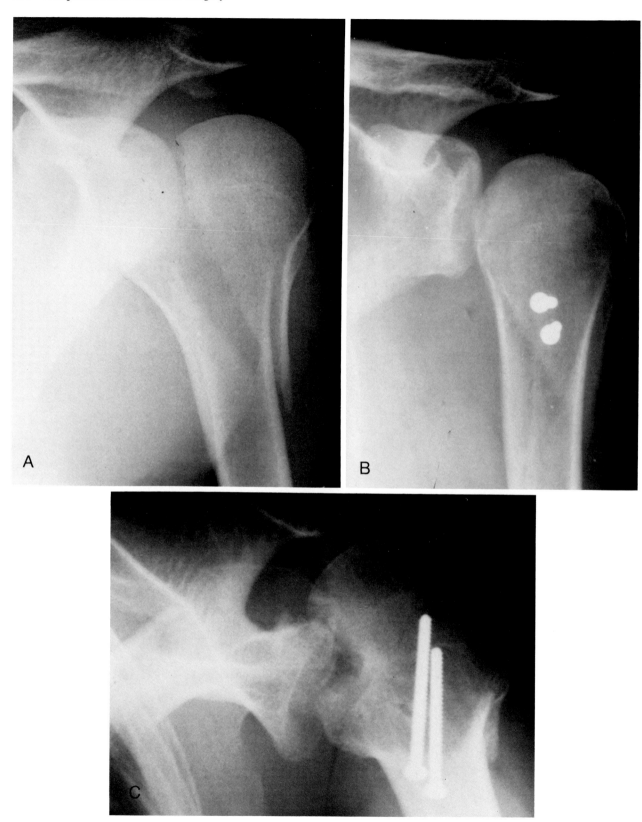

Figure 11.7.   A, This patient presented with a proximal humerus fracture. **B,** The patient was treated by open reduction and internal fixation, and followed for several months with AP views. **C,** But a velpeau axillary view (3) demonstrated that the internal fixation had converted a fracture-dislocation into a dislocation. A total shoulder replacement was required.

Table 11.2.   Results of Surgery for Chronic Anterior Shoulder Dislocations

Author	Date	Number	Procedure	Results
Neviaser (18)	1963	16[a]	OR[c] + Pin	7/16 elevation >90°
Hejna (12)	1969	4	3 OR, 1 HO	average incr elevation 55°
Schulz (25)	1969	16[b]	13 OR, 3 HE	85% satisfactory
Perniceni (20)	1982	3	OR + rib graft	good
Rowe (23)	1982	3	1 TSR, 1 OR, 1 HE	1E,1G,1F
Postacchini (21)	1987	1	1 HE	1G
Prichett (22)	1987	4	TSR/HHR	2G,2F
Bassey (1)	1988	4	OR + Bankart	50% unsatisfactory
Noack (19)	1988	4	OR + HO	3G,1F
Chen (4)	1990	3	OR + Bristow	1E,1G,1F
Neer (16)	1990	10	9 TSR, 1 OR	7E,2G,1S

[a] Includes anterior and posterior dislocations.
[b] Half with associated shoulder fractures.
[c] Abbreviations: OR = open reduction; Pin = metallic fixation; HO = (rotational) humeral osteotomy; HE = head excision; TSR = total shoulder replacement; E = excellent result; G = good result; F = fair result; and S = satisfactory result.

CONCLUSIONS

The best treatment of missed dislocations is to avoid them by proper diagnosis at the time of the initial injury. A careful history and physical, and routinely obtaining an axillary view are essential.

Some patients have little pain, and functional considerations play a role in deciding on whether surgical reconstruction should be considered. Common pathologic features such as humeral head impression defects, glenoid bone loss, rotator cuff tears, and extensive soft tissue distortions must be carefully evaluated if reconstruction is to be successful. If the articular surfaces are destroyed, replacement arthroplasty can be an effective treatment.

References

1. Bassey L. Alte und vernachlassigte Schulterluxationen als Indikation fur die Bankart'sche Operation. Unfallchir 1988; 91:85-90.
2. Bennett GE. Old dislocations of the shoulder. J Bone Joint Surg 1936;18:594-606.
3. Bloom MH, Obata WG. Diagnosis of posterior dislocation of the shoulder with use of velpeau axillary and angle-up roentgenographic views. J Bone Joint Surg 1967;49A:943-949.
4. Chen W. Modified Bristow-Helfet procedure in treatment of chronic unreduced anterior dislocation of the shoulder joint. In: Post M, Morrey BF, Hawkins RJ, eds. Surgery of the shoulder. St. Louis: Mosby Year Book, 1990:73-76.
5. Christophe K. A functioning false shoulder joint following an old dislocation. J Bone Joint Surg 1939;21:916-917.
6. Cooper A. Treatise on dislocations and fractures of the joints. 2nd Amer. ed. Boston: Lilly & Wait and Carter & Hendee, 1832.
7. Cubbins WR, Callahan JJ, Scuderi CS. The reduction of old or irreducible dislocations of the shoulder joint. Surg Gyn Obst 1934;58:129-135.
8. Delbet P. Des luxations anciennes et irreductibles de l'epaule. Arch Gen de Med 1893;31:19-39.
9. Flower WH. On the pathological changes produced in the shoulder-joint by traumatic dislocation, as derived from an examination of all the specimens illustrating this injury in the museums of London. Trans Path Soc London 1861; 12:179-200.
10. Ganel A, Horoszowski, Heim M, Engel J, Farine I. Persistent dislocation of the shoulder in elderly patients. J Am Geriatr Soc 1980;28:282-284.
11. Hawkins RJ. Unrecognized dislocations of the shoulder. AAOS Instructional Course Lectures 1985;34:258-263.
12. Hejna WF, Fossier CH, Goldstein TB, Ray RD. Ancient anterior dislocation of the shoulder. J Bone Joint Surg 1969; 51A:1030-1031.
13. Kirtland S, Resnick D, Sartoris DJ, Pate D, Greenway G. Chronic unreduced dislocations of the glenohumeral joint: imaging strategy and pathologic correlation. J Trauma 1988; 28:1622-1631.
14. Kummel BM. Fractures of the glenoid causing chronic dislocation of the shoulder. Clin Orthop 1970;69:189-191.
15. Litchfield JC, Subhedar VY, Beevers DG, Patel HT. Bilateral dislocations of the shoulders due to nocturnal hypoglycemia. Postgrad Med J 1988;64:450-452.
16. Neer CS II, Miller SR, Flatow EL. Chronic unreduced anterior dislocation of the shoulder. Orthop Trans 1990;14:596.
17. Neviaser JS. An operation for old dislocations of the shoulder. J Bone Joint Surg 1948;30A:997-1000.
18. Neviaser JS. The treatment of old unreduced dislocations of the shoulder. Surg Clin North Amer 1963;43:1671-1678.
19. Noack W, Strohmeier M. Die Behandlung der veralteten vorderen Schulterluxation. Unfallchir 1988;14:184-190.
20. Perniceni T, Augereau B, Apoil A. Traitement des luxations antero-internes anciennes de l'epaule par reduction sanglante et butee armee costale. A propos de trois cas. Ann Chir 1982;36:235-238.
21. Postacchini F, Facchini M. The treatment of unreduced dislocation of the shoulder. A review of twelve cases. Ital J Orthop Traumatol 1987;13:15-26.
22. Pritchett JW, Clark JM. Prosthetic replacement for chronic unreduced dislocations of the shoulder. Clin Orthop 1987; 216:89-93.

23. Rowe CR, Zarins B. Chronic unreduced dislocations of the shoulder. J Bone Joint Surg 1982;64A:494–505.
24. Rowe CR. Dislocations of the shoulder. In: Rowe CR, ed. The shoulder. New York: Churchill Livingstone, 1988:244–254.
25. Schulz TJ, Jacobs B, Patterson RL. Unrecognized dislocations of the shoulder. J Trauma 1969;9:1009–1023.
26. Souchon E. Operative treatment of irreducible dislocations of the shoulder joint, recent or old, simple or complicated. Trans Amer Surg Assoc 1897;15:311–451.
27. Steinman S, Bigliani LU, McIlveen SJ. Glenoid fractures associated with recurrent anterior dislocation of the shoulder. Presented at the American Academy of Orthopaedic Surgeons, Fifty-Seventh Annual Meeting, New Orleans, Louisiana, February, 1990.

12
Complications Following Repair of the Sternoclavicular Joint

"Better be wise by the misfortunes of others than by your own"
AESOP'S FABLES (6th century, B.C.)

Michael A. Wirth and Charles A. Rockwood, Jr.

INTRODUCTION

Since 1824, various reports have described the operative treatment of the unstable or degenerative sternoclavicular joint. The number of grave complications resulting from these surgical procedures have been startling.

In 1832, Sir Astley Cooper (8) described a posterior dislocation of the sternoclavicular joint in a patient who had such a severe scoliosis that, as the scapula advanced laterally around the chest wall, it pushed the medial end of the clavicle behind the sternum. The patient finally developed so much pressure on the esophagus and had such difficulty swallowing that Davie, a surgeon in Suffolk, resected the medial end of the clavicle with a scultetus saw (often called a Hey's saw). Familiar with the anatomy and concerned with potential complications, he protected the vital structures from the saw by introducing "a piece of well-beaten sole leather under the bone whilst he divided it" (8). Appreciating the difficulty of this operation and the possible complications that could follow, Cooper (8) wrote:

This case is extremely creditable to the knowledge, skill, and dexterity of Mr. Davie, surgeon at Bungay, in Suffolk; few would have thought of the mode of relief—very few would have dared to perform the operation—and a still smaller number would have had sufficient knowledge for its accomplishment.

The surgeon who is planning an operative procedure on or near the sternoclavicular joint should be completely knowledgeable about the vast array of anatomical structures immediately posterior to the sternoclavicular joint. There is a "curtain" of muscles—the sternohyoid, sternothyroid, and scaleni—which is posterior to the sternoclavicular joint and

the inner third of the clavicle. This curtain blocks the view of the vital structures. Some of these vital structures posterior to the protective curtain of muscles include the innominate artery, innominate vein, vagus nerve, phrenic nerve, internal jugular vein, trachea, and esophagus (Fig. 12.1). If one is considering stabilization of the sternoclavicular joint by running a pin down from the clavicle and into the sternum, it is important to remember that the arch of the aorta, the superior vena cava, and the right pulmonary artery are also very close at hand. Another structure to be aware of is the anterior jugular vein, which is between the clavicle and the curtain of muscles. The anatomy books state that it can be quite variable in size; we have seen it as large as 1.5 cm in diameter. This vein has no valves, and when it is nicked, it looks like someone has opened up the flood gates.

SPONTANEOUS ATRAUMATIC ANTERIOR SUBLUXATION OF THE STERNOCLAVICULAR JOINT

Some of the factors contributing to sternoclavicular joint stability are congenitally determined. These include the particular collagen makeup of the patient's ligaments, the arrangement of the sternoclavicular ligaments and their method of attachment, and the variation in bony anatomy of this saddle-type joint. As with classification of glenohumeral joint instability, the importance of distinguishing between traumatic and atraumatic instability of the sternoclavicular joint must be recognized if complications are to be avoided. Rowe (39) described several patients who have undergone one or more unsuccessful attempts to stabilize the sternoclavic-

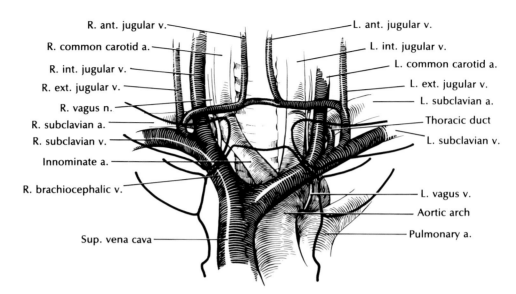

R. ant. jugular v.
R. common carotid a.
R. int. jugular v.
R. ext. jugular v.
R. vagus n.
R. subclavian a.
R. subclavian v.
Innominate a.
R. brachiocephalic v.
Sup. vena cava

L. ant. jugular v.
L. int. jugular v.
L. common carotid a.
L. ext. jugular v.
L. subclavian a.
Thoracic duct
L. subclavian v.
L. vagus v.
Aortic arch
Pulmonary a.

Figure 12.1. A diagram demonstrates the close proximity of the major vessels that are posterior to the sternoclavicular joint. (Reproduced with permission from Rockwood CA, Green DP, eds: Fractures (3 vols), 2nd ed. Philadelphia: JB Lippincott, 1984.)

ular joint. In all cases the patient was able to voluntarily dislocate the clavicle after surgery. In addition, he has described several young patients who were able to "flip the clavicle out and back in," without elevation of the arms (38).

In our experience, spontaneous atraumatic anterior subluxation of the sternoclavicular joint is a relatively rare problem that usually occurs in young people under the age of 20, and most often occurs in females. The senior author has evaluated 37 patients with this problem, and about the only symptom they have is that the medial end of the clavicle subluxes or dislocates anteriorly when they raise their arms over their heads (36). The dislocations occur spontaneously without any significant trauma. Some patients, when seen for another shoulder problem, are completely unaware that with the overhead motion the medial end of the clavicle subluxes or dislocates. We have never seen a posterior spontaneous subluxation of the sternoclavicular joint. Only occasionally does the patient with atraumatic anterior displacement complain of pain during the displacement. In the review by Rockwood and Odor of 37 patients with spontaneous atraumatic subluxation, 29 were managed without surgery and eight were treated with a surgical reconstruction elsewhere (36). With an average follow-up of more than 8 years, all of the 29 nonoperative patients were doing just fine, without limitations of activity or life-style. However, the eight patients who were treated with surgery had increased pain, a significant scar, limitation of activity, alteration of life-style, and persistent instability (Fig. 12.2).

As with voluntary, atraumatic subluxation of the glenohumeral joint, we agree with Rowe (39) that these patients can prove to be, if surgery is performed, a great embarrassment to the surgeon. Accordingly, nonoperative skillful neglect is advocated for this entity. The anatomy of the problem should be carefully explained to the patient and family. We explain further that surgery is hazardous and of little benefit, that they should discontinue the voluntary aspect of the dislocation, and that in time the symptoms will either disappear or they will completely forget that the dislocation is a problem.

RECURRENT SUBLUXATION AND DISLOCATION

Bearn (2) has shown that the capsular ligament is the most important structure in preventing superior displacement of the medial clavicle. This work has aided our understanding of the mechanisms of recurrent instability of the sternoclavicular joint following surgical repair. The lever arm of the upper extremity in the sternoclavicular joint approaches a ratio of 35:1. This inequality produces tremendous forces across the sternoclavicular joint as upper extremity motion is transferred proximally. In particular, the sternoclavicular ligaments are stressed with shoulder depression as the medial clavicle is levered superiorly over the fulcrum of the first rib (2). These findings help to explain the high incidence of recurrent subluxation and dislocation of the surgically treated sternoclavicular joint found in the literature.

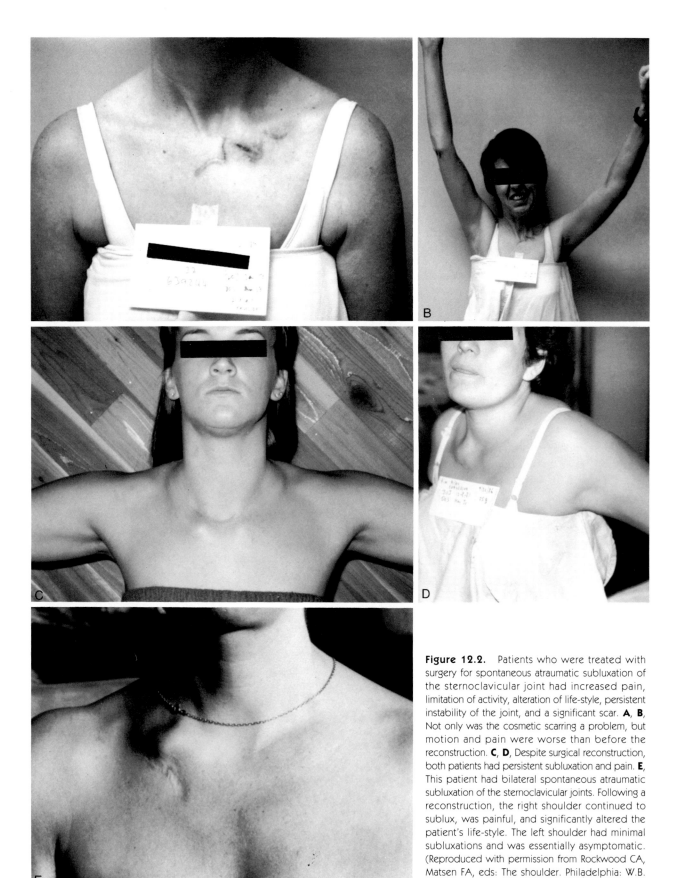

Figure 12.2. Patients who were treated with surgery for spontaneous atraumatic subluxation of the sternoclavicular joint had increased pain, limitation of activity, alteration of life-style, persistent instability of the joint, and a significant scar. **A, B,** Not only was the cosmetic scarring a problem, but motion and pain were worse than before the reconstruction. **C, D,** Despite surgical reconstruction, both patients had persistent subluxation and pain. **E,** This patient had bilateral spontaneous atraumatic subluxation of the sternoclavicular joints. Following a reconstruction, the right shoulder continued to sublux, was painful, and significantly altered the patient's life-style. The left shoulder had minimal subluxations and was essentially asymptomatic. (Reproduced with permission from Rockwood CA, Matsen FA, eds: The shoulder. Philadelphia: W.B. Saunders, 1990.)

In Omer's (31) review of case records with a minimum follow-up of 6 months, a 60% incidence of recurrent dislocation in patients treated with metallic fixation and a 66% incidence of recurrent dislocation with capsular ligament reconstruction was reported. We are in agreement with Omer's (31) observation:

Recurrent dislocation is a prolonged threat following surgical reduction of an anterior sternoclavicular dislocation because the entire upper extremity may act as a lever arm to disrupt the reconstruction in spite of external dressings or internal fixation.

Most patients with an unreduced and permanent anterior dislocation of the sternoclavicular joint are not very symptomatic, have almost a complete range of motion, and can work and even perform manual labor without many problems (Fig. 12.3). Because the articular contact of the clavicle to the manubrium is so small and incongruous and because the results we have seen in patients who have had attempted reconstructions are so miserable, a nonoperative skillful neglect type of treatment is recommended. In most instances of a failed previously attempted open reduction and internal fixation, the capsular ligament was repaired without reconstruction of the extra-articular coracoclavicular (rhomboid) ligament. The patient ends up with a painful joint that requires a major sternoclavicular arthroplasty, i.e., resection of the medial clavicle and reconstruction of a new costoclavicular ligament with fascia or Dacron graft.

PHYSEAL INJURIES

Although the clavicle is the first long bone of the body to ossify (5th intrauterine week), the epiphysis at the medial end of the clavicle is the last to close (Fig. 12.4) (13, 14, 33). The medial clavicular epiphysis does not ossify until the 18th–20th year, and fuses with the shaft of the clavicle around the 23rd–25th year (13).

In 1898, Poland (33) described in detail physeal injuries of the medial clavicle in his text entitled *Traumatic Separation of Epiphyses of the Upper Extremity.* This knowledge of the epiphysis is important to remember because many of the "dislocations of the sternoclavicular joint" are not dislocations but physeal injuries. Most of these injuries will heal and remodel with time, without surgical intervention. In time, the remodeling process eliminates any bone deformity or displacement. We believe that the operative complications are too great and the end results are too unsatisfactory to consider an open reduction.

Certainly in children, a nonoperative approach should be followed.

As with rare posterior sternoclavicular joint dislocations, the concern for late complications caused by pressure on the hilar structures with posterior physeal injuries has led many authors to recommend surgery after failure of closed reduction. The distinction between posterior sternoclavicular joint dislocations and posterior medial clavicle physeal injuries is paramount to ensuring proper treatment. Indeed, as with other childhood fractures, the potential for remodeling is significant and may extend until the 23rd–25th year. The senior author (37) has demonstrated a similar mechanism to support conservative treatment of adolescent acromioclavicular joint injuries or "pseudodislocation," in which there is a partial tear of the periosteal tube containing the distal clavicle. The coracoclavicular ligaments remain secured to the periosteal tube. Because of its high osteogenic potential, spontaneous healing and remodeling to the preinjury "reduced" position occur within this periosteal conduit. Zaslav et al. (48) have reported successful treatment of a posteriorly displaced medial clavicle physeal injury in an adolescent athlete with computerized axial tomography (CT) documentation of remodeling, most probably within an intact periosteal tube. Understanding this is critical, as explained earlier, and not merely for academic interest, as Denham and Dingley (9) would lead us to believe. While we agree that posterior physeal injuries in children and young adults under the age of 23 should have an attempted reduction, failure of reduction in the patient who is having no significant symptoms is a poor indication for surgery. On the other hand, when a posteriorly displaced medial clavicle physeal injury is symptomatic and cannot be reduced closed, the displacement must be reduced during surgery. Many authors have observed at the time of surgery that the intra-articular disc ligament stays with the sternum. In addition, we submit that the unossified or ossified epiphyseal disc, depending on the age of the patient, also stays with the sternum. Anatomically, the epiphysis is lateral to the articular disc ligament, and it is held in place by the capsular ligament and can be mistaken for the intra-articular disc ligament.

ARTHROPLASTY OF THE MEDIAL CLAVICLE

As with any surgical procedure on the sternoclavicular joint, careful preparation and appropriate precautions cannot be overstated. Medial clavicle ex-

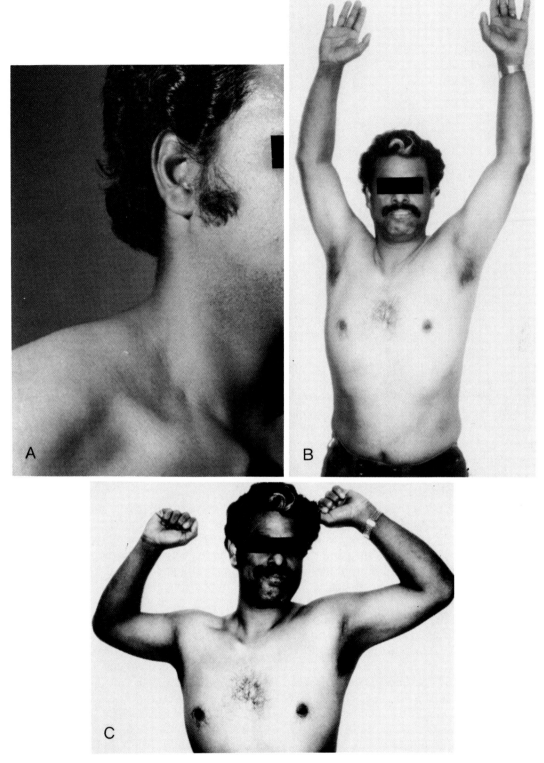

Figure 12.3. Unreduced anterior traumatic dislocation of the sternoclavicular joint. **A,** This patient suffered an unreduced traumatic anterior dislocation of his right shoulder following an automobile accident. At the time of the injury, the medial clavicle could be manually reduced, but it would not stay in position. **B, C,** Fifteen years later, the patient continues to have prominence of his right clavicle, but he works as a day laborer unloading and loading 50-lb. sacks of cement. (**A** reproduced with permission from Rockwood CA, Green DP, eds: Fractures (3 vols), 2nd ed. Philadelphia: JB Lippincott, 1984 . **B, C** reproduced with permission from Rockwood CA, Matsen FA, eds: The shoulder. Philadelphia: W.B. Saunders, 1990.)

Figure 12.4. Tomogram demonstrating the thin, waferlike disc of the epiphysis of the medial clavicle. (Reproduced with permission from Rockwood CA, Green DP, eds: Fractures (3 vols). 2nd ed. Philadelphia: JB Lippincott, 1984.)

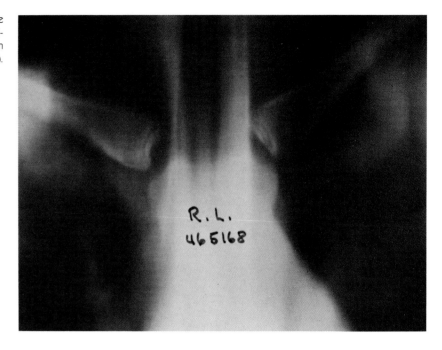

cision is a well-accepted procedure for the symptomatic sternoclavicular joint with degenerative changes. If the medial end of the clavicle is to be removed because of degenerative changes, the surgeon should be careful not to damage the costoclavicular ligament and to evaluate the residual stability of the remaining clavicle. If the ligaments are gone, the clavicle must be restabilized to the first rib. If too much clavicle is resected, or if the clavicle is not stabilized to the first rib, several complications may ensue (Fig. 12.5). Initially, there will be an improvement of pain and alleviation of crepitance, but this is usually short-lived. Subsequently, a return of mild to moderate symptoms occurs as the integral stabilizing role of the clavicle is lost. Functional deficits related to limited shoulder mobility, neurological symptoms, thoracic outlet syndrome, and fatigue have been reported (18, 22, 31, 36, 46).

The same analogy when resecting the distal clavicle for a chronic acromioclavicular joint problem applies here. If the coracoclavicular ligaments are intact, an excision of the proper amount of the distal clavicle is indicated and is successful. However, if the coracoclavicular ligaments are gone, then, in addition to the excision of the distal clavicle, the coracoclavicular ligaments must be reconstructed. If the costoclavicular ligaments are intact, the clavicle medial to the ligaments can be resected and beveled smooth (Fig. 12.6).

Just as problems may result from excessive medial clavicle excision, insufficient medial excision may also prove symptomatic. In many cases where the surgeon has attempted to resect the medial end of the clavicle, a portion of the posterior cortex of the medial clavicle has been left behind that continues to cause pain (Fig. 12.7). The senior author has also evaluated several patients, previously treated by resection of the medial clavicle, who later required additional medial clavicle resection because of posteriorly directed bony proliferation and degenerative spurring of the medial clavicle. This complication can be avoided by initially resecting enough bone, using bone wax at the osteotomy site, removing the proximal periosteum, and releasing the clavicular head of the sternocleidomastoid.

DEGENERATIVE ARTHRITIS OF THE STERNOCLAVICULAR JOINT

The sternoclavicular joint is a diarthrodial joint that forms the only bony connection of the shoulder girdle to the axial skeleton (35). The articular surface of the clavicle is much larger than its sternal counterpart, with less than half of the medial clavicle articulating with the upper angle of the sternum. An additional facet on the inferior aspect of the medial clavicle forms an articulation with the superior aspect of the first rib in 2.5% of patients (6). Patients may present with a stable sternoclavicular joint that is associated with a reproducible and painful clicking or popping sensation. Although rarely involved, injury to the intra-articular disc can be quite disabling (1). Although CT arthrography has been advocated as a diagnostic aid, 6% of intra-articular discs were found to be incomplete by DePalma (11). In patients refractory to conservative management, the joint can be injected with local anesthesia to confirm the source of pain. If the pain in the joint is obliterated, then at the time of arthrotomy a resection of the disc may eliminate the pain. If the pain is not relieved by this injection, further evaluation is indicated prior to surgical intervention. The differential diagnosis of a patient with a stable but seemingly symptomatic sternoclavicular joint must include possibilities that are extrinsic to the sternoclavicular joint itself. An example of this involved a 16-year-old female gymnast who noted the abrupt onset of pain about the upper sternum after performing a back hand-spring. Physical examination revealed marked tenderness upon medial clavicle compression, but further scrutiny on the part of the referring physician revealed maximum point tenderness about the distal manubrium. A lateral radiograph of the sternum confirmed a sternomanubrial separation (Fig. 12.8).

A potential complication of simple disc excision is failure to understand sternoclavicular joint articular anatomy. Initial inspection may fail to recognize degenerative changes at the inferior pole of the medial clavicle, where the true articular surface exists with the upper angle of the sternum. As with reconstructions for sternoclavicular instability, failure to address this aspect of the pathology will result in persistent symptoms. The management of patients with osteoarthritis of the sternoclavicular joint can usually be done with conservative nonoperative treatment, i.e., heat, anti-inflammatory agents, and rest (3, 5). However, the patient must be thoroughly evaluated to rule out other conditions that mimic the changes in the sternoclavicular joint, i.e., tumor, metabolic, infectious, or collagen disorders. Patients with post-traumatic arthritic changes in the sternoclavicular joint, which follow fractures of the sternoclavicular joint and previous attempts at reconstruction, may require a formal arthroplasty of the joint and careful stabilization of the remaining clavicle to the first rib.

If the patient has persistent symptoms of traumatic arthritis for 6–12 months, and if the symptoms can be completely relieved by injection of local anesthesia into the sternoclavicular joint region, we would perform an arthroplasty of the sternoclavicular joint. A diagnostic injection with local anesthesia is an important part of the evaluation because numerous studies have emphasized the astounding frequency with which radiographic findings were present in asymptomatic patients. This cannot be overstated, as we have seen several patients with radiographic degenerative changes of the sternoclavicular joint who remained symptomatic after medial clavicle resection for presumed post-traumatic arthritis. Following a thorough physical examination

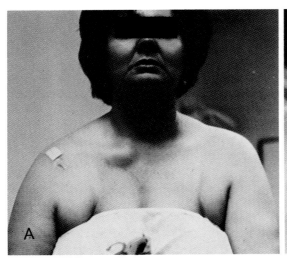 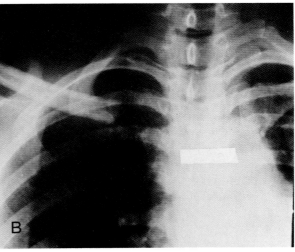

Figure 12.5. A, This postmenopausal right-hand dominant woman had a resection of the right medial clavicle because of a preoperative diagnosis of "possible tumor." The postoperative microscopic diagnosis was degenerative arthritis of the right medial clavicle. Following surgery, the patient complained of pain and discomfort, marked prominence, and gross instability of the right medial clavicle. **B**, An x-ray confirms that the excision of the medial clavicle extended lateral to the costoclavicular ligaments, hence the patient had an unstable medial clavicle. (Reproduced with permission from Rockwood CA, Green DP, eds: Fractures (3 vols). 2nd ed. Philadelphia: JB Lippincott, 1984.)

Figure 12.6. Technique of resecting the medial clavicle for degenerative arthritis. **A**, Care must be taken to remove only that part of the clavicle that is medial to the costoclavicular (rhomboid) ligaments. There must be adequate protection for vital structures that lie posterior to the medial end of the clavicle. **B**, **C**, An air drill with a side-cutting burr can be used to perform the osteotomy. **D**, When the fragment of bone has been removed, the dorsal and anterior borders of the clavicle should be smoothed down to give a better cosmetic appearance. (Reproduced with permission from Rockwood CA, Green DP, eds: Fractures (3 vols). 2nd ed. Philadelphia: JB Lippincott, 1984.)

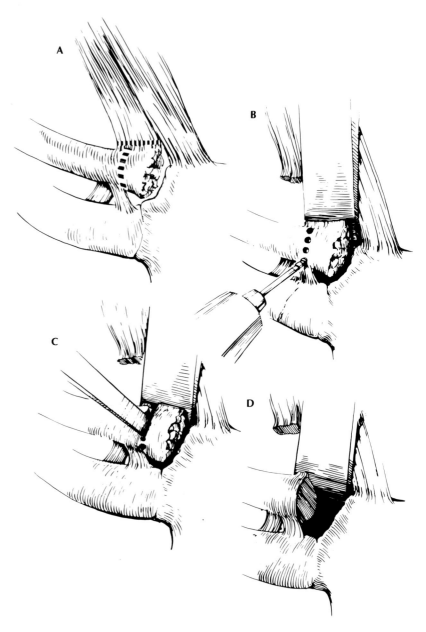

and injection of local anesthetic into the subacromial space for impingement syndrome, their symptoms were completely relieved. Just as acromioclavicular arthritis may both imitate and contribute to an impingement syndrome, the differential diagnosis of a symptomatic sternoclavicular joint must include referred pain from nearby sources. Surgery includes resection of that part of the clavicle that is medial to the costoclavicular ligament, a beveling of the superior and the anterior borders, and a debridement of the intra-articular disc ligament. If because of the previous surgery or injury the costoclavicular ligaments are absent, then the clavicle must be stabilized to the first rib with either fascia or 1.0-mm Dacron

tape. The clavicular head of the sternocleidomastoid should be released to temporarily resist the upward pull of the clavicle.

STERNOCLAVICULAR ARTHRODESIS

The sternoclavicular joint is freely movable and functions almost like a ball-and-socket joint in that the joint has motion in almost all planes, including rotation (15, 23). The clavicle, and therefore the sternoclavicular joint, in normal shoulder motion is capable of 30–35° of upward elevation, 35° of combined forward and backward movement, and 45–50° degrees of rotation around its long axis (Fig. 12.9). It

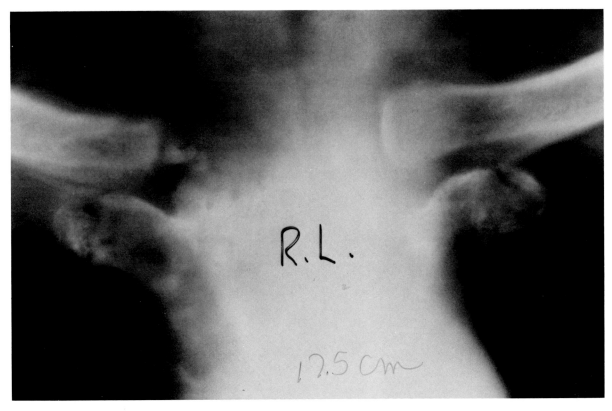

Figure 12.7. Tomogram showing retention of fragments after insufficient medial clavicle resection. A revision arthroplasty was required due to significant symptoms.

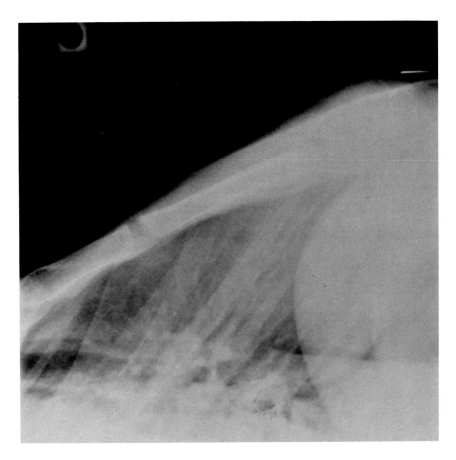

Figure 12.8. Lateral radiograph demonstrating a traumatic sternomanubrial separation in a 16-year-old gymnast.

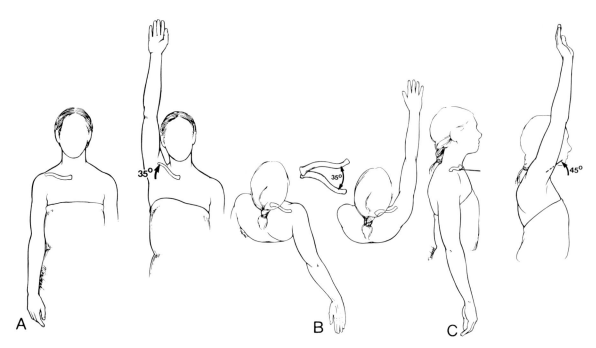

Figure 12.9.   Motions of the clavicle and the sternoclavicular joint. **A,** With full overhead elevation the clavicle elevates 35°. **B,** With adduction and extension, the clavicle displaces anteriorly and posteriorly 35°. **C,** The clavicle rotates on its long axis 45° as the arm is elevated to the full overhead position. (Reproduced with permission from Rockwood CA, Green DP, eds: Fractures (3 vols). 2nd ed. Philadelphia: JB Lippincott, 1984.)

is most likely the most frequently moved joint of the long bones in the body because almost any motion of the upper extremity is transferred proximally to the sternoclavicular joint.

There are several reports in the older literature advocating arthrodesis of the sternoclavicular joint for recurrent traumatic or atraumatic dislocation (16). In 1932, Rice (34) reported this as the procedure of choice. Rice stated: "Operative arthrodesis offers the only permanent cure for this condition (recurrent dislocation) and should be done when the condition causes any discomfort or disability."

However, it is now clear that an arthrodesis should not be performed because it prevents the previously described normal elevation, depression, and rotation of the clavicle. This produces a severe restriction of shoulder movement and subsequent function—a most debilitating complication (Fig. 12.10).

INFECTION OF THE STERNOCLAVICULAR JOINT

Most infections of the sternoclavicular joint are associated with intravenous drug abuse, bacteremia, local infection, rheumatoid arthritis, alcoholism, and chronic debilitating diseases. While these represent the majority of cases, wound dehiscence, pin tract infection, and osteomyelitis have all been reported. Infections of the sternoclavicular joint should be managed as they are in other joints, except that during aspiration and surgical drainage, great care and respect must be directed to the vital structures that lie posterior to the joint. If aspiration or a high index of suspicion demonstrates purulent material in the joint, a formal arthrotomy should be carried out. Occasionally, the infection will arise in the medial end of the clavicle or the manubrium, which will necessitate the resection of some of the necrotic bone. Depending on the status of the wound following the debridement, one can either close the wound loosely over a drain or pack the wound open and close it at a later time. Infections of the sternoclavicular joint are difficult to eradicate and may require several surgical debridements. The usual result is an unsightly scar, instability due to the amount of necrotic bone removed to provide an adequate resection, and chronic discomfort (Fig. 12.11).

PIN MIGRATION

As with arthroplasty of other joints, a host of creative procedures have been recommended for reconstruction of the sternoclavicular joint. Some of the older literature has recommended such unique materials as Kangaroo tendon xenograft (20, 34) and ivory fixation pegs (44) to stabilize the reconstruction; however, none has left a more ominous legacy of complications than Kirschner wires or Steinmann pins.

While most orthopaedic surgeons are aware of anecdotal accounts of the grave effects of pin migration, numerous pin-and-wire techniques continue to be used in the surgical management of the sternoclavicular joint. Various theories have been proposed to explain the propensity of pins to migrate from the region of the shoulder, but these remain obscure. Explanations have included muscular activity, respiratory movement, gravitational forces, capillary action, and the unrestricted motion of the upper extremity (19, 26, 45).

The perils of pin and wire migration have led to many recommendations by those who continue to use them for sternoclavicular joint surgery. These recommendations include *not* perforating the medial cortex of the manubrium, using smooth pins,

bending the pin ends at acute angles, leaving the pins in a palpable subcutaneous position, instructing patients not to elevate their arms above 90°, and the use of external supplementary bracing (10, 24, 39). However, it must be pointed out that smooth pins, threaded Kirschner wires, pins with bent ends, and Hagie pins have all been reported to migrate and cause serious complications including death (25, 30, 43) (Fig. 12.12). By 1984, four deaths (7, 21, 28, 41) and three near deaths (4, 32, 47) had been reported from complications of transfixing the sternoclavicular joint with Kirschner wires or Steinmann pins. The pins, either intact or broken, migrated into the heart, pulmonary artery, innominate artery, or into the aorta. Tremendous leverage force is applied to pins that cross the sternoclavicular joint, and fatigue breakage of the pins is common. Brown (4) reported an incidence of three complications in 10 operative cases: two from broken pins that had to be removed from a window in the sternum, and one, a near death, in which the pin penetrated the back of the sternum and entered into the right pulmonary artery. Nord-

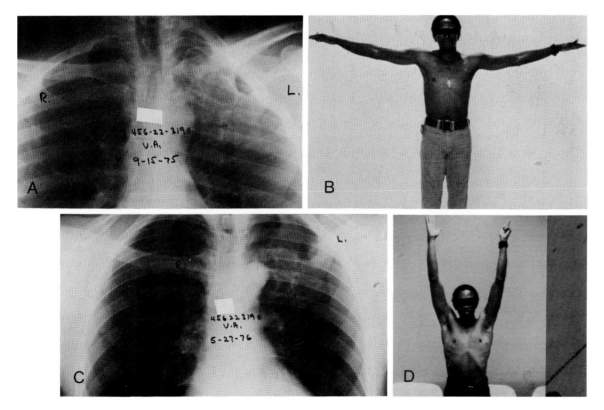

Figure 12.10.   The effect of an arthrodesis of the sternoclavicular joint on shoulder function. **A,** As a result of a military gunshot wound to the left sternoclavicular joint, this patient had a massive bony union of the left medial clavicle to the sternum and the upper three ribs. **B,** Shoulder motion was limited to 90° of flexion and abduction. **C,** An x-ray following resection of the bony mass, freeing up the medial clavicle. **D,** Function of the left shoulder was essentially normal following the elimination of the sternoclavicular arthrodesis. (Reproduced with permission from Rockwood CA, Green DP, eds: Fractures (3 vols). 2nd ed. Philadelphia: JB Lippincott, 1984.)

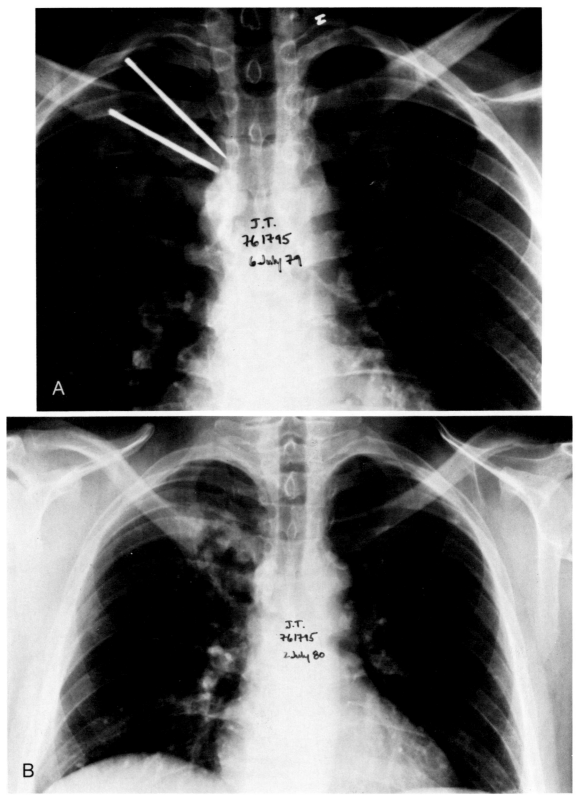

Figure 12.11.   A, This 32-year-old patient underwent ORIF of a right sternoclavicular joint sprain. **B**, Postoperative course was complicated by infection requiring multiple subsequent procedures that resulted in medial clavicle instability and chronic pain.

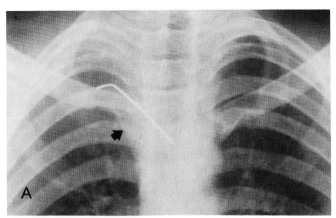

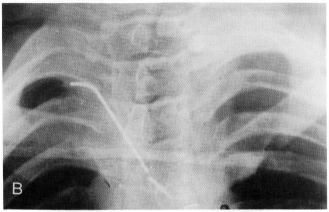

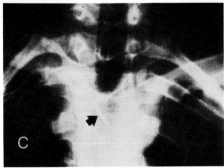

Figure 12.12. Complications with pins across the sternoclavicular joint. **A**, Postoperative anteroposterior x-ray with small-size Steinmann pins across the sternoclavicular joint. This dislocation occurred in a 13-year-old boy and probably was a type II epiphyseal injury. Note the fragment of the medial inferior clavicle in its normal relationship, and note that the joint has not been reduced (*arrow*). **B**, At 4 weeks, at the time of pin removal, a fracture of the pin was noted. **C**, Broken pins cannot be left in the manubrium because they may migrate into the mediastinum with serious consequences. (Reproduced with permission from Rockwood CA, Green DP (eds): Fractures (3 vols). 2nd ed. Philadelphia: JB Lippincott, 1984.)

back and Markkula (29) removed a pin that migrated completely inside the aorta. Jelesijevic and associates (17), Pate and Wilhite (32), Rubenstein and colleagues (40), and Schechter and Gilbert (42) reported cases where the pin migrated into the heart. Leonard and Gifford (21) reported on migration to the pulmonary artery. Sethi and Scott (43) reported on migration of the pin to lacerate the subclavian artery. Clark and associates (7), Nettles and Linscheid (28), and Salvatore (41) reported migration of pins into the aorta and resultant death. Grabski (12) reported on the migration of the pin to the opposite breast in a 37-year-old female. In addition, the senior author has treated patients in whom the pin has migrated into the chest and up into the base of the neck. Omer (31), in a review of 14 military hospitals, reported on 15 patients who had elective surgery for reduction and reconstruction of the sternoclavicular joint. Eight patients were followed by the same house staff for more than 6 months with the following complications: of the five patients who had internal fixation with metal, two developed osteomyelitis, two had fracture of the pin with recurrent dislocation, and one had migration of the pin into the mediastinum with recurrent dislocation. Omer commented on this series of complications: "It would seem that complications are common in this rare surgical problem."

In 1990, Lyons and Rockwood (24) reported on the complications of pins used in shoulder surgery. They reported on 45 instances where pins that were used in the fixation of the acromioclavicular joint, sternoclavicular joint, fracture of the proximal humerus, and arthrodesis of the shoulder had migrated to all parts of the patient's anatomy. Pins migrated into the heart, lung, spine, trachae, spleen, mammary gland, and even into the orbit. The important point is that eight deaths were reported, and all of them were associated with migration of pins from the sternoclavicular joint. On the basis of a review of the literature, we consider the risk of serious complications following fixation of the sternoclavicular joint with pins to be so grave as to contraindicate the use of pins in fixation of this joint.

References

1. Bateman JE. The shoulder and neck. Philadelphia: WB Saunders, 1972.

2. Bearn JG. Direct observations on the function of the capsule of the sternoclavicular joint in clavicular support. J Anat 1967;101:159-170.

3. Bonnin JG. Spontaneous subluxation of the sternoclavicular joint. Br Med J 1960;2:274-275.

4. Brown JE. Anterior sternoclavicular dislocation—a method of repair. Am J Orthop 1961;31:184-189.

5. Bremner RA. Nonarticular, non-infective subacute arthritis of the sternoclavicular joint. J Bone Joint Surg 1959;41B:749-753.

6. Cave AJE. The nature and morphology of the costoclavicular ligament. J Anat 1961;95:170-179.

7. Clark RL, Milgram JW, Yawn DH. Fatal aortic perforation and cardiac tamponade due to a Kirschner wire migrating from the right sternoclavicular joint. South Med J 1974;67:316-318.

8. Cooper A. A treatise on dislocations and fractures of the joints, 2nd American ed. from the 6th London ed. Boston: Lilly & Wait and Carter & Hendee, 1832.

9. Denham RH Jr, Dingley AF Jr. Epiphyseal separation of the medial end of the clavicle. J Bone Joint Surg 1967;49A:1179-1183.

10. DePalma AF. Surgery of the shoulder, 3rd ed. Philadelphia: JB Lippincott, 1983:460.

11. DePalma AF. Surgical anatomy of acromioclavicular and sternoclavicular joints. Surg Clin North Am 1963;43:1541-1550.

12. Grabski RS. Unusual dislocation of a fragment of Kirschner wire after fixation of the sternoclavicular joint. Wiad Lek 1987;40:630-632.

13. Grant JCB. Method of anatomy, 7th ed. Baltimore: Williams & Wilkins, 1965.

14. Gray H. Anatomy of the human body. 28th ed (CM Goss, ed). Philadelphia: Lea & Febiger, 1966:324-326.

15. Inman VT, Saunders JB, Abbott LC. Observations on the function of the shoulder joint. J Bone Joint Surg 1944;26:1-30.

16. Jean G. Habitual suprasternal dislocation of the clavicle treated by osteosynthesis. Bull et mem. Soc, November 7, 1923.

17. Jelsijevic V, Knoll D, Klinke F, et al. Penetrating injuries of the heart and intrapericardial blood vessels caused by migration of a Kirschner pin after osteosynthesis. Acta Chir Iugosl 1982;29:274.

18. Jupiter JB, Leffert RD. Nonunion of the clavicle. J Bone Joint Surg 1987;69A:753-760.

19. Kremens V, Glauser F. Unusual sequela following pinning of medial clavicular fracture. Am J Roentgenol 1956;76:1066-1069.

20. Lee HM. Sternoclavicular dislocations. Minn Med 1937;20:480-482.

21. Leonard JW, Gifford RW. Migration of a Kirschner wire from the clavicle into pulmonary artery. Am J Cardiol 1965;16:598-600.

22. Lipton HA, Jupiter JB. Nonunion of clavicular fractures: characteristics and surgical management. Surg Rounds Orthop 1988.

23. Lucas DB. Biomechanics of the shoulder joint. Arch Surg 1973;107:425-432.

24. Lyons FA, Rockwood CA Jr. Current concepts review: migration of pins used in operations on the shoulder. J Bone Joint Surg 1990;72A:1262-1267.

25. McCaughan JS Jr, Miller PR. Migration of Steinmann pin from shoulder to lung. JAMA 1969;207:1917.

26. Mazet R Jr. Migration of a Kirschner wire from the shoulder region into the lung. Report of two cases. J Bone Joint Surg 1943;25:477-483.

27. Neer CS II. Dislocations of the sternoclavicular joint in shoulder reconstruction. Philadelphia: WB Saunders, 1990;355-359.

28. Nettles JL, Linscheid R. Sternoclavicular dislocations. J Trauma 1968;8:158-164.

29. Nordback I, Markkula H. Migration of Kirschner pin from clavicle into ascending aorta. Acta Chir Scand 1985;151:177-179.

30. Norrell H Jr, Llewellyn RC. Migration of a threaded Steinmann pin from an acromioclavicular joint into the spinal canal. A case report. J Bone Joint Surg 1965;47A:1024-1026.

31. Omer GE Jr. Osteotomy of the clavicle in surgical reduction of anterior sternoclavicular dislocation. J Trauma 1967;7:584-590.

32. Pate JW, Wilhite J. Migration of a foreign body from the sternoclavicular joint to the heart: a case report. Am Surg 1969;35:448-449.

33. Poland J. Separation of the epiphyses of the clavicle. In: Traumatic separation of the epiphyses of the upper extremity. London: Smith, Elder, and Co., 1898:135-143.

34. Rice EE. Habitual dislocation of the sternoclavicular articulation: a case report. J Okla State Med Assoc 1932;25:34-35.

35. Rockwood CA Jr. Disorders of the sternoclavicular joint. In: Rockwood CA, Matsen FA, eds. The shoulder. Philadelphia: WB Saunders, 1990:477-525.

36. Rockwood CA Jr, Odor JM. Spontaneous atraumatic anterior subluxation of the sternoclavicular joint. J Bone Joint Surg 1989;71A:1280-1287.

37. Rockwood CA Jr. Injuries of the acromioclavicular joint. In: Fractures in children, Vol 3. 2nd ed. Philadelphia: JB Lippincott, 1984:631-645.

38. Rowe CR. personal communication, June 27, 1988.

39. Rowe CR. The shoulder. New York: Churchill Livingstone, 1988:313-327.

40. Rubenstein ZR, Moray B, Itzchak Y. Percutaneous removal of intravascular foreign bodies. Cardiovasc Intervent Radiol 1982;5:64–68.

41. Salvatore JE. Sternoclavicular joint dislocation. Clin Orthop 1968;58:51–54.

42. Schechter DC, Gilbert L. Injuries of the heart and great vessels due to pins and needles. Thorax 1969;24:246–253.

43. Sethi GK, Scott SM. Subclavian artery laceration due to migration of a hagie pin. Surgery 1976;80:644–646.

44. Speed K. A textbook of fractures and dislocations. 4th ed. Philadelphia: Lea & Febiger, 1942:282–290.

45. Tristan TA, Daughtridge TG. Migration of a metallic pin from the humerus into the lung. N Engl J Med 1964; 270:987–989.

46. Wilkins RM, Johnston RM. Ununited fracture of the clavicle. J Bone Joint Surg 1983;65A:773–778.

47. Worman LW, Leagus C. Intrathoracic injury following retrosternal dislocation of the clavicle. J Trauma 1967;7:416–423.

48. Zaslav KR, Ray S, Neer CS II. Conservative management of a displaced medial clavicular physeal injury in an adolescent athlete. Am J Sports Med 1989;17:833–836.

13
Complications of Clavicle Fractures

James S. Thompson

INTRODUCTION

The exceptionally important clavicle that Neer described as a "nonconformist bone" (21) does not receive the great respect it deserves. The clavicle (derived from the Latin "clavis," key) possesses many unique characteristics. It is the only long bone to form through intramembranous ossification, the first bone to ossify (5th week of fetal development), the last bone to completely ossify (18 years or older), and the most frequently fractured bone (10–12% of all skeletal fractures) (6). The clavicle serves as the anatomic strut between the axial skeleton and the shoulder girdle of the upper limb. The only true articulation between the upper limb and the axial skeleton is the sternoclavicular joint. Throughout the infinite positional changes of the upper limb, motion of the clavicle at the sternoclavicular joint is complex and multiplanar (18). It allows elevation and depression, protraction/retraction, and rotation (Fig. 13.1). The clavicle serves many important functions: (*a*) maintenance of the shoulder joint lateral to the chest wall—anatomical strut function, (*b*) provision of a stable point of attachment for multiple muscles and ligaments (Fig. 13.2); and (*c*) protection of neurovascular structures at the base of neck and within the thoracic outlet.

Physicians who treat clavicle fractures should critically review their experience to improve patient care recommendations. Published statistical analyses of clavicle fractures combine numbers for children and adults. This combination yields large numbers of fractures (the majority of which occur in children) and a low incidence of complications. The large numbers of fractures and reported low incidence of complications result in minor emphasis on clavicle fractures during orthopaedic residency training ("they all heal"), and it usually comes as a shock when a complication of a clavicle fracture oc-

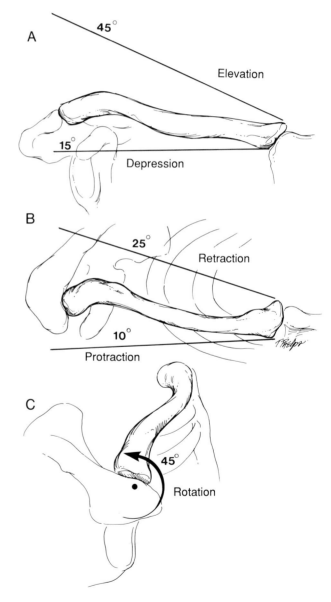

Figure 13.1. The three axes of motion of the clavicle: **A,** Elevation/depression. **B,** Protraction/retraction. **C,** Rotation.

154

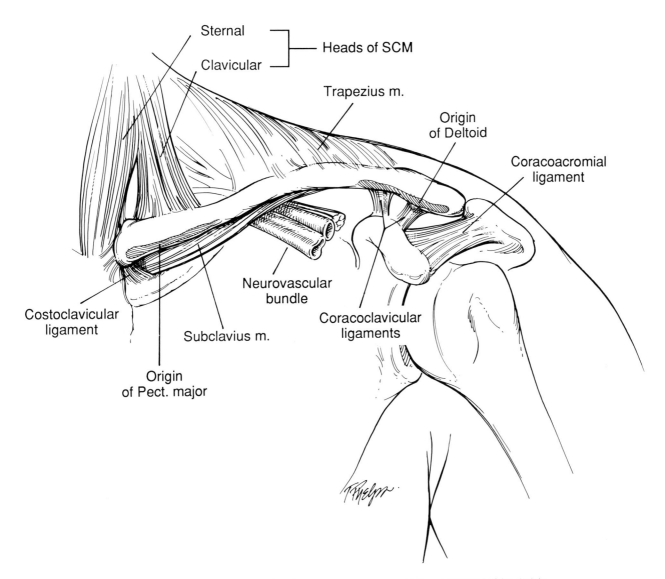

Figure 13.2. The neurovascular bundle to the arm passes beneath the middle third of the clavicle.

curs. This was clearly illustrated by Berkheiser in 1937 (4) when he wrote: "In a general way I believe that the present day treatment of clavicular fractures, particularly in adults, leaves a good deal to be desired." He wrote this after encountering nine cases of clavicular nonunion in adults over a "relatively short period."

Complications of clavicle fractures may be severe, dramatic, and even life-threatening. However, these instances are rare and treated operatively since the indications are clear—surgery is required to save a life or preserve a limb. The vast majority of complications of clavicle fractures are *not* acute (Table 13.1). These delayed complications are not as dramatic but the pain, dysfunction, and economic loss to patients are frequently devastating. This chapter

will deal with the complications of clavicle fractures as outlined in Table 13.1. One definition of a specialist is: "one who knows all the complications of a particular diagnosis or procedure and how to prevent them." This chapter is written as a contribution to the education of a "specialist."

ACUTE COMPLICATIONS

Neurovascular compromise, occurring at the time of clavicle fracture, is rare. When present, this complication of clavicle fracture demands operative intervention. The neurovascular bundle to the upper limb passes beneath the middle third of the clavicle (Fig. 13.2). Acute neurovascular compression is usually caused by displaced transverse or comminuted

Table 13.1.   Complications of Clavicle Fractures

ACUTE COMPLICATIONS
  Neurovascular compression
    Brachial plexus compression
    Subclavian vein thrombosis/laceration

  Pleural injury
    Pneumothorax
    Hemothorax

DELAYED COMPLICATIONS
  Complications of figure-of-eight bandages

  Malunion
    Scapulothoracic alteration
    Neurovascular compression
      Static
      Dynamic

  Nonunion
    Postfracture
      Hypertrophic
      Atrophic

  Surgical complications
    Cosmetically poor incisions
    Supraclavicular neuromata
    Neurovascular injury
    Intrathoracic injury
    Inadequate fixation techniques
    Nonunions
    Complications of clavicle excision

fractures of the middle third of the clavicle (9, 38) Suspicion of possible injury to subclavicular structures should be high if ipsilateral rib or scapular fractures are present (36). This fracture combination represents major high-energy trauma and is frequently associated with brachial plexus injuries, subclavian-axillary-brachial vascular injuries as well as hemopneumothorax (33).

The entire chest should be included in the initial radiographic examination of all patients with clavicle fractures. The lateral fragment of the clavicle is usually displaced posteriorly and inferiorly (Fig. 13.3A,B), compromising the costoclavicular space. Closed methods of reduction and immobilization of these clavicle fractures are not effective. The goals of surgical treatment are restoration of the costoclavicular space and reduction/removal of any comminuted fragments that are responsible for neurovascular compression. When stable fixation of the clavicle is obtained (Fig. 13.3C,D), primary union occurs without the need for autogenous bone grafting. Choice of fixation method and past reports of failed fixation will be discussed later. If surgery in cases of

acute neurovascular compression is carried out expeditiously by an experienced and skillful surgeon who is aware of both the potential complications of the procedure and how to prevent them, the results should be as satisfactory as they are for any other fractured bone that is treated by primary open reduction internal fixation (ORIF) (Fig. 13.3E).

DELAYED COMPLICATIONS

The very common delayed finding after clavicle fracture is an unsightly malunion with shortening of the clavicle, prominence of the fracture site, and alteration in the scapulothoracic articulation. With clavicular shortening, the upper limb is translated medially and inferiorly, changing the resting position of the scapula on the chest wall and altering periscapular muscle balance. Currently, this is not generally accepted as a "complication." However, patients do complain of the resultant shoulder asymmetry, plus fatigue and pain after exercise or strenuous activity. The significance of secondary scapular "winging" caused by an overriding malunion of the clavicle has recently been pointed out by Nakagawa et al. (20).

Malunion with neurovascular compression, either dynamic or static, is one of the most common complications of clavicle fractures in adults. Typically the fracture is midshaft, in bayonet apposition, and treated in standard nonoperative fashion. The use of a figure-of-eight bandage and/or a sling may rest the upper limb, but complete immobilization of a clavicle fracture by external means is impossible. Indeed, Rowe has demonstrated that a figure-of-eight bandage may increase fracture site deformity in midclavicular fractures (29). Andersen et al. (3) in a randomized comparison of simple sling vs. figure-of-eight bandage treatment of midclavicular fractures noted no difference in results, but complaints of impairment of agility and personal care, sleep disturbance, edema, and paresthesias of the arm were frequent in the figure-of-eight group. They also observed that neither a figure-of-eight bandage nor a sling will obtain or maintain reduction of a midclavicular fracture (3). Since motion at the fracture site is inevitable, caused by movement of the scapula on the chest wall, respiration, or ambulation, healing occurs through bridging callus formation. Depending upon the amount of displacement at the fracture site, the volume of callus formation and the available costoclavicular space, neurovascular compressive symptomatology may develop. Paresthesia, blanch-

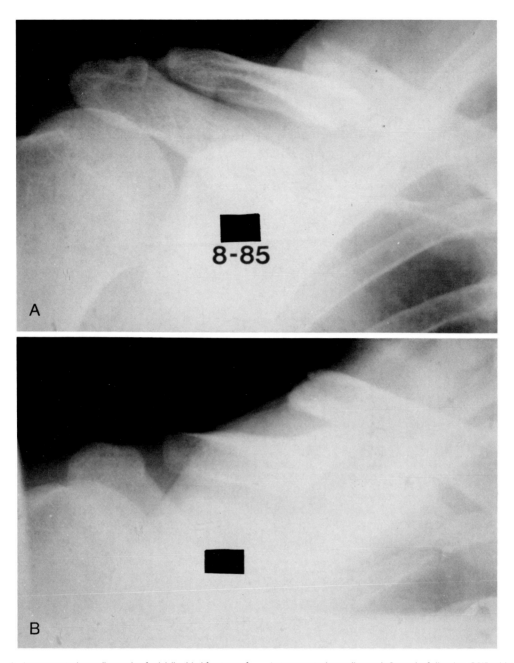

Figure 13.3. **A**, Anteroposterior radiograph of middle third fracture of the right clavicle in a 23-year-old cyclist and graduate student of music. Any movement or deep inspiration resulted in paresthesias and weakness in the right dominant upper limb. **B**, Lordotic radiograph of same fracture demonstrates posterior displacement of the lateral fragment. **C**, Anteroposterior radiograph 2 weeks following ORIF with compression plate and screws. **D**, Lordotic view demonstrates that anatomic reduction at fracture site (*arrow*) with a well-contoured 3.5 dynamic compression plate restores the costoclavicular space. **E**, Primary union complete and plate removed 7 months postfracture: normal function.

ing, cooling, and weakness of the upper limb may be positional and activity-related (dynamic subclavicular neurovascular compression) (Fig. 13.4) or constant and progressive (static subclavicular neurovascular compression) (Fig. 13.5). Chronic edema of the arm may indicate subclavian vein thrombosis. Surgical treatment is required to relieve neurovas-

cular pressure and enlarge the costoclavicular space, identical objectives as for primary open treatment of clavicle fractures with associated neurovascular compression. While the objectives are the same, the surgical realities are much different. Clavicular reconstruction with corrective osteotomy and brachial plexus decompression, months to years after the

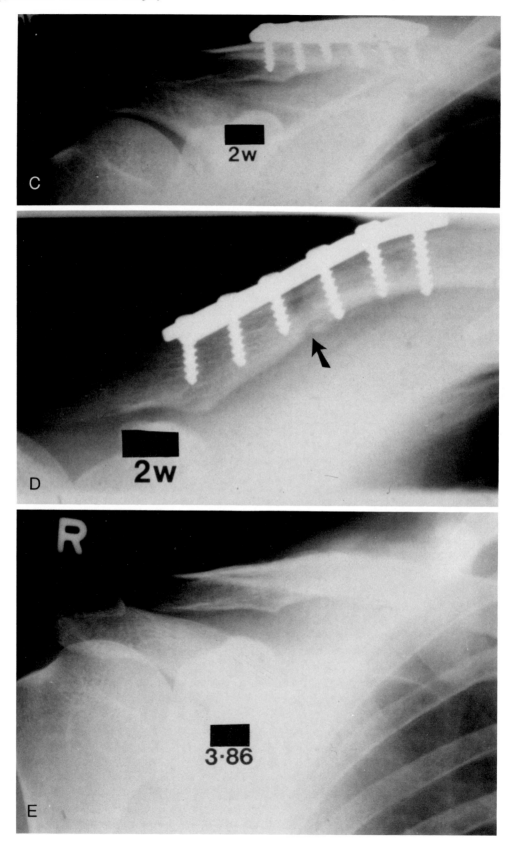

Figure 13.3.   C–E.

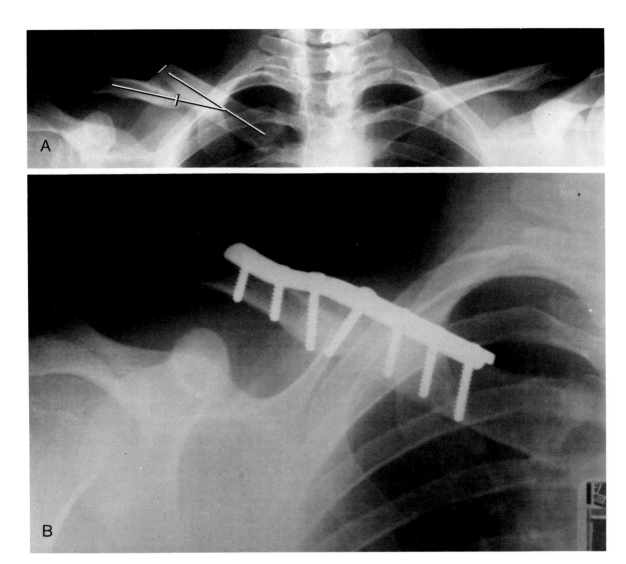

Figure 13.4. **A,** Anteroposterior radiograph of malunion 1 year post-right dominant midclavicle fracture in a 19-year-old student. Reaching down to lift or pull caused a "dead arm," weakness, and numbness. The clavicle is shortened 1.5–2.0 cm and angulated inferiorly 20–25°.

Depression of the clavicle resulted in dynamic costoclavicular compression. **B,** Corrective osteotomy restored length and elevated the distal fragment, restoring the costoclavicular space. Osteotomy healed and patient is asymptomatic.

fracture, is much more difficult than primary fixation of completely displaced clavicle fractures. Possible intraoperative complications, which can be dramatic, are discussed later.

Nonunion of the clavicle in an adult is *not* rare. Most orthopaedic surgeons have seen or cared for at least one adult patient with clavicular nonunion, usually in the middle one-third (15). Since 1937, the English literature contains 26 reports of descriptions and treatments of 523 clavicle nonunions (Table 13.2). If 523 cases have been published, many more have no doubt been observed or treated without being reported. Personal involvement in the treatment of 25 painful nonunions of the clavicle during

the past 15 years has yielded some observations. All of these cases were initially displaced fractures of the middle third, without bony contact (Fig. 13.6A). None of the patients had acute neurovascular compression, and all were treated in standard nonoperative fashion (Fig. 13.6B,C,D). While it is possible that nonunion of the clavicle may be asymptomatic (41), young active individuals are frequently disabled by weakness/pain with upper limb motion when a clavicle nonunion is present. The majority of these postfracture nonunions are hypertrophic in nature, indicating an attempt to bridge the defect with callus (Fig. 13.7). While atrophic nonunions do occur, they are usually seen in the elderly or in patients with se-

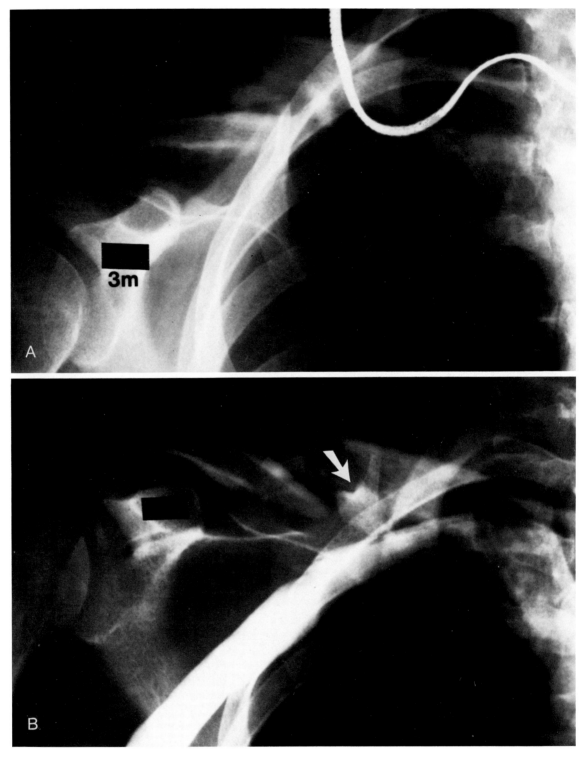

Figure 13.5. **A**, Comminuted displaced midshaft right dominant clavicle fracture in a 33-year-old female tennis player, 3 months postinjury. Weakness, numbness, coolness of right arm and hand had been progressive since injury. **B**, Venogram demonstrates compression of subclavian vein by rotated comminuted fragment (*arrow*). **C**, CT scan demonstrates costoclavicular compromise by the comminuted fragment (*arrow*). **D**, Clavicle healed after removal of comminuted fragment and anatomic clavicle reduction, which decompressed the costoclavicular space. The brachial plexus was not scarred; patient was asymptomatic.

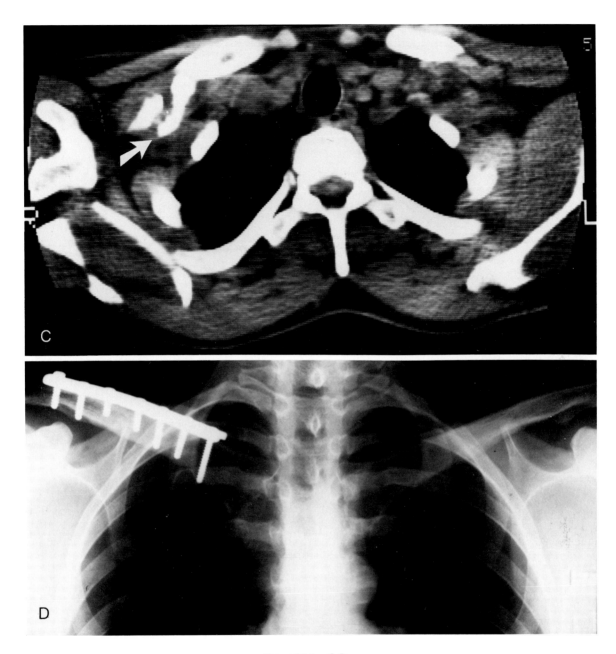

Figure 13.5. C–D.

vere injuries, poorly performed prior surgery, or postirradiation. An example of atrophic nonunion will be illustrated in the section of this chapter devoted to postsurgical complications. Painful hypertrophic postfracture clavicle nonunions should be treated by open reduction, internal fixation, and bone grafting with the usually available and abundant local fracture callus (Fig. 13.8). Several methods of internal fixation have been described and reported as successful including internal fixation by intramedullary Knowles pin (24, 32), ex-

ternal fixation (31) and cortical onlay/massive cancellous bone grafts (4, 7). The proven (1, 4, 10, 11, 14, 39, 41) and personally preferred method is compression plating with a well-contoured 3.5 dynamic compression plate and autogenous bone grafting either from local hypertrophic callus or, in cases of atrophic nonunion, iliac crest. This method provides the most stable fixation for resisting the tension, bending, and torque forces exerted on the clavicle. At least six screws with bicortical purchase should be used (Fig. 13.8).

Table 13.2.   Clavicle Nonunions: English Literature Reports

Date	Author	# Cases	Date	Author	# Cases
1937	Berkheiser	9	1976	Weber	18
1941	Ghormley	20	1976	Tregonning	42
1944	Le Cocq	4	1977	Thompson, A.G.	2
1946	Storen	1	1977	Edvardsen	6
1948	Annersten	5	1978	Pyper	3
1951	Moore	3	1979	Aepli	99
1952	Powell	2	1979	Raaymakers	7
1960	Neer	18	1983	Wilkens	33
1961	Sakellarides	20	1985	Manske	10
1963	Johnson	69	1986	Eskola	24
1965	Mayer	1	1987	Jupiter	23
1969	Taylor	31	1988	Schuind	20
1970	Marsh	28	1990	Thompson, J.S.	25
		211			312

Total Cases
523

After treating a series of clavicle nonunion cases and observing the initial fracture pattern, a repetitive scenario was recognized. The initial fractures were similar, treatments similar, and the months/years of patient disability/economic loss were similar. How could these nonunions have been prevented? What clear predictive indicators existed that would have improved the initial care of these patients destined for clavicle nonunion?

The 1968 classification of clavicle fractures, proposed by Neer (23), addressed only the distal third. Neer recommended primary ORIF with transacromial wires for displaced fractures of the distal third with detachment of the coracoclavicular ligaments from the medial fragment (23). While this classification has been useful for the specific fracture type described, the majority of fractures of the clavicle do not occur in the distal third (21).

In order for any classification system to be useful, it must be comprehensive yet simple. In 1985, a comprehensive clavicle fracture classification was devised (Table 13.3). The clavicle is divided into five anatomic zones (Zones I–V) (Fig. 13.9A), including the acromioclavicular and sternoclavicular joints and modifiers (A,B,C) are used to designate the magnitude of fracture displacement or presence of neurovascular compression (Fig. 13.9B).

When the reports listed in Table 13.2 were reviewed for description of original fractures, 11 reports containing adequate information on 111 clavicle fractures were found. The original fractures were grouped using the clavicle fracture classification, and it was noted that 93 (84%) were type IIIB

fractures. All of the 25 postfracture nonunions in the personal series were type IIIB fractures. The fracture of the middle third of the clavicle in an adult with greater than 100% displacement, no osseous contact, with or without a comminuted interposed fragment, accounts for 87% of the nonunions in the analysis of 136 total nonunions. The remaining 13% were displaced fractures of the lateral one-third, type IIB, which corresponds to the Neer type II fractures described in 1968 (23). All 136 nonunions occurred as the result of either a type IIB or IIIB fracture. These types of fractures are relatively rare, accounting for approximately 3–4% of all clavicle fractures. It is this small percentage of all clavicle fractures that accounts for most, if not all, clavicle nonunions. Since 1985, primary ORIF has been recommended for type IIB and IIIB clavicle fractures, if they cannot be reduced and maintained in a position of bony contact. Following initial displacement caused by the injury, several factors contribute to difficulty in achieving and maintaining a closed reduction in these fracture types: (a) upward pull of the sternocleidomastoid on the medial fragment; (b) downward and posterior pull of the weight of the upper limb on the lateral fragment, which allows scapular retraction and maintains periosteal stripping of the lateral end of the medial fragment; (c) embedding of the end of the medial fragment into the trapezius muscle or actual trapezius muscle interposition at the fracture site; and (d) medial pull of the pectoralis major and latissimus dorsi muscles (Fig. 13.10).

Clearly, a classification that identifies those clavicle fractures in adults most likely to progress to nonunion could have a major influence on clarifying operative indications for a certain selected group of patients (35).

SURGICAL COMPLICATIONS

When considering surgical treatment of the clavicle, the approach should be carefully planned. A gentle infraclavicular curvilinear incision has provided the most extensile exposure and cosmetic scar. The location of the scar below the clavicle, care in closure of the platysma as a separate layer after the deltotrapezius fascia, and use of a subcuticular suture with adhesive skin closure reinforcement, all combine to provide excellent coverage for the plate and screws plus a cosmetically acceptable scar.

The supraclavicular nerves (Fig. 13.11), which are deep to the platysma at the level of the clavicle, should be carefully protected. There are two significant branches that cross the clavicle, the medial and the intermediate supraclavicular nerves (8). Iatrogenic neuromata of these nerves can be painful and extremely distressful to the patient, compromising an otherwise satisfactory result.

The brachial plexus, subclavian vessels, and pleural dome are all in close proximity and potentially injured during surgery about the clavicle (Fig. 13.12). In 1940, Murray (19) correctly characterized surgery of the clavicle when he wrote: ". . . in the hands of careless operators there might be grave dangers." A case has been reported (5) in which a single patient sustained four different complications at surgery: pneumothorax, subclavian vein injury, air embolism, and transient brachial plexus damage. Knowledge of anatomy and a few technical safeguards will prevent these complications. A pad posterior to the scapula on the operative side will result in protraction of the shoulder girdle, increasing the distance between the clavicle and the apex of the lung. When drilling the clavicle, it is possible to place a small flat retractor subperiosteally at the exit site of each hole to protect adjacent structures and prevent plunging of the drill bit.

Some orthopaedic surgeons may feel that any surgical treatment of clavicle fractures contributes to nonunion. That general statement is false. Even Neer, whose classic paper (21) is often quoted in support of the notion that surgery contributes to clavicle nonunion, stated: ". . . the most important causal factor in nonunion of fractures of the middle third [of the clavicle] has been *improper* open surgery." The improper surgery that was done in these cases (between 1936 and 1959) was use of inadequate fixation techniques,

usually simple wire loops through the ends of the clavicle. High nonunion rates have also been reported when catgut sutures, Parham bands, cerclage wires, screws, and kangaroo tendon have been used for fixation (7, 16, 30). These methods (Fig. 13.13) are inadequate and if used will predictably fail. In a review of 99 nonunions of the clavicle documented by the AO group between 1968–1976, Aepli and Burch (1) found that 73% had been treated nonoperatively and 27% had been treated with inadequate surgical fixation. Surgical treatment itself does not contribute to clavicle nonunion (37). *The cause of clavicle nonunion is inadequate reduction and insufficient stabilization of the fracture, regardless of the method of primary treatment.* The 4.4% nonunion rate that was reported (21) after surgery resulted from two nonunions in 45 cases treated by primary ORIF. The true incidence of nonunion in adults after closed treatment of clavicle fractures is unknown since all statistics available are drawn from totals that include children.

There are at least 120 cases of primary ORIF of clavicle fractures that have been reported (2, 19, 20, 23, 24, 34, 41) in which no nonunions occurred (Table 13.4). The successful fixation methods utilized in these patients were either intramedullary devices or compression plates and screws. If intramedullary fixation is not stable, rotational movement at the fracture site is possible, and small smooth pins may migrate (25, 29). There are several reports of intrathoracic migration of smooth, headless intramedullary pins, which had been used in open reduction of clavicle fractures and were directed inferiorly and medially (12, 17, 25, 27). These devices and that method *should not be used* as a surgical treatment for clavicle fractures. Knowles pins have been reported as the most satisfactory intramedullary fixation (20, 24, 41) since they have threads for compression at the fracture site and a head that prevents possible migration of the pin in the direction of the point. Plates and screws, while a personal preference, are not immune to complications if certain precautions are not taken. Semitubular plates do not have the strength of dynamic compression plates (Fig. 13.14) and should not be used. Even if satisfactory compression plating has been done, patients should be placed in a sling for at least 2 weeks and not allowed overhead activities or lifting for 6–8 weeks. Unrestricted athletic activities and heavy lifting should not be allowed for 3–4 months (Fig. 13.15). If certain clavicle fractures meet carefully applied operative indications, the singular act of surgical treatment does not contribute to nonunion. However, the method of surgical treatment and postoperative management may definitely contribute to nonunion.

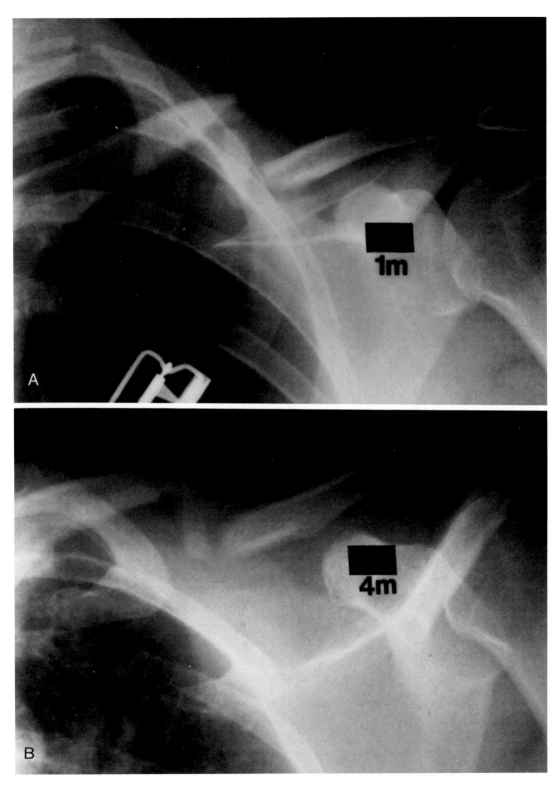

Figure 13.6. **A,** Comminuted displaced left nondominant midclavicle fracture in a 35-year-old tractor-trailer driver, 1 month postinjury. **B,** Four months postinjury. **C,** Nine months postinjury; has used external electro-magnetic coil for 4 months. **D,** Thirteen months postinjury; 8 months of electrostimulation. Patient has pain with any motion; no work since injury.

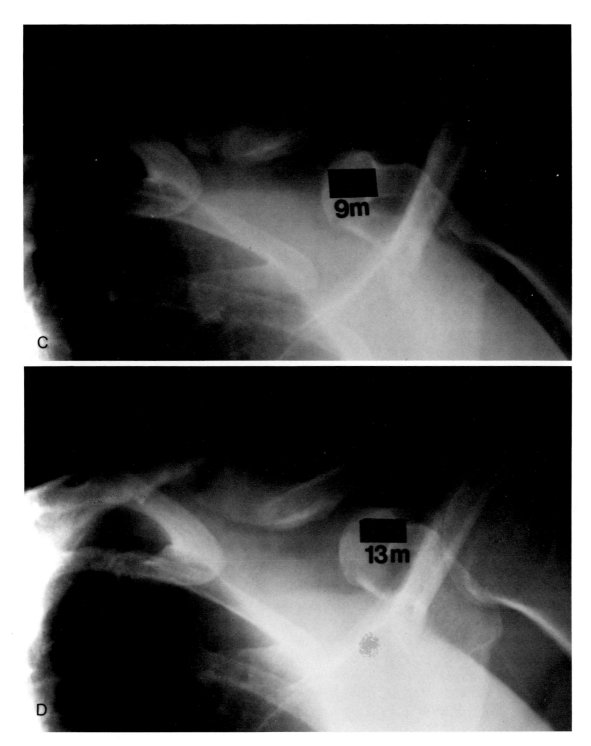

Figure 13.6. C–D.

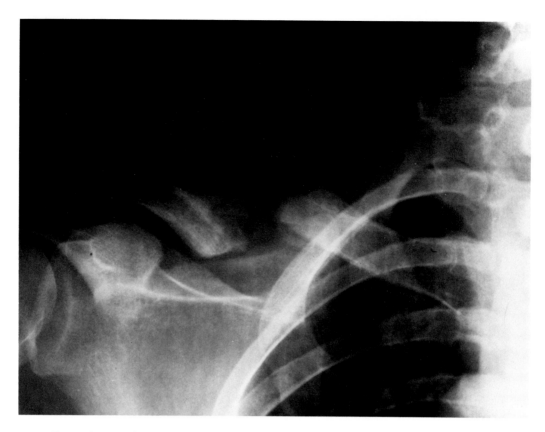

Figure 13.7. Painful hypertrophic nonunion midshaft right dominant clavicle in a 40-year-old veteran.

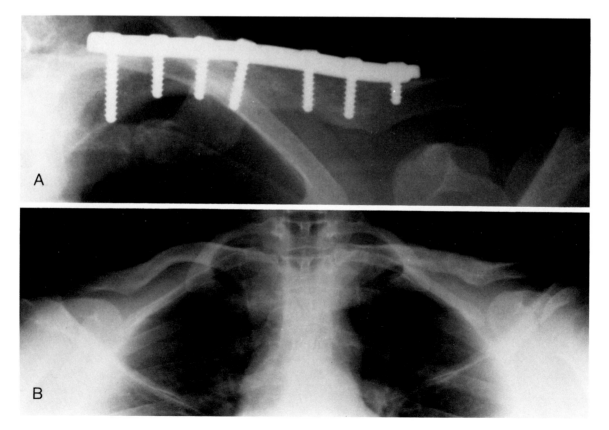

Figure 13.8. **A**, Same patient shown in Figure 14.6. Nonunion healed 3 months post-ORIF, and patient is back to work. **B**, Anteroposterior radiograph of bilateral clavicles after plate removed, 1 year post-ORIF.

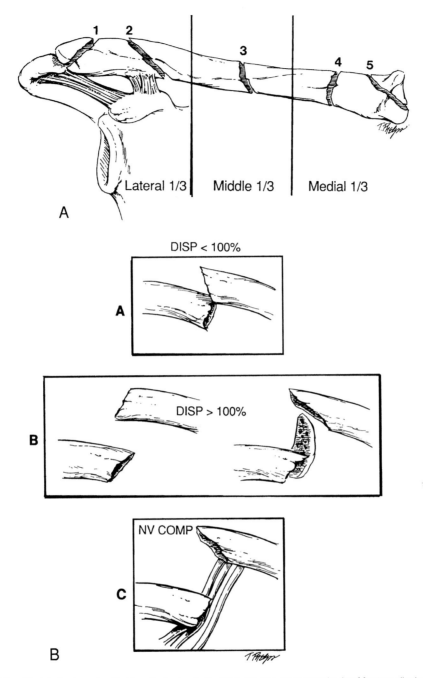

Figure 13.9. Clavicle fracture classification. **A**, Anatomic location, zones I–IV. **B**, Magnitude of fracture displacement or presence of neurovascular compression, types A–C.

Clavicle excision as a treatment for clavicle fractures should be mentioned only for the sake of completeness and as a procedure to be avoided. Excision of the lateral clavicle in cases of lateral one-third fractures with rupture of the coracoclavicular ligaments has failed (22, 28). Excision of the middle portion always allows clavicular shortening with resulting shoulder asymmetry, possible neurovascular compression, or painful shoulder motion due to the mobile converging clavicular ends. Medial clavicular excision has not proven to be predictably beneficial (28).

Table 13.3.   Clavicle Fracture Classification

Type	Location		Type	Location
I	A–C Joint			FRACTURE PATTERN
II	Lateral 1/3			
III	Middle 1/3		A	Bony contact
IV	Medial 1/3		B	No bony contact With or without comminuted fragment
V	S–C Joint		C	Neurovascular compression

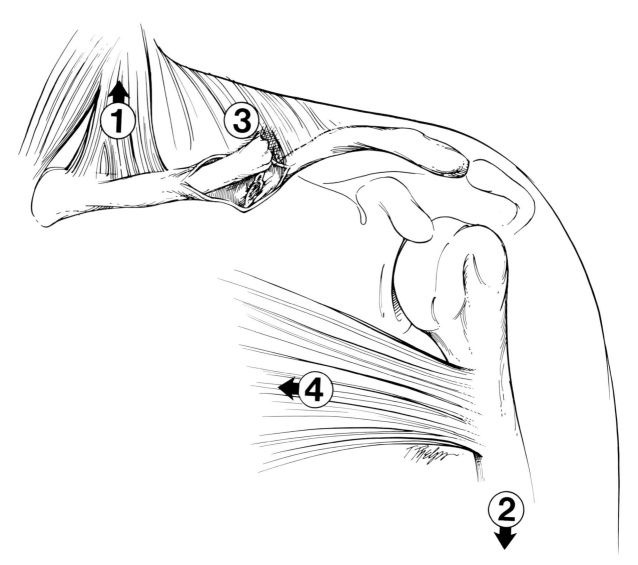

Figure 13.10.   Factors contributing to difficulty in achievement and maintenance of reduction of IIIB clavicle fractures: 1. upward pull of sternocleidomastoid on medial fragment; 2. downward and posterior pull of upper limb weight; 3. embedding of the end of the medial fragment, which is stripped of periosteum, into the trapezius muscle that remains inserted on the lateral fragment; 4. medial pull of pectoris major and latissimus dorsi muscles.

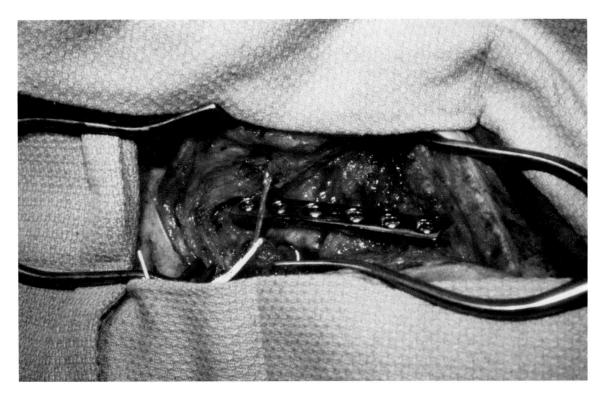

Figure 13.11. Operative photograph of isolated and preserved medial supraclavicular nerve (*arrow*).

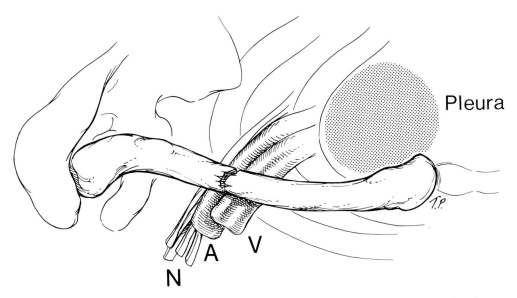

Figure 13.12. Axial view of relationship between the clavicle, pleural dome, and neurovascular bundle.

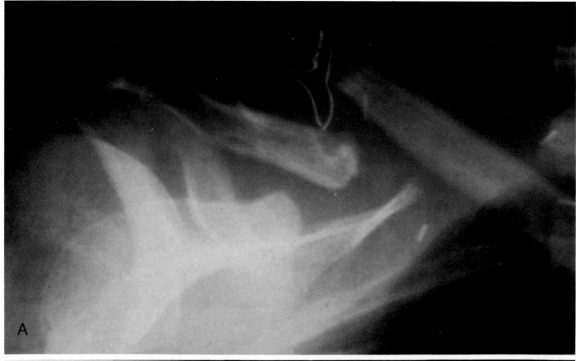

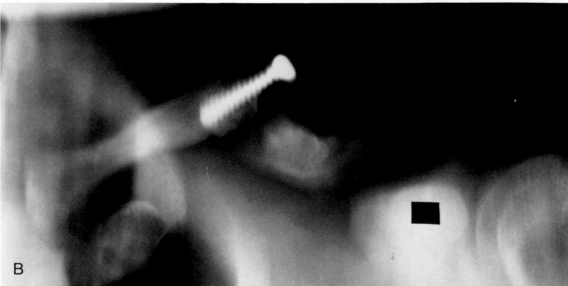

Figure 13.13. **A**, Atrophic nonunion, postirradiation, following resection of chest wall fibrosarcoma. The clavicle was "repaired" with interosseous wire. **B**, Nonunion after fixation of iliac bone graft with single screw.

Table 13.4.   Reports of Primary ORIF Certain Clavicle Fractures

Year	Author	# Cases	Nonunions
1940	Murray (19)	29	0
1968	Neer (23)	7	0
1975	Neviaser (24)	7	0
1978	Ali Khan (2)	20	0
1981	Zenni (42)	25	0
1988	Thompson (35)	5	0
1989	Nakagawa (20)	27	0
	TOTAL CASES	120	TOTAL NONUNIONS 0

CONCLUSION

This chapter has been written in an attempt to reduce the incidence of complications that occur either as a result of a clavicle fracture or its treatment. A well-trained orthopaedic surgeon should be prepared, on occasion, to treat clavicle fractures surgically. If indications for primary surgical treatment are well established and the surgery is done properly, medical care will be improved. At the same time, patient suffering and societal cost will be decreased for those who sustain these injuries.

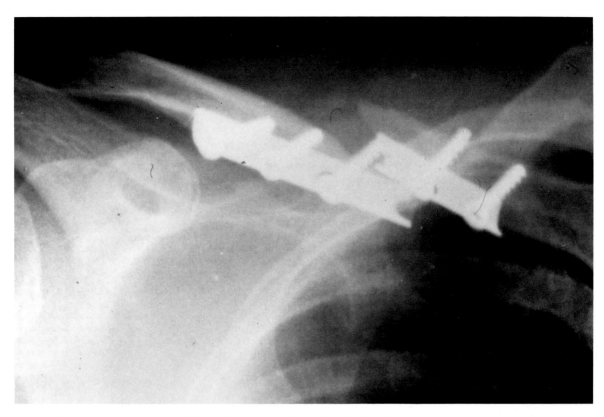

Figure 13.14.   Fracture through hole of anteriorly applied semitubular plate. Photo supplied by Louis U. Bigliani, M.D.

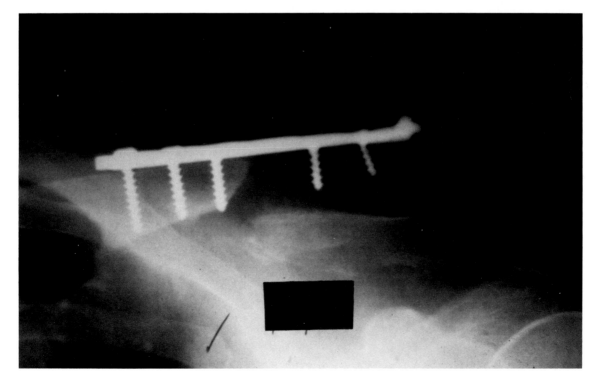

Figure 13.15.   Failure of compression plate fixation: plate not contoured, inadequate screw fixation on lateral fragment, and patient allowed to lift at 5 weeks following surgery. A longer contoured plate with stable fixation on the lateral fragment plus careful postoperative management resulted in union and full painless function.

ACKNOWLEDGMENTS

Special thanks to Timothy H. Phelps, M.A., A.M.I. for the superb illustrations that add visual clarification to this chapter. As usual, manuscript preparation was carried out with speed, skill, and patience by Shari T. Clatterbuck, A.M.S. No one could expect a finer medical secretary.

References

1. Aepli L, Burch HB. Study on the pseudarthrosis of the clavicle. In: Chapchal G, ed. Pseudarthroses and their treatment. Eighth international symposium on topical problems in orthopaedic surgery. Stuttgart: Thieme, 1979:188–189.

2. Ali Khan MA, Lucas HK. Plating of fractures of the middle third of the clavicle. Injury 1978;9:263–267.

3. Andersen K, Jensen PO, Lauritzen J. Treatment of clavicular fractures: figure-of-eight bandage versus a simple sling. Acta Orthop Scand 1987;57:71–74.

4. Berkheiser EJ. Old ununited clavicular fractures in the adult. Surg Gynecol Obstet 1937;64:1064–1072.

5. Eskola A, Vainionpaa S, Myllynen P, Patiala H, Rokkanen P. Surgery for ununited clavicular fracture. Acta Orthop Scand 1986;57:366–367.

6. Eskola A. Fractures and dislocations of the clavicle [thesis]. Helsinki, Finland: Helsinki University Department of Orthopaedics and Traumatology 1989:81 pp.

7. Ghormley RK, Black JR, Cherry JH. Ununited fractures of the clavicle. Am J Surg 1941;51:343–349.

8. Grant JCB. Grant's atlas of anatomy. AMR Agur, ed. Baltimore: Williams & Wilkins, 1991:552.

9. Howard FM, Shafer SJ. Injuries to the clavicle with neurovascular complications. J Bone Joint Surg 1965;47A:1335–1346.

10. Jupiter JB, Leffert RD. Nonunion of the clavicle. J Bone Joint Surg 1987;69A:753–760.

11. Jupiter JB. Nonunion of the clavicle. Complications in Orthopedics 1989;Jan/Feb:29–32.

12. Kremens V, Glauser F. Unusual sequela following pinning of medial clavicular fracture. Amer J Roentgen 1956;76:1066.

13. Lim EVA, Day LJ. Subclavian vein thrombosis following fracture of the clavicle. Orthopaedics 1987;10:349–351.

14. Manske DJ, Szabo RM. The operative treatment of midshaft clavicular nonunions. J Bone Joint Surg 1985;67A:1367–1371.

15. Marsh HO, Hazarian E. Pseudarthrosis of the clavicle. J Bone Joint Surg 1970;52B:793.

16. Mayer JH. Nonunion of fractured clavicle. Proc Roy Soc Med 1965;58:182.

17. Mazet R Jr. Migration of Kirschner wire from shoulder region. J Bone Joint Surg 1943;25:477.

18. Mosely HF. The clavicle: its anatomy and function. Clin Orthop Rel Res 1968;58:17–27.

19. Murray G. A method of fixation for fracture of the clavicle. J Bone Joint Surg 1940;22:616–620.

20. Nakagawa Y, Ozaki J, Tamai S, Masuhara K. Knowles pin fixation of clavicular fractures. Proceedings of the Fourth International Conference on Surgery of the Shoulder. New York, 1989.

21. Neer CS. Nonunion of the clavicle. JAMA 1960;172:1006–1011.

22. Neer CS. Fracture of the distal clavicle with detachment of the coracoclavicular ligaments in adults. J Trauma 1963;3:99–110.

23. Neer CS. Fractures of the distal third of clavicle. Clin Orthop Rel Res 1968;58:43–50.

24. Neviaser RJ, Neviaser JS, Neviaser TJ, Neviaser JS. A simple technique for internal fixation of the clavicle. Clin Orthop Rel Res 1975;75:103–107.

25. Paffen PJ, Jansen EWL. Surgical treatment of clavicular fractures with Kirschner wires. A comparative study. Arch Chir Neerlandicum 1978;30:43–53.

26. Penn I. The vascular complications of fractures of the clavicle. J Trauma 1964;4:819–831.

27. Rey-Baltar E, Errazu D. Unusual outcome of Steinmann wire. Arch Surg 1963:1024–1025.

28. Rockwood CA, Odor JM. Spontaneous atraumatic anterior subluxation of the sternoclavicular joint. J Bone Joint Surg 1989;71A:1280–1288.

29. Rowe CR. An atlas of anatomy and treatment of midclavicular fractures. Clin Orthop Rel Res 1968;58:29–42.

30. Sakellarides H. Pseudarthrosis of the clavicle. J Bone Joint Surg 1961;43A:130–138.

31. Schuind F, Pay-Pay E, Andrianne Y, Donkerwolcke M, Rasquin C, Burny F. External fixation of the clavicle for fracture or nonunion in adults. J Bone Joint Surg 1988;70A:692–695.

32. Taylor AR. Non-union of fractures of the clavicle: a review of thirty-one cases. J Bone Joint Surg 1969;51B:568–569.

33. Thompson DA, Flynn TC, Miller TC, Fischer RP. The significance of scapular fractures. J Trauma 1985;25:974–977.

34. Thompson JS. Operative treatment of certain clavicle fractures. An orthopaedic controversy. Orthop Trans 1988;12:141.

35. Thompson JS. Classification of clavicle fractures has an impact on operative indications [abstract]. Proceedings of the Fourth International Conference on Surgery of the Shoulder. New York, 1989.

36. Thompson JS. Shoulder girdle injuries. In: Champion HR, Robbs JV, Trunkey DD, eds. Rob and Smiths operative surgery. Trauma surgery. 4th ed. London: Butterworth 1989:913–924.

37. Tregonning G, MacNab I. Post-traumatic pseudarthrosis of the clavicle. J Bone Joint Surg 1976;58B:264.

38. Van Vlack, HG. Comminuted fracture of clavicle with pressure on brachial plexus. J Bone Joint Surg 1940:446–447.

39. Weber BG, Cech O. Pseudarthrosis. New York: Grune & Stratton, 1976:104–107.

40. Wilkins RM, Johnston RM. Ununited fractures of the clavicle. J Bone Joint Surg 1983;65A:773–778.

41. Zenni EJ, Krieg JK, Rosen MJ. Open reduction and internal fixation of clavicular fractures. J Bone Joint Surg 1981;63A:147–151.

14
Humeral Shaft Nonunions

Joseph D. Zuckerman, Carl Giordano, and Howard Rosen

INTRODUCTION

Humeral shaft fractures are one of the most common fractures encountered by orthopaedic surgeons. A variety of treatment methods have been successfully utilized ranging from a swing and swathe to internal fixation with plates and screws. The complication rate following humeral shaft fractures is quite low and generally includes nonunion, malunion, radial nerve injury, and infection (after open fractures or following open treatment of closed fractures). However, nonunion remains the most common complication of humeral shaft fractures. A review of the many different series reported in the literature shows an overall nonunion rate ranging from 0–13% with most series reporting less than 5% (1, 17, 10). Interestingly, higher rates of nonunion have been reported following operative treatment than following nonoperative management (17) (Figs. 14.1 and 14.2). In this chapter we will discuss the classification of healing disturbances following humeral shaft fractures, the factors implicated in the development of healing disturbances, and the treatment options based upon careful evaluation of the problem.

Healing disturbances following humeral shaft fracture include delayed unions and nonunions. Since most humeral shaft fractures heal within 12 weeks, any fracture that does not show evidence of significant healing in that time could be considered a delayed union. Although some disagreement exists, most authors agree that delayed union should be reserved for those fractures that do not show evidence of clinical union within 4 months. Nonunion should be reserved for fractures without evidence of clinical healing 8 months after injury.

Humeral nonunions are most commonly classified based upon location, presence or absence of callus, and presence or absence of infection. Nonunions may be midshaft in location, thereby providing a reasonable length of bone proximal and distal for fixation. However, nonunions at the proximal and distal portions of the shaft have limited area for internal fixation within the metaphysis where, in addition, bone quality is often poor. Fractures that have attempted to heal with significant callus formation are considered hypertrophic or vascular nonunions (Fig. 14.3); the absence of callus is considered an atrophic or hypovascular nonunion (Fig. 14.4). The presence of infection may be active as evidenced by drainage, erythema, swelling, and systemic symptoms. However, infection may also be quiescent with a paucity of clinical findings. The treatment approach utilized will depend, in large part, on the type of nonunion being treated.

ETIOLOGY

Nonunions develop more commonly in association with specific factors. These include injury factors (displacement, location, fracture pattern, open versus closed injury), treatment factors (reduction, type and duration of mobilization, adequacy of open reduction internal fixation, presence of postoperative complications), and patient factors (age, bone quality, ability to participate in the prescribed treatment program). Each of these factors will be discussed individually. However, it is important to recognize that the development of healing disturbances should be considered a multifactorial problem. While any one factor may contribute to the development of a delayed union or nonunion, ultimately it is caused by combination of these factors.

Injury factors include fracture location, pattern and displacement, and associated soft tissue injuries (open versus closed). In general, fractures of the mid-third (13, 16, 17) and those at the junction of

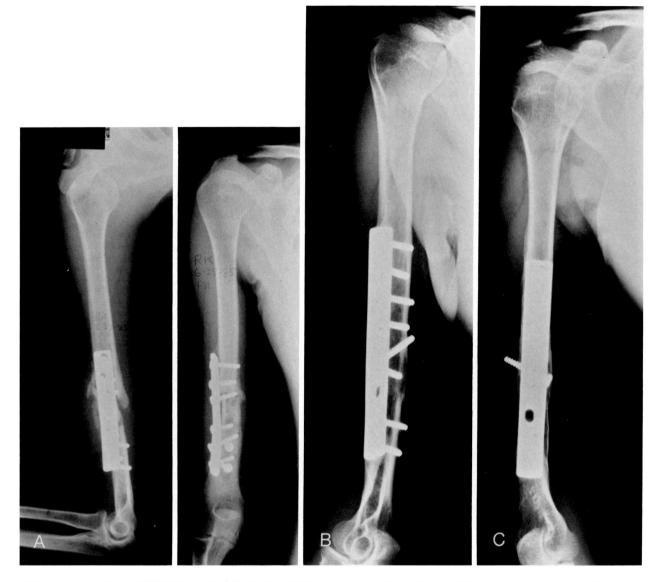

Figure 14.1. **A,** A 30-year-old female 7 months following primary plating of a midshaft humerus fracture. She has continued pain with radiographic evidence of nonunion. Note the placement of a screw in the fracture site with only four cortices of fixation in the proximal fragment. The patient underwent removal of the plate and screws, open reduction, and internal fixation using a broad DC plate with interfragmentary fixation and cancellous autograft. **B** and **C,** Follow-up radiographs taken 8 months after surgery show healing of the nonunion. The patient regained full range of motion of the shoulder and elbow.

the proximal third and mid-third (9, 10, 12) more commonly result in nonunion. However, fracture location has to be considered in the context of fracture pattern. Transverse and short oblique patterns, particularly in the mid-shaft have been most commonly reported (10, 16, 17, 29). The reasons for this may be the limited area of bony contact possible compared with long oblique or spiral fracture patterns. This may be further compromised by any treatment approach that results in fracture distraction. In addition, the nutrient artery to the humerus enters at the medial aspect of the distal portion of the mid-third region. Fractures in this area may result in compromise of the blood supply, further increasing the risk of healing disturbances (13, 16, 20).

Fracture comminution has consistently been reported as an important factor in the development of nonunion (1, 17). This raises an important aspect of associated soft tissue injuries. It is well known that fracture healing relies on an adequate blood supply and that devascularized bone has reduced healing potential. Comminuted fractures or those with significant displacement represent much higher energy injuries than long oblique or spiral fractures that result from relatively minor trauma. The resulting disruption in the soft tissue envelope vascularity results in a slower healing process, possibly leading to nonunion. In addition, significantly displaced fracture fragments raise the possibility of soft tissue interposition as an impediment to healing (12, 14). Muscle is the most common offending structure. The deltoid may be involved in proximal third fractures or the biceps, brachialis, or triceps in mid-shaft fractures. The interposed muscle interferes with the healing process by maintaining the fracture ends in a displaced position and exceeding the gap over which bone healing is possible.

Open fractures are at higher risk for nonunion because of a combination of factors. First, the open injury itself represents a much higher energy injury than most closed fractures. This results in significant soft tissue injury and vascular compromise. Second, the open wound increases the risk of infection because of contamination of the tissues and fracture site. Numerous authors have cited open fractures, particularly when they are complicated by infection, as having significant increased risk of nonunion (1, 5, 12, 13, 16, 17, 28, 29, 32).

Treatment factors include the choice of treatment approach, adequacy of the reduction, type and duration of immobilization, adequacy of open reduction and internal fixation, and the development of postoperative complications. The type of treatment—nonoperative versus operative—has been identified as an important factor in the development of healing disturbances. Operative management has consistently resulted in a higher nonunion rate than nonoperative management (16, 17, 29). In one large series compiled by the Pennsylvania Orthopaedic Society, closed treatment resulted in a 5% nonunion rate compared with 12% for operative management (12). It is difficult to isolate operative management as the primary factor since none of the series reported had a prospective, randomized design. The cases treated operatively were chosen for operative management, which represents a treatment bias. Very possibly, they may represent fractures for which a closed reduction could not be obtained, more comminuted and unstable fractures or open injuries. All of these are factors that predispose to healing disturbances. However, surgery itself, even if done properly, will have the effect of interfering with the fracture hematoma, possibly devascularizing bone ends, and, in general, disrupting the fracture "milieu." When operative management is performed improperly, these negative effects are compounded many times, as will be discussed.

The ability to obtain an adequate reduction is important for a variety of reasons. Certainly, an adequate reduction in terms of angulation and rotation is important to prevent a malunion that may interfere with function. However, angulation or malrotation have not been shown to increase the risk of nonunion. Rather, distraction and displacement of the fracture fragments are much more important factors. Closed reduction should result in acceptable alignment of the humerus with the fracture surfaces at least within 1 cm of each other. This is more important for transverse and short oblique fractures than for long oblique or spiral fractures because of the reduced surface area for healing. Failure to obtain and maintain an adequate reduction by closed means is generally considered an indication for operative management.

The type and duration of immobilization may also be important factors. A variety of nonoperative immobilization techniques have been used successfully, including the hanging arm cast, coaptation splints, shoulder spica, collar and cuff, simple sling, sling and swathe, and functional bracing (11, 22, 25, 33). The method chosen is generally based upon the fracture pattern and location and the experience and preference of the treating physician. There is no doubt that all of these methods can be effective when used properly. However, the one nonoperative approach that has consistently been problematic is any technique that results in distraction of the fracture ends (13, 17, 29). This has most commonly been encountered with the use of a hanging arm cast, especially with transverse fracture patterns.

In one large series of humeral shaft fractures treated with hanging casts, the nonunion rate was 6%. However, 11 of the 18 nonunions were felt to be secondary to distraction at the fracture site (1). Another important factor is duration of immobilization, particularly with respect to the initiation of a therapeutic range of motion program (13). Immobilization is necessary to promote fracture healing. However, this has to be balanced with the need for a functional range of motion of the elbow and shoulder. Problems can arise when range of motion exercises are begun too early or pursued too vigorously. Before a program is initiated, fracture healing should be sufficient to withstand the stresses produced by the exercises. These can be minimized by using proper techniques, but most importantly, they should not be

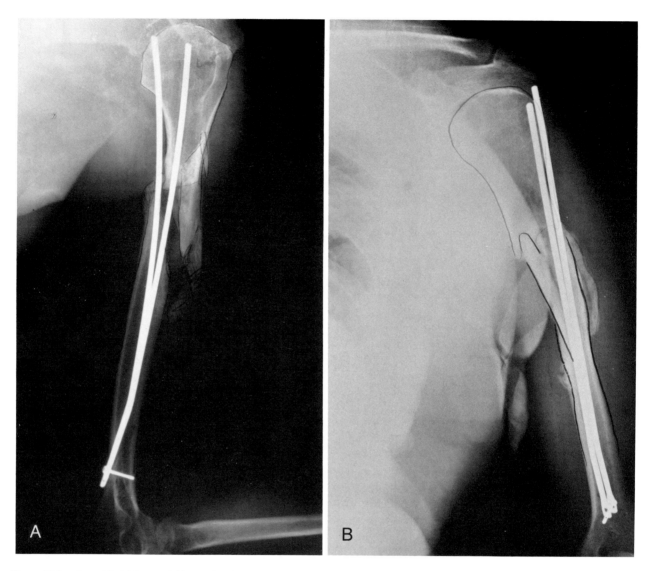

Figure 14.2. **A**, and **B**, A 70-year-old female fell off a chair and sustained a comminuted fracture of the proximal-third of the humerus. Initial treatment consisted of retrograde insertion of two Ender nails with locking. Ten months later, pain persisted and radiographs show a nonunion with a lateral butterfly healed to the proximal fragment. The Ender nails have not been securely placed in the proximal fragment. **C**, Following careful preoperative planning, the patient underwent removal of Ender nails, open reduction, and internal fixation of the nonunion with a 10-hole dynamic compression plate including lag screw placement. Prominent callus was used as bone graft. **D** and **E**, Radiographs obtained 8 months later show a well-healed nonunion. (Reproduced with permission from Rosen H. The treatment of nonunions and pseudarthrosis of the humeral shaft. Orthop Clin North Am 1990;21:725–742.)

started until there is evidence of early clinical union. Clinical union can be documented by a careful examination for motion at the fracture site in combination with the interpretation of serial radiographs.

When operative management is performed, improper technique will only increase the already increased risk of nonunion associated with operative management (1, 12, 17). Examples of improper technique include inadequate reduction (particularly with distraction of the fracture site), inability to achieve compression at the fracture site, misplaced

or misdirected internal fixation (Fig. 14.2), and inability to achieve a stable reduction and secure internal fixation (Fig. 14.1). In one study of operative management using the principles of internal fixation according to the AO/ASIF group (the Swiss association for the study of internal fixation), union was achieved in 33 of 34 cases (30). This series was particularly challenging because it included 16 comminuted fractures, 13 open fractures, and 10 with ipsilateral upper extremity injuries. In a similar series of 39 fractures in multiple trauma patients (14

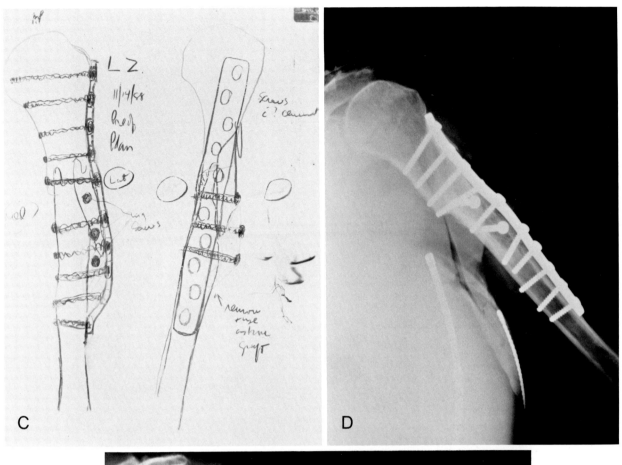

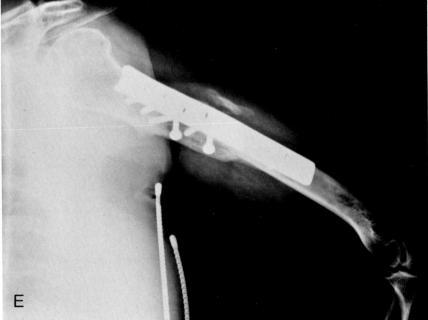

Figure 14.2.   C–E.

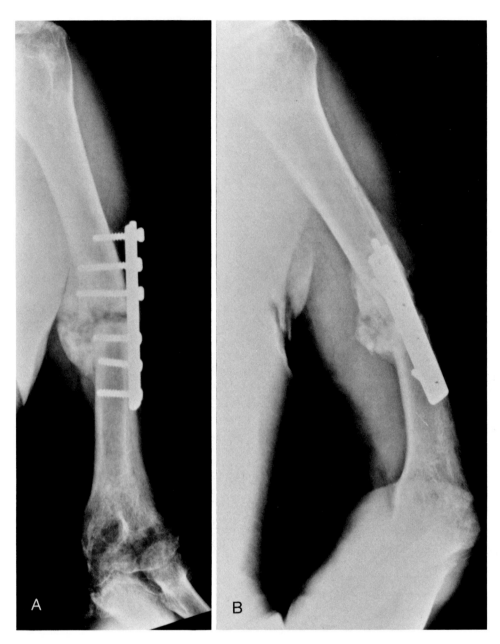

Figure 14.3.   **A** and **B**, A 65-year-old male 7 months following primary open reduction and internal fixation of a midshaft humerus fracture. Radiographs show a hypertrophic nonunion with loss of fixation in the proximal fragment. **C** and **D**, The patient underwent removal of hard-ware, open reduction, and internal fixation using an 8-hole broad DC plate with morselized callus as bone graft. **E**, Radiograph taken 1 year later shows complete healing of the nonunion.

open fractures, 20 comminuted fractures), plating resulted in a 97% union rate (4).

The development of postoperative complications, particularly infection, will compromise the results of operative management. This has been consistently reported by numerous authors (7, 12, 17, 29). Infection contributes to the development of nonunion by: (*a*) causing osteolysis of bone ends, thereby increasing the fracture gap; (*b*) producing se-questrum formation of devitalized bone; and (*c*) causing loosening of implants by replacement of bone by infected granulation tissue (24).

Patient factors that contribute to nonunion include bone quality, age, nutritional status, and compliance with postoperative instructions. Bone quality can be compromised by any process that interferes with its structural integrity. Osteopenia, defined as a decrease in bone mass, can be caused by

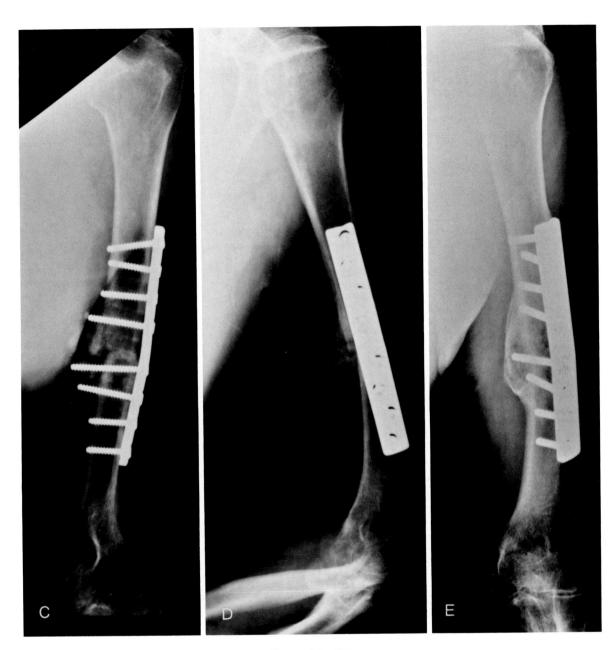

Figure 14.3. C–E.

many different conditions including senile osteoporosis, hyperparathyroidism, Cushings disease, exogenous steroid use, osteomalacia, and tumors (34). All of these conditions result in a reduced fracture healing response of varying degrees. Senile osteoporosis becomes more significant as patient age increases. Osteomalacia, although very uncommon, is important to recognize because it is a treatable cause of osteopenia (34). The reduced healing response associated with these causes of osteopenia might make one consider operative management. However, this can be even more problematic because of the diffi-

culty of achieving secure fixation in osteopenic bone. This will be discussed in the section on treatment.

Patient age has been reported to be a significant risk factor. In one large series of humeral shaft fractures, all delayed unions and nonunions occurred in patients between 50–70 years of age (10). Inadequate nutrition is also associated with the development of healing disturbances (21). This is frequently encountered in alcoholics, a subgroup of patients that also pose problems with compliance.

Patient compliance is an important aspect of both nonoperative and operative treatment (12, 17).

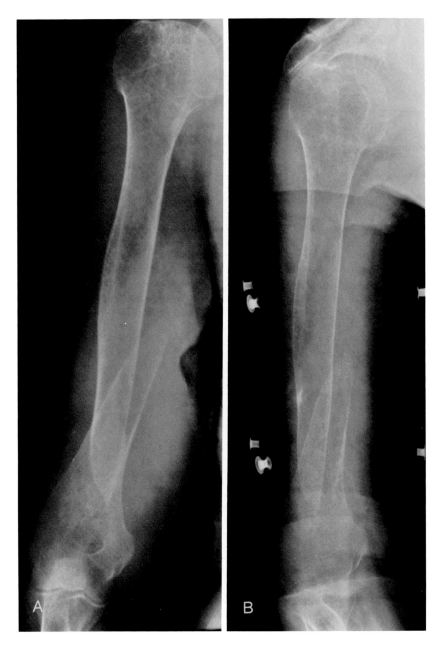

Figure 14.4. **A** and **B**, A 76-year-old female fell at home, sustaining a closed spiral fracture of the distal humerus with an associated radial nerve palsy. Initial treatment consisted of coaptation splints followed by a humeral fracture sleeve. Six months later, the patient has significant pain and gross motion. Radial nerve function had returned but paresthesias persisted, and wrist and digit dorsiflexion were graded 4 out of 5. Radiographs showed an atrophic nonunion with significant osteoporosis. **C** and **D**, The patient underwent open reduction and internal fixation using a 10-hole 4.5-mm pelvic reconstruction plate with autograft and fresh-frozen cancellous allograft. Methylmethacrylate was used for six of the screw holes to augment fixation. Care was taken to prevent any extravasation of cement into the nonunion site. The radial nerve was found to be adherent to the nonunion site. It was mobilized and a neurolysis performed. **E** and **F**, Radiographs taken 10 months later show healing of the nonunion. Elbow range of motion was 15–125° flexion/extension and 70° pronation, 80° supination. Radial nerve paresthesia had resolved, and muscle power was normal.

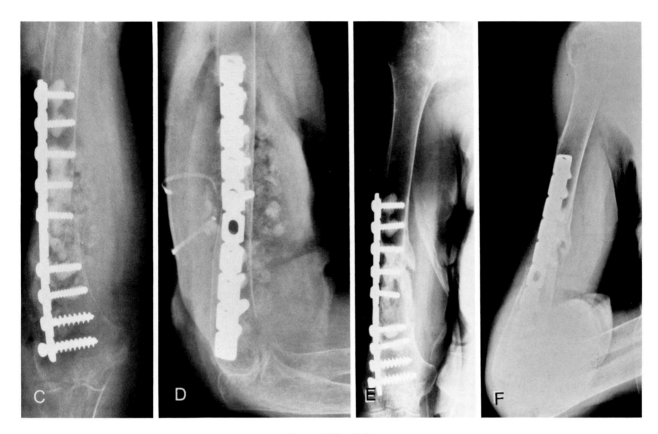

Figure 14.4.   C–F.

A successful outcome is not possible if patients do not follow instructions. Most of these problems arise from failure to maintain proper immobilization, excessive use of the shoulder and elbow during mobilization, or premature return to activities of daily living. It is often difficult to determine the level of patient compliance early in the treatment plan. However, it is important that the degree of patient participation required by the closed treatment approach not exceed the patient's ability to comply.

TREATMENT

Treatment of humeral shaft nonunions depends on the careful evaluation of many factors including the type and location of the nonunion, bone quality, level of pain and dysfunction, patient's expectations, and the experience of the treating surgeon. In general, the first choice to be made is between nonoperative and operative management. If operative management is chosen, various techniques are available, each with specific advantages and disadvantages. In this section, we will discuss the principles of the treatment of these nonunions, with specific reference to our preferred approach.

NONOPERATIVE MANAGEMENT

Nonoperative management may be preferred to operative management in two types of situations. The first is the case of nonunions associated with only minimal pain and dysfunction (10) (Fig. 14.5). In this situation, operative intervention, even if completely successful, would not significantly improve the patient's overall function. The second is the case in which although significant disability exists, there are specific contraindications to surgical management. These may include inadequate bone quality or anticipated problems with patient compliance.

In some situations, mostly in elderly patients, nonunions may be associated with minimal pain (Fig. 14.5). Although some dysfunction is present (restricted range of motion of the shoulder and/or elbow and inability to use the upper extremity for activities of daily living), it is not significant enough to justify an extensive surgical procedure that, even in the best circumstances, may not result in significant functional improvement. In some cases, the nonunion is hypertrophic and has some inherent stability. In others, where gross motion is present, the use of a light-weight plastic arm orthosis with Velcro

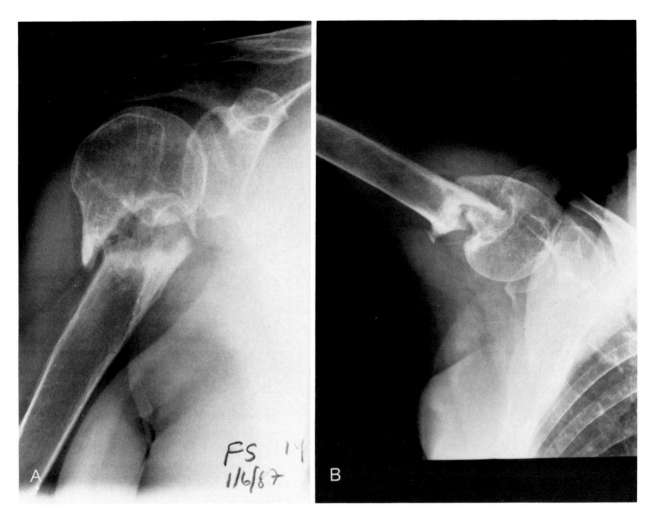

Figure 14.5. **A**, A 75-year-old female 2 years after closed treatment of a proximal humerus fracture has a painless nonunion with reasonably good function. **B**, Abduction radiograph shows slight motion at the nonunion, but most motion is at the glenohumeral joint. (Reproduced with permission from Rosen H. Management of nonunions and malunions in long bone fractures. In: Zuckerman JD, ed. Comprehensive care of orthopaedic injuries in the elderly. Baltimore: Urban & Schwarzenberg, 1990:490.)

straps may provide sufficient stability to improve overall function and decrease discomfort. In the experience of one of us (H.R.), over 40 patients have been successfully treated using this type of orthosis.

Nonoperative management is also preferred in cases where there is a contraindication to surgical management. Most often, this involves poor bone quality, such that secure internal fixation would not be possible using the techniques available. Also, the presence of significant medical problems may make it unsafe to proceed with anesthesia and surgery. Certain risk factors can be identified. Patients on chronic renal dialysis have poor bone quality and reduced healing secondary to renal osteodystrophy. Alcoholics have poor nutritional status, which further compromises the bone quality and can cause problems with wound healing. In addition, patient

compliance can be significantly problematic in alcoholics.

Electrical stimulation has been advocated by some for the treatment of humeral shaft nonunions. Although it would seem to be an attractive alternative to operative management, the clinical results have been disappointing. In one large series using constant direct current with percutaneously placed electrodes, union was achieved in only 46% of cases (13). Most of the successes were in patients that had preexisting secure internal fixation (66% union). In those cases without internal fixation, electrical stimulation resulted in a 22% success rate. In another series, also using direct current, all four humeral nonunions failed to unite (2). The problems using electrical stimulation for the treatment of humeral shaft nonunions involve: (a) the difficulty of achieving proper immobilization; (*b*) the frequency of bony gaps exceeding 1 cm; (*c*) the presence of synovial pseudarthroses; and (*d*) the prevalence of osteoporosis, avascular fragments, dense fibrous tissue, or interposed soft tissue. In general, electrical stimulation should not be considered a useful treatment option.

OPERATIVE MANAGEMENT

Operative management will be preferred for the treatment of the majority of humeral shaft nonunions when significant pain and disability are present. The goals of operative management are as follows: (*a*) achieving union; (*b*) correction of deformity; and (*c*) restoration of shoulder and elbow function. As with any operative procedure, the first step is proper preoperative evaluation and planning. This should be done carefully and should include the following areas:

1. Evaluation of the extremity including assessment of range of motion of the shoulder and elbow; neurological status, especially radial nerve function; vascular status, particularly if there is a history of open fracture with significant soft tissue injury; condition of the skin including location of previous incisions; presence of infection including active drainage and sinus tracts.

2. Completion of all necessary diagnostic tests, which may include standard radiographs with oblique views to assess nonunion geometry; technetium bone scan and/or indium scan for cases of suspected infection; culture and sensitivity for both aerobic and anaerobic organisms when drainage is present; aspiration of the nonunion site for suspected infection; electrodiagnostic tests to evaluate nerve function; angiogram if vascular compromise is suspected.

3. Careful planning of the surgical procedure that will be performed including surgical approach, internal fixation device to be used, and use of bone graft or adjunctive fixation with methylmethacrylate; the need for special postoperative immobilization devices.

Attention to these specific points during preoperative planning will undoubtedly increase the chance of a successful result. However, neglect of these important points may further complicate the problem and the goals of operative management.

SURGICAL APPROACH

Adequate exposure of the nonunions is a central part of operative management. The extensile approach as described by Henry can be used to expose the entire humeral shaft, including both the proximal and distal metaphyseal-diaphyseal junctions. Proximal exposure is obtained through a deltopectoral approach that often requires partial detachment of the deltoid insertion, which should be repaired during closure. The midshaft region is approached by blunt dissection through the brachialis muscle. The musculocutaneous nerve can be identified and mobilized in the interval between the biceps and brachialis muscles. The branch that forms the lateral cutaneous nerve of the forearm can be identified in this interval at the lower end of the biceps. The distal portion of the skin incision curves anteriorly and medially into the anterolateral aspect of the antecubital fossa. At the lower end of the incision, the interval between the brachialis and brachioradialis should be developed to expose the radial nerve. Dissection can be performed in a distal to proximal direction tracing the nerve back to the point that it passes through the lateral intermuscular septum. This approach allows exposure of the entire humeral shaft, as well as exposure of the musculocutaneous and radial nerves for decompression or immobilization during the procedure.

As noted, obtaining union is the most important goal of operative management. This is generally performed in conjunction with correction of deformity and release of contractures of adjacent joints. To achieve these goals, the following guidelines should be followed:

1. Resect all soft tissue at the nonunion site, including synovial pseudarthrosis tissue, so that bony surfaces are exposed;
2. Modify the end of the exposed bone with shortening if necessary, to achieve maximal apposition of well-vascularized bone;
3. Drill or shingle sclerotic areas to promote revascularization;
4. Correct angulation, rotation, and reduction of any gap that may exist between the bone ends;
5. Obtain secure internal fixation including compression across the nonunion site;
6. Promote bony healing by the use of cancellous bone grafts, especially in atrophic nonunions;
7. Release adhesions of adjacent joints, particularly for diaphyseal-metaphyseal nonunions.

TECHNIQUES

Many different techniques have been used for the treatment of humeral shaft nonunions, but the two most common ones are intramedullary devices (1, 6, 14, 15, 23, 28, 31) and plate and screw devices (1, 3, 7, 14, 24, 29). External fixation has been used infrequently and generally only for initial stabilization in the treatment of infected nonunions (8, 32).

Intramedullary devices include rigid nails inserted either retrograde or antegrade after reaming (Kuntscher-type nails) or flexible nails inserted either retrograde or antegrade without reaming (Ender nails). In general, they have been used successfully in the treatment of acute fractures in the middle third of the humeral shaft, especially for transverse or oblique patterns. Locked intramedullary nails have extended the indications in acute fractures to long oblique, spiral, and comminuted fractures covering the middle third (26). However, the experience with intramedullary devices for nonunions has been much less extensive, with significantly less predictable results (6, 14, 28, 31). Foster et al. reported a 73% union rate for 11 nonunions treated by antegrade Kuntscher nailing (14). They specifically cited frequent problems with subacromial impingement secondary to prominence of the nail at the insertion point. Other authors have reported a 56% incidence of adhesive capsulitis following antegrade nailing (28). A locked intramedullary nail has been used in a small series of six patients (31) with a union obtained in 83%. However, open bone grafts were used in four of the five cases that united, and adjunctive cerclage wires were used in four of the six cases. These additional measures represent another treatment variable that makes it difficult to determine the efficacy of the nailing itself. Flexible intramedullary nails inserted using a retrograde technique were used to treat 10 humeral shaft nonunions (23). Bone grafts were not used, nor was the fracture site opened. Union was achieved in nine cases using this technique (23).

In spite of the degree of success reported by some authors, in principle, intramedullary devices have significant limitations in the treatment of humeral shaft nonunions. First, they cannot be used for nonunions located at the proximal or distal portions of the diaphysis. Second, insertion by closed technique is commonly not possible because of the need to reduce displaced, overriding, or angulated fragments; the need to perform bone grafting; or the need to expose adjacent nerves. Third, rigid fixation, particularly in rotation, is difficult, if not impossible to achieve. And fourth, compression across the nonunion site can, at best, be achieved to only a limited degree even using locked intramedullary devices.

The use of compression plating is generally considered to be the treatment of choice for humeral shaft nonunion (Figs. 14.1, 14.2, and 14.3). Numerous authors have reported excellent results using a broad AO dynamic compression plate in combination with cancellous bone grafting (1, 3, 7, 14, 17, 21, 29). In some cases, methylmethacrylate has been used for adjunctive fixation as well (3, 24, 29). Healey et al. reported union in 24 of 25 nonunions treated by compression plating (17). All of the healed nonunions had concurrent bone grafting performed. Foster et al. reported an 80% success rate in 10 nonunions using similar treatment principles (14). Barquet et al. used a "uniform therapeutic protocol" consisting of decortication, internal fixation with a broad straight ASIF dynamic compression plate, and autologous bone grafting to achieve union in 24 of 25 cases (3). Our results using a similar approach achieved a success rate of over 90% (24).

AUTHORS' PREFERRED APPROACH

After careful evaluation of the patient and deciding that operative management is indicated, preoperative planning in accordance with the principles discussed is completed. An operative plan is drawn on the preoperative radiographs including the type and length of plate anticipated. Specific requests for the necessary internal fixation are made with the operating room, and its availability is confirmed in advance of the day of surgery. Patients should have 2 units of blood available, and every effort is made to use autologous or donor-directed blood. For a proximal one-third shaft nonunion, we prefer the beach chair position with the arm of the side of the table, resting on a sterile Mayo stand, if necessary. For mid- and distal third shaft nonunions, the supine position is used with an armboard. A sterile tourniquet should be used to allow proper draping of the operative site and for hemostasis during the initial dissection. We prefer to prep the opposite anterior iliac crest for cancellous bone graft, if it has not been used previously. This allows a second team, if available, to harvest the graft while the nonunion is prepared. The ipsilateral anterior crest can be used, although it is less convenient. If both anterior crests have been previously harvested, we will use the posterior crest and harvest the graft during the first part of the procedure with the patient in the prone or side-lying position. If there is concern about the availability or adequacy of autogenous cancellous graft, arrangements should be made to have allograft available. We prefer fresh frozen cancellous allograft, but will use freeze-dried material if necessary.

The extensile anterolateral approach of Henry, as discussed, is utilized. For proximal nonunions, the musculocutaneous nerve should be identified; for distal nonunions, the radial nerve is identified; for midshaft nonunions, both nerves are identified. A small penrose drain or similar marker should be passed around the nerve for easy identification and to allow mobilization without direct contact with the nerve. In any case with a preoperative radial nerve deficit, exposure of the nerve is mandatory. Plans should be made to proceed with neurolysis, nerve repair, or grafting with appropriate surgical consultants and equipment, as needed, depending on the findings at the time of exploration. If nerve grafting is anticipated, the preferred harvest site should be prepped at the start of the procedure.

As the nonunion site is exposed, care must be taken to minimize the degree of soft tissue stripping. The bone should be handled very carefully to avoid fracture. All soft tissue at the nonunion site should be excised so that the nonunion surfaces are completely exposed. In cases of midshaft nonunions, a sleeve of posterior soft tissue should be maintained to prevent injury to the radial nerve as it passes along the posterior aspect of the humerus. In mid- and distal shaft nonunions, the radial nerve may be caught up in the nonunion site. This can occur in cases with completely intact radial nerve function and serves to emphasize the importance of careful dissection and mobilization of the radial nerve.

When the nonunion site is exposed, the bone should be prepared for reduction. It is important that all avascular bone be removed so that the vascular surfaces can be placed in apposition. Additional preparation of the nonunion will be necessary, depending on the deformity present, the type of nonunion, and its geometry. In general, deformity should be corrected such that there is maximal opposition of bone surfaces. Often, the ends of the bone can be modified to obtain a stable, interlocking fit that will facilitate the application of compression during internal fixation. When significant overriding or deformity is present, the bone may have to be shortened to obtain a reduction without excessive tension on the neurovascular structures. Correction of valgus or recurvatum deformities may place significant stress on the radial nerve. This should be evaluated carefully with additional mobilization of the nerve, if necessary. Any vascular bone that is removed during shortening should be morselized and

saved for bone grafting. In hypertrophic nonunions, contouring of the nonunion site for reduction and plate placement may require removal of callus. This should also be saved for use as bone graft. All sclerotic bone is drilled to promote a vascular response. If the intramedullary canals are closed, we prefer to open them by drilling. Shingling of the bone—raising small flaps of cortical bone—should be performed with a small sharp osteotome for 3–4 cm on both sides of the nonunion. In atrophic nonunions, the bone is very fragile and must be handled carefully. The intramedullary canal should be opened by drilling. Shingling should not be performed because of the fragility of the bone. Rather, after fixation, "petaling" of the exposed bone is recommended. "Petaling" consists of raising small osteal, periosteal "petals" that remain attached to the bone at their base. It is performed by hand, using a small osteotome or gouge.

The next step is deciding the exact type of internal fixation to be used and preparing it for insertion. In general, the broad 4.5 mm AO dynamic compression plate is preferred (Figs. 14.1, 14.2, and 14.3). This plate has a staggered screwhole pattern that permits insertion of the fixation screws in multiple planes. This prevents propagation of cortical fractures between adjacent screwholes, which would compromise fixation. A narrow 4.5 mm AO dynamic compression plate or a 4.5-mm pelvic reconstruction plate (Fig. 14.4) can be used if the diameter of the humeral shaft is too small for the broad plate. These plates may also be more suitable for distal third nonunions because of the size and shape of the humerus in the supracondylar region. A T or L can be used for very proximal shaft nonunions if additional fixation of the proximal humerus is needed. However, this is a weaker, noncompression plate, and is not recommended if use of a compression plate is possible. For most nonunions, we prefer to place the plate on the anterolateral surface of the humerus. However, this may not always be possible. In some situations, the contour of callus or the presence of healed butterfly or segmental fragments prevents anterolateral placement. In these situations, the plate should be placed wherever the best fit can be obtained. This is often the posterior surface or, less frequently, the anterior surface of the humerus. For proximal third nonunions, the plate should be placed lateral to the bicipital groove with care taken to avoid proximal placement that encroaches on the subacromial space. For distal third nonunions, the plate is often placed posteriorly. In this situation, care must be taken to avoid encroachment of the olecranon fossa, which would limit elbow extension. If encroachment is a concern, it is often helpful to resect the tip of the olecranon to increase the available clearance.

An essential part of the internal fixation is achieving compression at the nonunion site. This can usually be achieved in all but the most atrophic nonunions. It can be accomplished by four techniques—prestressing the plate, external compression device, interfragmentary screws, and insertion of "loaded" plate screws. Prestressing of the plate refers to overcontouring of the plate at the fracture site by approximately 1 mm, thereby giving a slight varus contour. This overcontouring will provide compression to the medial side of the nonunion, when a compression is applied to the anterolaterally placed plate. Compression can be applied to the plate by placement of "loaded" screws or use of the external compression device. One or two eccentrically "loaded" screws can be placed through the plate on either side of the nonunion after one or two standard screws have been placed to stabilize the plate to the shaft. The external compression device can be used

instead of the "loaded screws." It is generally attached to the end of the plate on the longer fragment. In short oblique fractures, the fragments should be compressed into the axilla created by the oblique fracture pattern and the plate. When compression is achieved, a 4.5-mm interfragmentary cortical screw can be placed across the nonunion site (for oblique patterns), or screws can be placed through the plate to fix the plate to the shaft and maintain a compression achieved.

In general, the goal is to achieve at least six and preferably eight cortices of secure fixation on each side of the nonunion. This can generally be achieved by use of a 9-hole plate. However, in atrophic nonunions, a slightly longer plate—10 or 11 holes—can be used (Fig. 14.4). This would allow five or more screws on either side of the nonunion. Even with the use of a longer plate, the bone is often of such poor quality that eight cortices of secure fixation cannot be obtained by standard means. Therefore, methylmethacrylate is often used to enhance screw fixation (Fig. 14.6). Loose screws should be removed, except those at the end of the plate, and directly adjacent to

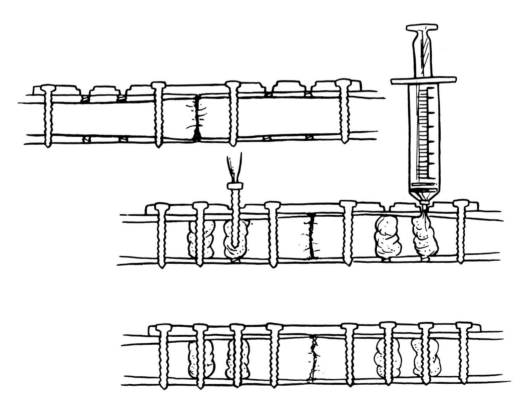

Figure 14.6. Technique for using methylmethacrylate cement to gain purchase for loose screws in osteoporotic bone. The loose screws are removed. Liquid cement (1–2 minutes after mixing) is injected into these holes with a syringe. Screws are then replaced in their proper holes while the cement is soft. They are finally tightened only after the cement has set. Cement should not enter the fracture site. If there is extruded cement around the bone, it should be removed. (Reproduced with permission from Rosen H. Management of nonunions and malunions in long bone fractures. In: Zuckerman JD, ed. Comprehensive care of orthopaedic injuries in the elderly. Baltimore: Urban & Schwarzenberg, 1990:499.)

the nonunion. The position of the removed screws should be clearly marked for later reinsertion. A batch of methylmethacrylate is mixed, and in approximately one minute, it is loaded into a 20-cc syringe with the tip that fits directly into the screwhole. The cement is injected into each screwhole, and when possible, the hole in the opposite cortex is covered to prevent cement extravasation. As each hole is filled with cement, the screws are reinserted by the first assistant, and excess cement is removed. The screws can usually be pushed into place, and when necessary, a screwdriver can be used. Care must be taken to prevent any extravasation of cement into the nonunion site. After the cement is completely hardened, the screws are tightened for final fixation. This usually requires no more than one or two turns.

After fixation is completed, cancellous bone graft should be applied. It is generally placed circumferentially around the nonunion site, as well as throughout the areas of petaling and shingling. Although some authors feel that bone graft is optional in hypertrophic nonunions, in general, it is a safer policy to graft all humeral shaft nonunions.

There is often significant stiffness of the shoulder and elbow present preoperatively. This generally results from the prolonged periods of immobilization. At the time of surgery, it is important to address this specific problem. For the shoulder, this usually involves mobilization of the subacromial space by passing a blunt Darrach elevator over the supraspinatus and infraspinatus muscles. The coracoacromial ligament should be excised along with any hypertrophic bursa that may be adherent to the underside of the acromion. The coracoacromial ligament (originating from the base of the coracoid and inserting into the rotator interval) should be divided, particularly if there is restriction of external rotation. If significant restriction of motion remains, additional steps can be taken. A "Z" lengthening of the subscapularis tendon will improve external rotation. Abduction can be improved by release of the inferior capsule and the pectoralis major insertion to the proximal portion of the humeral shaft. Gentle manipulation can be performed only after completion of all soft tissue releases. Any manipulation should not stress the fixation, but rather should involve only the proximal humerus with as short a lever arm as possible.

For significant elbow stiffness, a similar approach is used. This generally requires elevation and possible release of the brachialis anteriorly and the triceps posteriorly. A gentle manipulation can be performed, but in our experience, anterior capsular releases are often necessary to gain improved extension. A lateral capsulotomy should be made to expose the joint and release any articular adhesions. The anterior capsule can be released in two ways: First, by releasing its attachment to the anterior aspect of the distal humerus, or second, by separating it from the overlying soft tissues and resecting a central portion. This should be done with care because of the location of the neurovascular structures.

After all releases have been completed, the range of motion of the shoulder and elbow should be assessed. In addition, while determining the range of motion, the stability of the fixation should also be assessed. This information is essential to provide specific guidelines and limitations for the mobilization program to be followed postoperatively.

During closure of the wound, particular attention should be given to the radial nerve. To avoid scarring of the nerve to the anterolaterally placed plate, soft tissue should be interposed to protect the nerve. The brachialis muscle is most suitable for this. This is most easily accomplished during the initial exposure of the radial nerve. A portion of the brachialis muscle should always be preserved medial to the nerve to provide the necessary soft tissue interpositioning. Suction drains are generally used. Muscle layers are allowed to fall back together, and a routine closure of the subcutaneous tissue and skin is completed. If secure stable fixation is achieved, a simple sling will be sufficient immobilization. However, additional support in the form of a humeral fracture sleeve or light-weight hinged cast brace will be necessary if patient reliability is a concern or when fixation is less than adequate. Mobilization consisting of active and gentle assisted range of motion of the shoulder and elbow can be started postoperatively based upon the assessment performed intraoperatively. The sling or brace should be worn until union and bone graft incorporation is evident radiographically.

SPECIAL SITUATIONS

The presence of infection significantly increases the difficulty of obtaining a successful outcome (8, 32). The principles discussed thus far also apply to infected nonunions. However, some important modifications are needed. Appropriate bacteriological studies should be performed to identify the organisms involved so that appropriate antibiotic therapy can be initiated. We feel that antibiotics are most important as an adjunct to operative debridement.

Therefore, the next step in management is an extensive debridement of all infected and nonviable tissue. This includes skin, sinus tracts, muscle, fascia, and bone. After the initial debridement, a decision must be made concerning the type of immobilization needed. This decision should be based on an assessment of the need for dressing changes, additional debridements, soft tissue coverage procedures, and bone grafting. In most situations, an external fixation device will be necessary to stabilize the nonunion and maintain alignment. In some situations in which the extent of soft tissue involvement is limited and the wound is small, a posterior splint can be used in anticipation of the ability to proceed with internal fixation relatively early in the process. Debridement and definitive treatment of a nonunion should not be performed as a one-stage procedure because of the risk of continued infection.

After the initial debridement, the wound should remain open and packed to eliminate any dead space. For large wounds, antibiotic impregnated beads may be useful, but in general, we prefer Betadine-soaked 4 × 4s. Dressing changes are begun the day after the debridement and continued until a clean, healthy granulation tissue bed is evident. The goal of obtaining a clean, healthy wound may require serial surgical debridements and daily whirlpool treatments, in addition to frequent dressing changes.

When a clean, granulating wound is achieved, definitive treatment can be performed. If the external fixation device is providing sufficient immobilization and alignment of the bone ends, this should be left in place and used as the "definitive stable" fixation in combination of preparation of the bone ends and extensive bone grafting. If an external fixator has not been used or if fixation is inadequate, plating and bone grafting should be performed as previously described. At the same time, as the definitive bony procedure, any soft tissue procedures (local or free flaps, split-thickness skin graft) should be performed to obtain adequate soft tissue cover.

In some cases, particularly infected nonunions or in nonunions following severe open fractures with extensive bone or soft tissue injury, large areas of bone loss may be present. In these situations, two options are available. In the past, vascularized bone grafts (i.e., fibula or iliac crest) have been used with some success (27). More recently, ring external fixators (Ilizarov) have been used for stabilizations of nonunions in combination with lengthening of the humerus by proximal or distal corticotomy and bone transport to achieve compression at the nonunion site (18, 19). The early results with this technique have been quite good, and it is an important addition to the treatment armamentarium. However, procedures of this type—Ilizarov and vascularized bone grafts—are technically difficult, labor-intensive techniques that require significant expertise and a very high degree of patient compliance and cooperation to achieve successful outcome.

References

1. Abdel-Fattah H, Halawa E, Shaft TH. Nonunion of the humeral shaft: a report on 25 cases. Injury 1981;14:255-262.
2. Ahl T, Anderson G, Herberts P, Kalen R. Electrical treatment of nonunited fractures. Acta Orthop Scand 1984;55:585-588.
3. Barquet A, Fernandez A, Luvizio J, Mashah R. A combined therapeutic protocol for aseptic nonunion of the humeral shaft: a report of 25 cases. J Trauma 1989;29:95-98.
4. Bell MJ, Beachamb CG, Kellam JK, McMurty RY. The results of plating humeral shaft fractures in patients with multiple injuries. J Bone Joint Surg 1985;67B:293-296.
5. Bostman O, Bakalim G, Vainionpaa S, et al. Radial palsy shaft fracture of the humerus. Acta Orthop Scand 1986;57:316-319.
6. Christiansen NO. Kuntscher intramedullary reaming and nail fixation for nonunion of the humerus. Clin Orthop 1976;116:222-228.
7. Collie LP, Cooney WP, Kelly PJ. Nonunions of the humeral shaft. Orthop Trans 1983;6:517.
8. Coong P, Griffiths J. External fixation of complex open humeral fractures. Aust N Z J Surg 1988;58:137-142.
9. Coventry MB, Laurnen EL. Ununited fractures of the middle and upper humerus. Clin Orthop 1970;69:192-198.
10. Dameron TB, Gnubb SA. Humeral shaft fractures in adults. South Med J 1981;74:1461-1467.
11. Epps CH, Cotler JM. Complications of treatment of fractures of the humeral shaft. In: Epps CH, ed. Complications in Orthopaedic Surgery. 2nd ed. Philadelphia: J.B. Lippincott, 1986:277-304.
12. Epps CH. Nonunions of the humerus. In: Instructional Course Lectures. Park Ridge, IL: American Academy of Orthopaedic Surgeons, 1988;37:161-166.
13. Esterhal JL, Brighton CT, Heppenstall RB, Thrower A. Nonunion of the humerus. Clin Orthop 1986;211:228-234.
14. Foster RJ, Dixon GL, Bach A, et al. Internal fixation of fractures and nonunions of the humeral shaft. J Bone Joint Surg 1985;67A:857-864.
15. Gupta R, Gaur S, Tiwari R, Varma B, Gupta R. Treatment of ununited fractures of the shaft of the humerus with bent nail. Injury 1985;16:276-280.
16. Hall RF, Pankovich AM. Ender nailing of acute fractures of the humerus. J Bone Joint Surg 1987;69A:558-567.
17. Healey W, White G, Mick C, et al. Nonunion of the humeral shaft. Clin Orthop 1987;219:206-213.
18. Ilizarov GA. The principles of the Ilizarov method. Bull Hosp J Dis 1988;48:1-11.
19. Ilizarov GA, Devyatov A, Kamenin V. Plastic reconstruction of longitudinal bone defects by means of compression and subsequent distraction. Acta Chir Plast 1980;22:32-40.
20. Klenerman L. Fractures of the shaft of the humerus. J Bone Joint Surg 1966;48B:105-111.
21. Loomer R, Kokan P. Nonunion in fractures of the humeral shaft. Injury 1974;7:274-278.

22. Post M. Fractures of the shaft of the humerus. In: Post M, ed. The shoulder: surgical and nonsurgical management. 2nd ed. Philadelphia: Lea & Febiger, 1988:488–517.

23. Pritchett JW. Delayed union of humeral shaft fractures treated by closed flexible intramedullary nailing. J Bone Joint Surg 1985;67B:715–718.

24. Rosen H. The treatment of nonunions and pseudarthrosis of the humeral shaft. Orthop Clin North Am 1990;21:725–742.

25. Sarmiento A, Kinman PB, Murphy RB, Phillips JG. Treatment of ulnar fractures by functional bracing. J Bone Joint Surg 1976;58A:1104–1107.

26. Seidel H. Humeral locking nail: a preliminary report. Orthopaedics 1989;12:2, 219–226.

27. Solonen KA. Free-vascularized bone graft in the treatment of pseudarthrosis. Int Orthop 1982;6:9–13.

28. Stern PJ, Mattingly DA, Pomeroy DL, Zenni EJ, Kreig JK. Intramedullary fixation of humeral shaft fractures. J Bone Joint Surg 1989;66A:639–646.

29. Tratter DH, Dobozi W. Nonunion of the humerus: rigid fixation, bone grafting, and adjunctive bone cement. Clin Orthop 1986;204:162–168.

30. Vandergriend R, Tomasin J, Ward EF. Open reduction and internal fixation of humeral shaft fractures. J Bone Joint Surg 1986;68A:430–433.

31. Ward EF, White JL. Interlocked intramedullary nailing of the humerus. Orthopaedics 1989;12:1353–141.

32. Zinghi GF, Specchia L, Borsani S, Galli G. Surgical treatment of infected pseudoarthrosis of the humerus. 3rd Surgical Division, Rizzoli Orthopaedic Institute, Bologna.

33. Zuckerman JD, Lubliner J. Arm, elbow and forearm injuries. In: Zuckerman JD, ed. Comprehensive care of orthopaedic injuries in the elderly. Baltimore: Urban & Schwarzenberg, 1990:345–409.

34. Zuckerman JD, Perry C. Principles of fracture treatment. In: Zuckerman, JD, ed. Comprehensive care of orthopaedic injuries in the elderly. Baltimore: Urban & Schwarzenberg, 1990:15–23.

15
Complications of Internal Fixation of Proximal Humeral Fractures

Keith C. Watson

INTRODUCTION

Fortunately for orthopaedic surgeons and their patients, displaced fractures of the proximal humerus requiring operative intervention are infrequent (20% of all proximal humerus fractures) (12). Fortunately, too, the shoulder is a rather forgiving joint when it comes to recovering function following such trauma. However, this requires a combination of adequate anatomic restoration, appropriate rehabilitation, and patient selection. DePalma addressed the importance of early rehabilitation in 1950:

Most essential to a complete and rapid recovery is preservation of the gliding mechanism between the soft tissue layers of the shoulder. To attain this, motion must be started early ... (3).

Therefore, one of the primary goals of an orthopaedic surgeon is the restoration of anatomy with adequate fixation to allow early passive range of motion. Codman, however, recognized that this enthusiasm did not always bode well for the patient. He argued that improper fixation causes most delays and failures in restoring normal function (2).

Indeed, the ease with which we are often able to treat 80% of proximal humerus fractures may lull us into a false sense of confidence when it comes to the treatment of these more unusual fractures that the orthopaedist may encounter infrequently.

Numerous factors must be considered when deciding to repair a fracture. Inappropriate selection of any one factor can result in failure. There are a variety of fixation devices to choose from including pins, screws, wire, suture, staples, plates, IM rods and combinations of all of these. Each device has an appropriate place in the treatment of these fractures. In addition, the character of the fracture will have a direct bearing on the applicability of certain devices (e.g., surgical neck, two, three, four-part, or comminution). Finally, the patient's general condition must be taken into consideration (elderly osteoporotic vs. young active, alcoholism, multitrauma, etc.).

DEVICE-SPECIFIC CONCERNS

Pins

Pins are applied either at the time of an open procedure or percutaneously. Percutaneous pin fixation is deceptively difficult and carries with it the concern for pin tract complications (Fig. 15.1A), premature loosening, and loss of fixation (9). The majority of pins, however, are inserted at the time of open reduction, and have been widely used. Comminution of fragments, which is often poorly appreciated on radiographs, minimizes applicability of pin fixation. Surprisingly, serious complications unrelated to the healing of the fracture have been identified with the use of pins (Fig. 15.1B). This implies that the use of pins obligates the patient to future surgery for removal. Recent examination of the magnitude of pin migration by Lyons has produced six guidelines to be followed when using pins about the shoulder (11).

1. Pins must be used with caution, if at all, in the shoulder girdle;
2. The patient must be instructed regarding the importance of follow-up evaluation;
3. The ends of pins must be bent;
4. Radiographs should be made immediately postoperatively, and follow-up x-rays every 4 weeks until the pins are removed;
5. Patients should be followed closely, clinically and radiographically until conclusion of therapy, at which time all pins should be removed; and

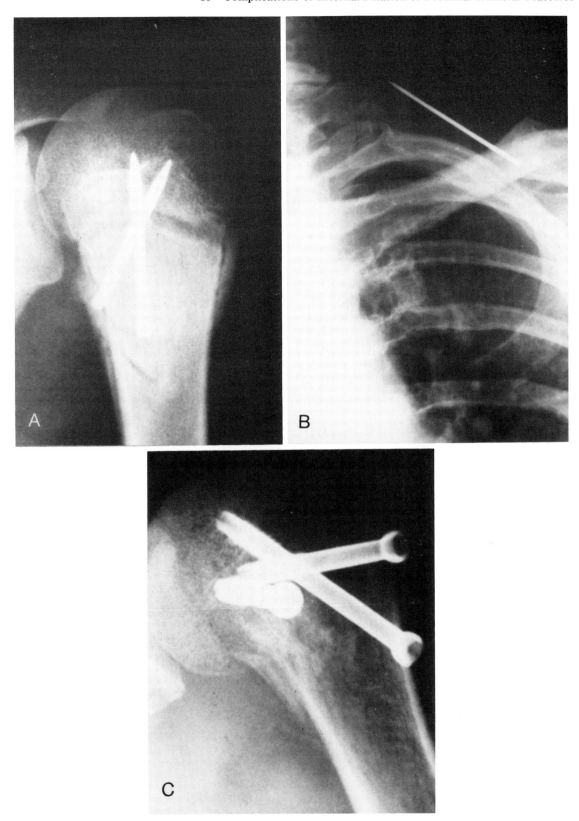

Figure 15.1. **A**, Percutaneous pin fixation effective in good quality bone without comminution. **B**, Dangerous pin migration occurs frequently demanding extremely close monitoring of the patients and aggressive efforts to assure removal after healing. **C**, Use of cannulated screws offers a hybrid approach which may be an advantage in some situations.

6. If a pin migrates, it must be removed as a matter of urgency, regardless of the lack of symptoms. (The development of bioabsorbable pins may improve their applicability in the future.)

Screws

Screw fixation for shoulder fractures is attractive because screws are relatively easily placed and can provide stable fixation. However, certain conditions must be present for these devices to work properly. Again, comminution must be minimal, and the bone must be sturdy. There is nothing so disheartening as to have the head of the screw sink into the cortex of the greater tuberosity like butter, or have the screw spin without purchase in the cobweb-like trabeculae of a 75-year-old humeral head. In the young and active patient with good bone stock, such fixation can be quite adequate. Interestingly, reports of screws migrating following fracture repair are conspicuously absent in the literature (11, 15). The advent of smaller caliber cannulated screws may broaden the indications for the use of screws in the future (Fig. 15.1C).

Staples

The use of staples about the shoulder has been popular since the beginning of this century, but their use in fracture fixation has been limited. The bone of the tuberosities and humeral head will not provide as secure anchoring as that of the glenoid neck. The same constraints regarding bone quality—no comminution and high density—are necessary for good staple fixation, while the method of insertion makes the use of these devices more difficult for fractures about the shoulder (Fig. 15.2).

Wire

Wire is one of the most widely used fixation devices for shoulder fractures because it is malleable and presents a low profile, avoiding impingement against the acromion. Therefore, it can used to secure small fragments, compress the fracture site, and provide reasonable fixation without extensive dissection. Also, the wire can be woven through the soft tissues (rotator cuff), which may provide better fixation than the osteoporotic bone. Unfortunately, these same qualities contribute to problems with wire fixation. At times, the fracture is not rigidly fixed, allowing sufficient motion to result in either a

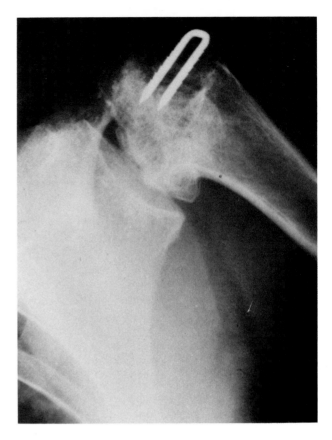

Figure 15.2. Despite use of a staple (minimal tissue dissection) there is subsequent avascular necrosis.

fibrous union or breakage of the wire (Fig. 15.3A). This tendency for wire to break may occur even in the face of a well-healed fracture. Unfortunately, broken wire tends to migrate toward the joint, requiring additional surgery for removal (Fig. 15.3B). Attempts to secure reduction with wire in osteoporotic bone may result in the wire actually cutting through, causing loss of fixation. Wire is most useful in conjunction with intramedullary fixation to provide an axial compression, thereby controlling rotation (5).

Suture

Large (#2 or #5) nonabsorbable suture has become a popular alternative to wire in many instances where there is comminution and adequate soft tissue purchase (e.g., the tuberosities) (7). While suture does not have the compressive abilities of tension band wiring, it can achieve satisfactory fracture control and has the advantage of being radiolucent. If the suture breaks, there is no need for reoperation to remove it (Fig. 15.3C).

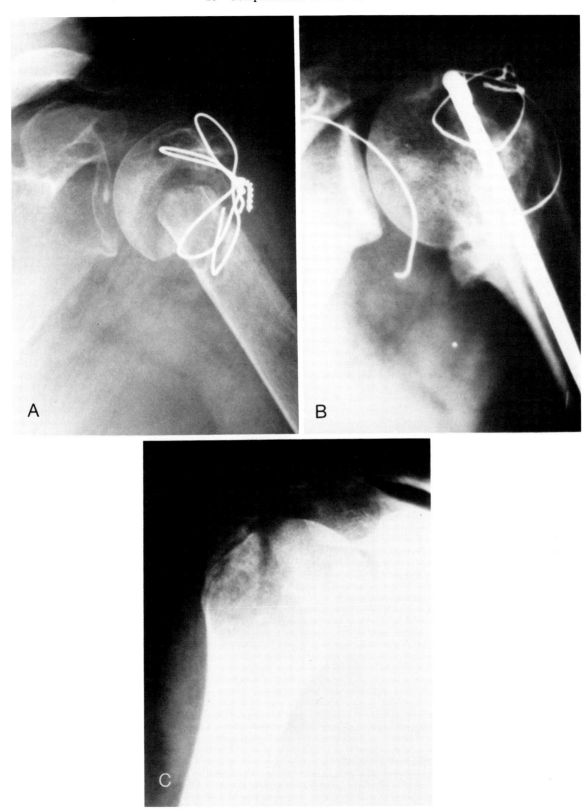

Figure 15.3. A, Inadequate fixation with wire allows excessive motion at fracture site promoting non-union. **B,** Typical late complication of wire fixation with migration toward joint. Much more extensive dissection may be necessary to retrieve these pieces after migration occurs. **C,** Greater tuberosity fracture adequately repaired with nonabsorbable suture. Avoids need for reoperation to remove fixation.

Plates

Fracture fixation using plates and screws has been advocated by the AO Group. Severely displaced fractures can be remarkably restored with this technique, but it requires extensive soft tissue dissection, which has been reported to increase the incidence of avascular necrosis (Fig. 15.4A and B). Proximal positioning of the device is a common error, causing impingement under the acromion, promoting loosening, and requiring additional surgery for premature removal. Certainly, with good bone stock, this approach can be very effective, but the indications for this method should be carefully considered in the elderly with osteoporotic bone, for there is a high risk for complications (Fig. 15.4C) (14).

Intramedullary (IM) Rods

Intramedullary devices for fixation of proximal humeral fractures have been extensively employed. Biomechanically, the IM rod enjoys an advantage over the plate devices. The most familiar intramedullary device is the Rush rod which was introduced in the 1950s. Other devices have been utilized as well (e.g., Ender's rods) with equal success. There are several inherent problems to be aware of when utilizing one of these devices (10). Rotational control is inadequate as there is no compression at the fracture site. These devices commonly migrate proximally, impinging on the acromion and requiring early removal. They may also interfere with rehabilitation (Fig. 15.5). These devices are most often used in combination with additional fixation and, therefore, their isolated use must be in a special fracture pattern. It is tempting to just "drop a rod" in a proximal humeral fracture, but often this technique does not provide the rotational stability that is necessary.

FRACTURE-SPECIFIC CONCERNS

The choice of fixation device is dependent in part on the fracture pattern as well. There are complications unique to each type of fracture.

Anatomical Neck

This fracture is extremely rare, and since it occurs more frequently in the younger age range, problems with internal fixation have not been reported. Unfortunately, due to the unique character of the fracture, resulting in the disruption of blood flow to the humeral head, the incidence of avascular necrosis is quite high despite treatment efforts (Fig. 15.6).

Tuberosity Fractures

Internal fixation with a screw can be satisfactorily accomplished if there is no comminution and there is adequate bone stock in the head for screw head fixation. However, often there is comminution and osteoporosis, and a nonabsorbable suture technique is preferred, incorporating a portion of the rotator cuff tendon as well (Fig. 15.3C) (8). This is the only fracture for which a superior deltoid-splitting approach is recommended. This approach is fairly straightforward and appealing, but is not without risk from denervation of the deltoid if the split extends too far distally and violates the axillary nerve. Generally, a safe zone is 4–5 cm. from the anterior lateral tip of the acromion.

Surgical Neck (Subtuberous) Fractures

These are the most commonly encountered two-part fractures, and accordingly, the ones most likely to develop a nonunion (11). Factors shown to contribute to the development of a nonunion include osteopenia, poor initial reduction, soft tissue interposition, distraction of fracture fragments, premature motion, and inadequate ORIF. Single-method fixation is commonly employed and may result in inadequate stabilization when early mobilization is attempted. With good bone stock, almost any fixation device will be successful, but when there is significant osteoporosis, a combination of IM rod and tension band wire (TBW) can achieve very secure control of these fractures with limited dissection (Fig. 15.7).

Three-Part Fractures

Three-part fractures can present the most challenging of proximal humeral fractures because they are more likely to be candidates for internal fixation than even four-part fractures, which most often require primary hemiarthroplasty. These patients are often older having osteoporotic bone, limiting the choice of fixation devices (Fig. 15.8A). Intramedullary fixation to the proximal articular segment may be tenuous because of comminution. Furthermore, screw fixation can be precarious as well, due to osteoporosis (4). This fracture will most often be amenable to some combination of techniques including an intramedullary rod in conjunc-

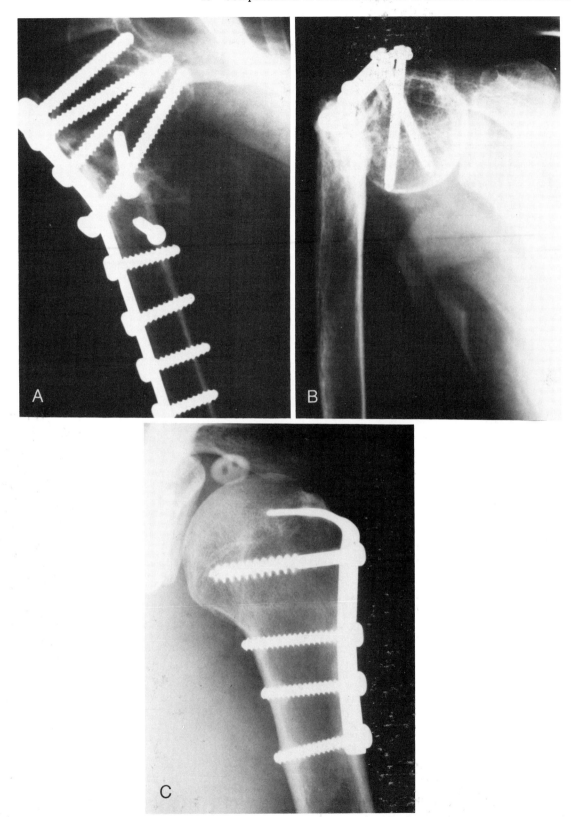

Figure 15.4. **A**, Proximal prominence of plate limits motion due to impingement. Also note penetration of head fragment by large screws. **B**, Biomechanically plates are at a disadvantage compared to axial (intramedullary) fixation. In osteoporotic patients this can result in failure. **C**, Extremely satisfying results can be achieved with plate fixation if bone is of good quality and there is minimal comminution.

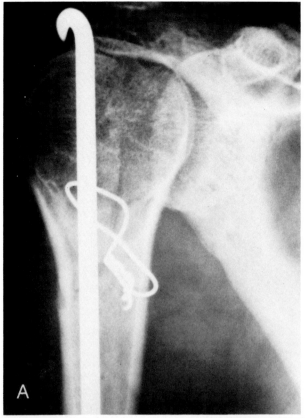

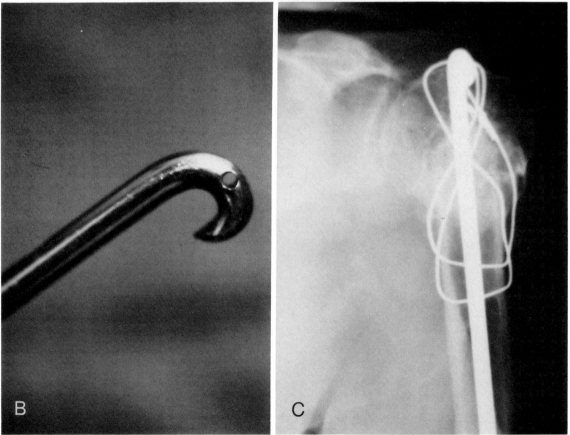

Figure 15.5. **A**, Intramedullary fixation with Rush rod frequently requires compression by wire augmentation to control rotation. Note proximal migration of rod which frequently results in impingement interfering with rehabilitation. **B** and **C**, Alteration of proximal end of device to allow passage of tension band wire and prevent migration.

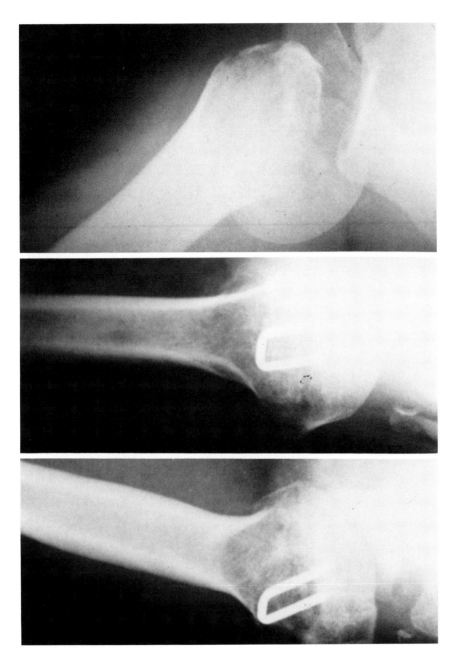

Figure 15.6. Uncommon displaced anatomic neck fracture repaired anatomically with minimal tissue dissection yet proceeds to avascular necrosis.

tion with heavy nonabsorbable suture or wire. We prefer Enders rods because of the curve that allows three-point fixation. In these fractures, the treatment of the soft tissues is often the difference between a good and poor result (Fig. 15.8B and C).

Four-Part Fractures

Internal fixation of four-part fractures, should be reserved for the rare young patient in whom there is still some significant degree of soft tissue attached to the articular segment. Even with good technique, follow-up shows an extremely high rate of avascular necrosis (Fig. 15.9) (6). Therefore, hemiarthroplasty is probably the procedure of choice.

Patient-Specific Concerns

Of the three factors to be considered in the treatment of proximal humerus fractures—the

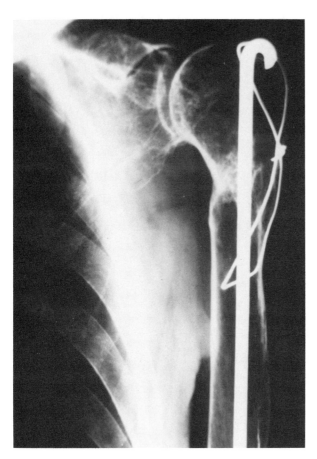

Figure 15.7. Adequate union in osteoporotic subtuberous fracture with combination of intramedullary device and tension band wire.

device, the fracture pattern, and the patient's condition—this is the one that is the most difficult for surgeons because they have so little control over it. The medical condition of the patient has been shown to have a significant effect on the quality of healing and ability to rehabilitate the injury (10).

Multitrauma patients, particularly those with closed head injuries, are prone to form extensive heterotopic bone. Special consideration must be given to the nonambulatory patient who will undoubtedly attempt to transfer following surgery, thereby subjecting the repair to higher stresses than typically experienced in an ideal situation. Such conditions may require longer hospitalization, home health care, special instructions to the family, and earlier than normal follow-up. Medically impaired patients, such as alcoholics and those with seizure disorders, may stress the repair beyond the capacity of any fixation device, or may fail to follow through with rehabilitation instructions. Adhesions and loss of shoulder motion could result.

NONSPECIFIC CONCERNS

Infection

While not unique to surgical treatment of fractures about the shoulder, infections do occur with greater frequency following internal fixation. Overall, the shoulder enjoys a better environment than the hip and knee with regard to the potential for surgical infection. These injuries are rarely compound, the area is distant from excretory orifices, circulatory compromise is extremely rare, and dependency of the extremity is unlikely. Still, when infection occurs, it is extremely serious and requires strict attention to principles of treating infected wounds. Careful isolation of the offending organism, debridement of all devitalized tissues, removal of all foreign bodies (hardware), adequate drainage and then appropriate antimicrobial chemotherapy are essential. The problem with infection in the shoulder is the extensive fibrosis that occurs with healing, which obliterates the subdeltoid and subacromial spaces and prevents recovery of mobility. Still, a stiff comfortable shoulder following infection is better than a painful weak shoulder with a draining sinus. Also, occult infection following ORIF for fracture is one of the most common causes of infection following total shoulder arthroplasty for posttraumatic arthrosis (6). Be wary of the patient who has a history of postoperative drainage, slow incisional healing, or "spitting" of sutures (Fig. 15.10).

Stiffness

Although stiffness is not a problem specific to proximal humeral fractures treated by internal fixation, the presence of the hardware may be a contributory factor in some cases (e.g., the prominent rod or plate impinging under the acromion and preventing full rehabilitation). In these circumstances, the decision to remove the hardware (after healing of the fracture has occurred) provides an opportunity to release subdeltoid and subacromial adhesions (including the often contracted coracohumeral ligament). In addition, because at that point there is no worry of displacing a tenuously fixed fracture, mobilization can be pursued aggressively. Closed manipulation under anesthesia for posttraumatic stiffness is rarely rewarding and carries with it the real risk of refracturing relatively immature bone. If stiffness is due to heterotopic bone formation, aggressive intervention should be delayed until there is evidence by bone scan that the area is no longer "active" (6).

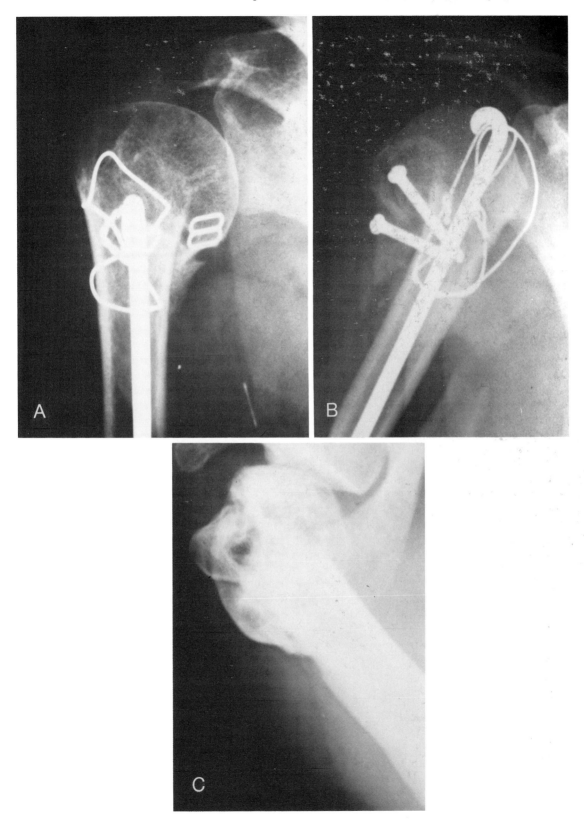

Figure 15.8.   A, Intramedullary rod (through lesser tuberosity) in combination with tension band wire gives good result in three-part fracture. **B** and **C**, Union achieved in comminuted three-part fracture using multiple fixation devices. Avascular necrosis developed following removal of hardware.

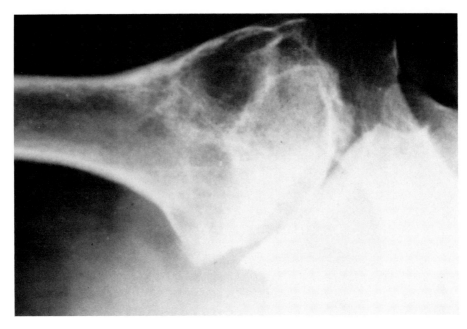

Figure 15.9.   Avascular necrosis following meticulous repair of four-part fracture in 36-year-old patient.

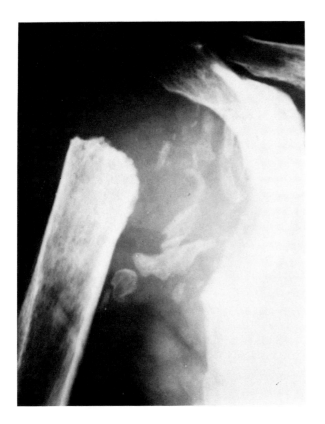

Figure 15.10.   Extensive debridement (multiple) required to control infection in unfortunate patient.

CONCLUSION

Fracture repair about the shoulder demands the same meticulous attention to technique as fractures in other parts of the body. In addition, the surgeon must combine those techniques in a way to successfully address the anatomical restrictions demanded by the shoulder. Specifically, this means that fixation must be secure enough in small bones or bone parts to allow an extreme amount of motion without interfering with the gliding mechanisms encompassing the shoulder. Clearly, this cannot be accomplished 100% of the time, and alternatives in the optimum treatment protocol will be necessary. It is not practical to treat all proximal humeral fractures in the same way. Orthopaedic surgeons must have a variety of modalities at their disposal to optimize the subsequent result. Four areas should be addressed to minimize complications: (a) the operating surgeon should have a good understanding of the strengths and weaknesses of different modalities in different situations; (b) precise knowledge of fracture characteristics (number of fragments, comminution, displacement, osteoporosis) prior to surgery is essential; (c) there should be a good operative plan that is flexible enough to allow for alterations when the intraoperative findings differ from the preoperative assessment; and, (d) one must establish and maintain a close clinical and radiographic follow-up in the healing period.

References

1. Bigliani LU. Fractures of the shoulder. In: Rockwood, Green, Bucholz, eds. Fractures. Philadelphia: JB Lippincott, 1991.
2. Codman EA. The shoulder. Malabar, Florida: Robert E. Kreiger Publishing Co., 1934.
3. DePalma AF. Surgery of the shoulder, 3rd ed. Philadelphia: JB Lippincott, 1983.
4. Flatow EL, et al. Open reduction and internal fixation of two-part displaced fractures. J Bone Joint Surg 1991;73A: 1213–1218.
5. Gibb TP, et al. The effect of capsular venting on glenohumeral laxity. CORR 1991;268:120–127.
6. Hawkins RJ, et al. The three-part fracture of the proximal part of the humerus. J Bone Joint Surg 1986;68A:1410–1414.
7. Hawkins RJ, Kiefer GN. Internal fixation techniques for proximal humeral fractures. CORR 1987;223:77–85.
8. Healy WL, et al. Nonunion of the proximal humerus surgery of the shoulder. Post, Morrey, Hawkins, eds. St. Louis: CV Mosby, 1990:59–62.
9. Jaberg H, et al. Percutaneous stabilization of unstable fractures of the humerus. J Bone Joint Surg 1992;74A:508–515.
10. Kristiansen B, Christensen SW. Plate fixation of proximal humeral fractures. Acta Orthop Scand 1986;57:320–323.
11. Lyons FA, Rockwood CA. Migration of pins used in operations on the shoulder. J Bone Joint Surg 1990;72A: 1262–1267.
12. Neer CS. Displaced proximal humeral fractures, Part I and II. J Bone Joint Surg 1970;52A:1077–1103.
13. Neer CS II. Shoulder reconstruction. Philadelphia: WB Saunders, 1990.
14. Sturznegger M, et al. Results of surgical treatment of multifragmented fractures of the humeral head. Arch Orthop Trauma Surg 1982;100:249.
15. Zuckerman JD, et al. Complications about the glenohumeral joint related to the use of screws and staples. J Bone Joint Surg 1984;66A:175–180.

16
Shoulder Infections

Thomas P. Goss

INTRODUCTION

Infections about the shoulder region, although uncommon, are capable of causing serious morbidity. Microorganisms can gain access to the area via direct inoculation, direct extension from a nearby infected focus, or hematogenous/lymphatic seeding from a distant site. Many predisposing factors have been described, but most important are: (*a*) lowered host resistance in general and/or in the local area; and (*b*) the virulence and number of microorganisms gaining access to the area. Prognosis is also dependent upon many factors, but a successful outcome is most likely if the diagnosis is made early and treatment is appropriate, expeditious, and aggressive (2, 3, 8–11).

ACUTE HEMATOGENOUS OSTEOMYELITIS

This bacteremia-induced infection of bone marrow is primarily a disorder of childhood; however, this discussion will be limited to the occurrence of acute hematogenous osteomyelitis in adults. *Staphylococcus aureus* is the most common infective organism (90%), followed by the various *Streptococcus* species, and then a variety of other organisms.

In the adult age group, acute hematogenous osteomyelitis of long bones is uncommon, and rarely seen in the humerus. An increased risk of involvement of the humerus, clavicle, and sternoclavicular joint has been reported, however, in intravenous drug abusers—infective organisms include *S. aureus, Pseudomonas, Serratia,* and others. When it does occur, the process is characterized by rapid spread along the entire length of bone and frequent implication of the adjacent joints due to the unbroken vascular connections. Large sequestra and involucra tend not to form, but extraperiosteal abscesses and

chronic sinuses may develop. Rapid and progressive cortical resorption may occur, resulting in pathologic fracture. The reparative capacity is diminished in adults, thus favoring chronicity. Chronic marrow and cortical infection as well as joint destruction are the main devastating results.

Clinical Manifestations

In the early stages, an intense local inflammatory response is present, including heat, swelling, erythema, tenderness, and muscle splinting. Pain is intense and localized to the area of involvement. If the limb is handled gently, range of motion of the glenohumeral joint is relatively normal. The synovium of the adjacent articulation, however, often responds to the inflammation with an outpouring of sterile synovial fluid. Systemic features are usually present and include chills, malaise, toxicity, high fever, and gastrointestinal (GI) disturbances.

Laboratory Tests

In the very early stages (24–36 hours) the diagnosis is made from clinical features. After 48 hours, laboratory tests give valuable information for both diagnosis and guiding management. Blood cultures should be taken before any specific treatment is begun, and will be positive in half the cases. The white blood cell count (WBC) is usually greater than $10,000/mm^3$ with a predominance of neutrophils and a shift to the left. The WBC rises as the disease progresses. The erythrocyte sedimentation rate (ESR) is usually greater than 20 mm/hour and rises over the next 7–8 days. Anemia may appear and progress rapidly. As toxicity increases, electrolyte imbalance supervenes.

X-rays

Initial x-ray findings of soft tissue swelling and obliteration of bone/muscle/fat planes are usually seen between the 2nd and 4th days. By the 5th–7th days, subperiosteal reaction is visible in most untreated, full-blown cases (Fig. 16.1). Later, destruction of the metaphysis and diaphysis occurs, with the formation of sequestra and new subperiosteal bone. Bone scanning with a short-lived isotope such as ^{99m}Tc polyphosphate will detect foci of infection long before they are seen radiographically. Accuracy is approximately 90%.

Biopsy

If the presence of osteomyelitis is strongly suspected, the area should be biopsied under sterile conditions. If septic arthritis is suspected, the joint

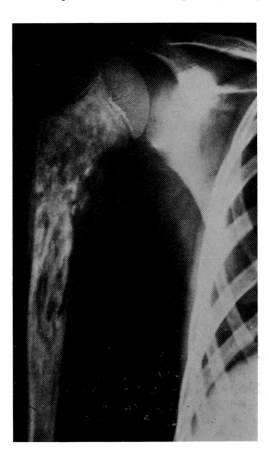

Figure 16.1. An 11-year-old child with a *Staphylococcus aureus* osteomyelitis of the humerus. The x-ray was taken 6 weeks following onset of the process. Note the large sequestrum formation. (Reproduced with permission from Post M. The shoulder: surgical and nonsurgical management. 2nd ed. Philadelphia: Lea & Febiger, 1988:141.)

should be aspirated first to avoid cross-contamination. Fluid is sent for culture and sensitivity (C/S), and if additional fluid is present, a Gram's stain is obtained.

Treatment

Treatment is governed by the stage of the disease.

EARLY

In the early stage (24–36 hours after infection), one wants to prevent intramedullary abscess formation, transcortical extension, and subperiosteal stripping. Since the most common infective organism is *S. aureus,* initial antibiotic treatment should be directed against it. The antibiotic should be given via the intravenous route and in doses sufficient to obtain high blood levels and high concentration in the local area of involvement. As soon as the bacterial diagnosis is established and sensitivities determined, the most efficacious antibiotic is ordered. Antibiotics are also continued if no organisms are discovered on the initial cultures, but the patient responds satisfactorily. Intravenous antibiotics should be administered for at least 4–6 weeks, or at least 3 weeks after there is clear clinical evidence that the infection has been controlled (normal general condition, no toxicity, normal temperature, decreasing/normal ESR, decreasing/normal WBC). The author usually favors a full 6-week course. Supportive measures include IV hydration, blood transfusions for significant anemia, and splintage to reduce pain and prevent pathologic fracture. Gentle progressive use of the shoulder and range of motion exercises are encouraged when signs of infection have resolved. If diagnosed early and appropriate treatment is instituted promptly, complete recovery is likely. If the patient does not respond favorably within the first 24–36 hours (increasing temperature, elevated or increasing ESR, elevated or increasing WBC, general condition not improving), the antibiotic is not effective and pus is forming. One must then assume the intermediate stage has been reached.

INTERMEDIATE

Usually, if treatment has been delayed 48–72 hours, or if treatment has been inadequate, pus will form, causing periosteal elevation and increased intramedullary pressure. One must then provide a site for pus drainage to reduce intramedullary pressure and prevent subperiosteal stripping. An incision is made over the point of maximal tenderness. If pus is found under the periosteum, it should be evacuated and irrigated thoroughly with saline. The cortex should be windowed, and the interior of the bone explored and curetted. Material for C/S should be obtained. The wound is closed either loosely over a drain or tightly around a closed intramedullary suction/irrigation system (CSI). Controversy exists, but the author's preference is to maintain the CSI for no more than 48–72 hours, fearing the development of a superinfection. The author also prefers to use sterile saline as an irrigant, since only mechanical debridement of the involved area is desired. Appropriate intravenous antibiotic therapy should be instituted and maintained according to the principles detailed earlier (early-stage osteomyelitis). With this regimen, the cure rate is quite high.

LATE/CHRONIC

This is usually the result of no treatment or inadequate treatment. Despite the rather guarded prognosis when this stage has been reached, at least one good all-out attempt at eradication of the infection should be considered. The goal is to rid the bone of infectious material while preserving/restoring cortical integrity and preserving the articular cartilage. This generally involves decompression/debridement of the bone and adequate drainage, often using the closed suction/irrigation technique. Occasionally, the wound is packed open and closed at a later date, or allowed to granulate in. Areas of sequestration and necrotic debris are potential sites for reactivation of the disease process and should therefore be removed. Following debridement, the humerus may need to be supported with some sort of external fixation/splintage/casting. In some patients, multiple debridements are needed before all of the necrotic bone and debris are removed and the infection obliterated. The author favors a 6-week course of appropriate intravenous antibiotics following the surgical debridement. If the infection cannot be eradicated, therapeutic options and goals change significantly, but such a discussion is beyond the scope of this chapter.

Prognosis

Prognosis is obviously dependent upon whether the bone infection can be eradicated and the degree of damage to the cortical cylinder, the adjacent joint, and the periarticular soft tissues. As always, early diagnosis and expeditious, appropriate, aggressive treatment are critical.

SEPTIC ARTHRITIS

As with acute hematogenous osteomyelitis, this discussion will be limited to the occurrence of septic arthritis in adults (1, 4–7, 13). This is a far more devastating disease and can result in rapid joint destruction. Consequently, immediate attention is extremely important. Sepsis of the glenohumeral joint is uncommon in adults and rare in young and/or healthy individuals. It may be due to direct inoculation at the time of trauma or surgery, hematogenous spread from a distant infected focus, or direct extension of an adjacent metaphyseal osteomyelitis. S. aureus is the most common infective organism by far, followed by a variety of other bacteria. A less common but preventable cause of sepsis in and about the glenohumeral joint is careless injection and aspiration procedures (Fig. 16.2). The skin in the local area should be carefully prepared, strict sterile technique should be practiced, and use of materials contained in multidose vials should be avoided.

Clinical Features

In the adult, septic arthritis is often a difficult diagnosis to make, and unfortunately, the diagnosis is usually delayed. There is a wide range of variation in the presenting signs and symptoms and septic arthritis may be difficult to differentiate from an adjacent osteomyelitis as well as many noninfectious shoulder disorders. Pain and diminished range of motion are generally present but other local features (swelling, increased skin temperature) are often absent. Signs and symptoms consistent with an acute systemic infection including an elevated temperature may or may not be present.

Laboratory Tests

Diagnosis requires a joint fluid aspiration for Gram's stain and C/S. An elevated/increasing WBC with neutrophils predominant and a shift to the left may or may not be present; however, an elevated/increasing ESR (steady and rapid rise) is always noted. Blood cultures should be obtained in all individuals with clinical manifestations and are positive in approximately 50%.

X-rays

X-rays are not reliable in making an early diagnosis. The earliest changes are limited to the soft tissues—swelling, joint distention, loss of muscle

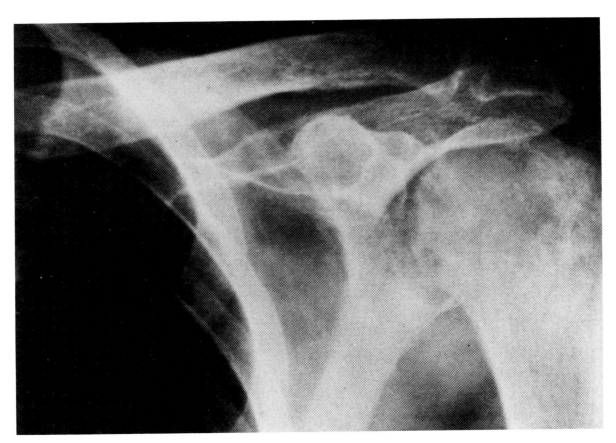

Figure 16.2. Destruction of the glenohumeral joint by a pyogenic infection that followed an intra-articular corticosteroid injection. (Repro- duced with permission from DePalma AF. Surgery of the shoulder. 3rd ed. Philadelphia: JB Lippincott, 1983:338.)

planes—and juxta-articular osteoporosis secondary to hyperemia. If due to an adjacent osteomyelitis, a destructive focus and the usual subsequent progres- sion may be seen in the metaphysis. Bone scans are also unreliable and not very helpful, although they may show some periarticular uptake. Initial bone changes (subchondral resorption and decalcification of the epiphysis and metaphysis) are usually not evi- dent before 1 week and frequently not before 10–14 days. Periarticular subchondral erosions and joint space narrowing occur still later, as do other changes consistent with joint destruction. As the process is brought under control, some remineralization occurs at the articular surface but the joint space is not restored.

Aspiration

If the diagnosis of septic arthritis is suspected, an arthrocentesis under strict sterile conditions should be performed. An immediate Gram's stain and C/S should be performed on the fluid obtained. If the Gram's stain and/or C/S are negative but other clinical indicators strongly point to septic ar- thritis, either an arthroscopic examination or a formal open arthrotomy should be performed. If frank pus is withdrawn, immediate surgical interven- tion is indicated. A WBC of the aspirate should be obtained and, if 10,000 to 100,000 cells/mm^3 are found, an active pyogenic infection is present. A sig- nificant number of individuals with septic arthritis will have negative C/S results. Occasionally, an un- usual organism is responsible, necessitating special serologic testing.

Treatment

Appropriate, expeditious, and aggressive treat- ment is the most important factor in the final func- tional capacity of the limb. Treatment includes adequate drainage, debridement, antibiotics, immo- bilization, and rehabilitation following eradication of the infective process. Once the diagnosis is made, or if clinical findings strongly point to septic arthritis, many will open the joint via a formal incision. The joint is meticulously cleared of purulent material/

debris and irrigated, the capsule left open, and the area closed over drains or closed-suction irrigation (CSI) instituted. If CSI is chosen, the author's preference is to leave this in place for no longer than 48–72 hours for fear of a superinfection, and sterile saline is used as the irrigant. Appropriate intravenous antibiotics are given for 4–6 weeks or at least 3 weeks after all indicators are normal.

Others feel that most joints can be adequately treated by needle aspiration or arthroscopic lavage as often as deemed necessary to keep pus and necrotic debris from accumulating. Arthroscopy allows direct visualization of the articular surfaces; debridement and evacuation of necrotic and inflamed tissue/lesions/fibrous accumulation; biopsy of the synovium; placement of CSI prn; and elimination of purulent material from recesses while avoiding the scarring and adhesions that occur with open procedures. If no response is noted within 48 hours or if there is any doubt about the adequacy of the needle/arthroscopic treatment, open surgical drainage should be instituted.

After fluid for Gram's stain and C/S has been obtained, an antistaphylococcal antibiotic should be started. The definitive antibiotic, however, is based upon the results of the C/S. The extremity is immobilized until the infective process is under control and pain and swelling have subsided. Gentle range of motion exercises without overstressing the joint are then begun. Once range of motion is adequate, exercises to regain strength are instituted. The patient can gradually increase the functional use of his shoulder as symptoms allow.

Prognosis

Prognosis is related to many factors but ultimately is dependent upon whether the infection can be eradicated and the degree of residual damage to the articular surfaces and the periarticular soft tissues. Early diagnosis and appropriate aggressive treatment are critical to a favorable outcome, and since the diagnosis of glenohumeral septic arthritis is difficult to make, a high index of suspicion is a necessity. Should symptomatic postsepsis degenerative joint disease occur, one's options are rather limited. Assuming that nonoperative therapeutic modalities are inadequate in alleviating pain and limiting disability, operative choices include: (a) arthrodesis; (b) prosthetic arthroplasty; and (c) humeral head excision. Arthrodesis generally provides significant pain relief and improvement in function, but the prolonged postoperative immobilization and rehabilita-

tion as well as loss of glenohumeral motion make it rather unpopular. Prosthetic arthroplasty can potentially give excellent relief of discomfort and restore near-normal function; however, one must be certain the infection has been eradicated, and even then there is the risk that the procedure will reactivate the infective process. Humeral head excision is at best a salvage procedure. If all else fails, it can be performed to provide significant pain relief, but for all intents and purposes, the patient is left with a flail shoulder.

SICKLE CELL AND SALMONELLA OSTEOMYELITIS/SEPTIC ARTHRITIS

Several inherited combinations of abnormal hemoglobin associated with significant implication of the skeletal system occur, including hemoglobin SC, hemoglobin SS (sickle cell anemia), hemoglobin SA (sickle cell trait), and hemoglobin S-thalassemia. Erythrocytes containing these abnormal hemoglobins assume a sickle shape if oxygen tension is low, and hemoglobin SS produces the most severe sickling. This results in increased blood viscosity, stasis, and finally, thrombosis and infarction. Bone involvement is common, with pain secondary to infarction. These areas of bony infarction may become secondarily infected by hematogenous seeding, and for various reasons, *Salmonella* is the most common infective organism.

Diagnosis

Pain secondary to acute bony crisis/infarction is more common, but osteomyelitis may develop insidiously and must be recognized since superimposed infection greatly increases morbidity and complicates recovery. It may be difficult to distinguish between the two. Both demonstrate fever, bone tenderness, severe acute pain, swelling, and similar radiologic bony changes (bone destruction, sequestration, involucra, and dense new bone formation).

Patients with osteomyelitis often display a spiking fever and a persistently elevated WBC. The shoulder may swell dramatically, and the patient may become toxic. Unfortunately, radiologic changes secondary to osteomyelitis are not seen for 1–3 weeks after onset, and one must differentiate these changes from those secondary to infarction. Generally, there is diffuse thickening of the bony trabeculae and endosteal sclerosis as well as narrowing of the intramedullary canal by new endosteal bone, resulting in an irregular but generalized sclerotic pattern (Fig. 16.3). Osteomyelitic lesions are often multiple and frequently involve the diaphysis of long bones. One must often rely on the results of blood and stool cultures as well as those of pathologic tissues, but all may be negative. Osteomyelitis, as opposed to infarction, will respond to appropriate antibiotic treatment.

Treatment

Treatment is usually conservative, consisting of appropriate antibiotic therapy. Surgery is performed only for drainage of obvious localized abscesses, followed by immediate closure or secondary closure after a short period. If appropriate antibiotics fail to control the process, one must consider surgical decompression of the involved bone. If the bone is significantly infarcted and multiple sites of osteomyelitis are present, surgery may be fruitless. If the adjacent joint is involved, prompt and adequate debridement, irrigation, and drainage, either by aspi-

ration, arthroscopic, or open techniques, is indicated as well as appropriate antibiotic treatment.

TUBERCULOSIS

Although uncommon, the incidence of skeletal tuberculosis in the United States may be rising. Many mycobacteria are capable of implicating the skeletal system, but *Mycobacterium* tuberculosis is the most common. Skeletal tuberculosis occurs most frequently during the first three decades of life, but this discussion will deal only with the occurrence in skeletally mature individuals. Spread is usually via the hematogenous route but occasionally via the lymphatics. There is a predilection for the metaphyseal/epiphyseal portion of the major bones, including the proximal humerus, and weightbearing joints are more commonly involved. The essential lesion in most patients is a combination of osteomyelitis and septic arthritis. The joint space is invaded either by the hematogenous route or from an infected focus

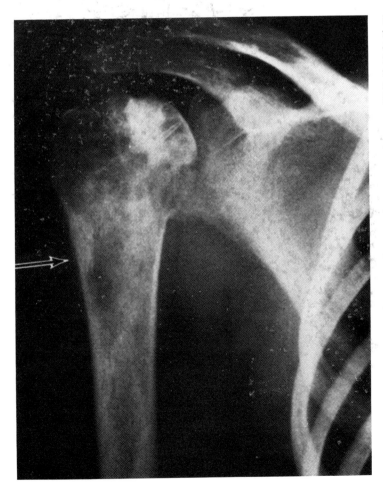

Figure 16.3. A 24-year-old female with sickle cell disease who developed a *Salmonella* osteomyelitis and septic arthritis. Note the periosteal reaction changes (*arrow*) and the osteonecrotic areas in the humeral head. (Reproduced with permission from Post M. The shoulder: surgical and nonsurgical management. 2nd ed. Philadelphia: Lea & Febiger, 1988:151.)

within the adjacent epiphysis or metaphysis, especially if the metaphysis lies partially within the joint cavity, as is the case with the proximal humerus. Bacilli lodge at the ends of bone or in the synovium and produce an inflammatory granulation tissue, which is highly destructive. As destruction progresses, caseation and liquefaction result, creating abscesses that contain necrotic and caseous debris, WBCs, and bacilli. If the lesion becomes quiescent and inactive, the abscesses become fibrotic, contract, and calcify. In more aggressive lesions, paraosseous cold abscesses and soft tissue necrosis may develop, giving rise to draining sinuses with ulceration, liquefaction, and even secondary infection.

Intra-articularly, the development of synovial lesions and a pannus of granulation tissue result in hyperemia and destruction of the hyaline cartilage. Peripheral erosion occurs first, followed by a slow, progressive destruction of the entire joint surface as well as destruction of the underlying subchondral and cancellous bone, generalized demineralization,

caseation, necrosis, and abscess formation (Fig. 16.4). In time, fibrous tissue forms, resulting in joint stiffness. If the disease is overcome, reactive fibrosis develops, and the reparative process begins. Functional capacity of the extremity is then dependent upon the degree of residual bone, joint, and periarticular soft tissue damage. Most involved joints show at least some stiffness and diminished range of motion, although bony ankylosis is rare.

Clinical Features

Skeletal tuberculosis usually follows an indolent, chronic, and insidious course. Occasionally, however, the disease is fulminant with fever, toxicity, severe pain, local erythema/redness, local swelling, and an elevated WBC. There is usually a sustained increased temperature, as well as some swelling and diminished functional capacity of the involved joint/limb.

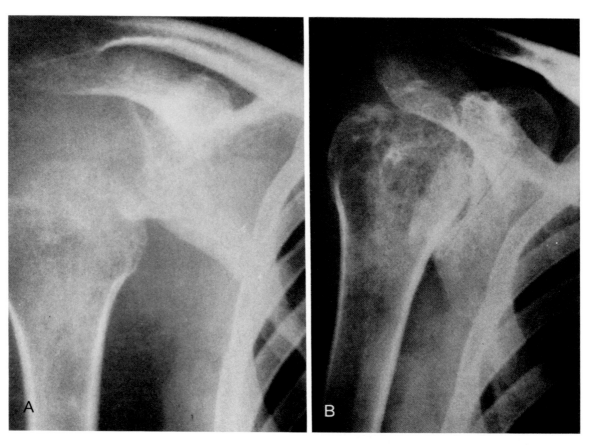

Figure 16.4. Tuberculosis of the glenohumeral joint. **A**, The process is very active. Note the demineralization of the bones, destruction of the articular surfaces, and dislocation of the joint. **B**, Same joint 8 months later, after immobilization and antitubercular therapy. There is complete destruction of the articular surfaces. The joint was eventually fused. (Reproduced with permission from DePalma AF. Surgery of the shoulder. 3rd ed. Philadelphia: JB Lippincott, 1983:343.)

Diagnosis

A positive diagnosis can only be made by a culture or guinea pig inoculation of the aspirated joint fluid or fluid obtained from the infected area. One may need to biopsy the involved tissues (bone or synovium).

Treatment

In the early stages, appropriate chemotherapy and immobilization of the involved area controls most cases, salvages most joints, and precludes surgical intervention. In late cases, synovectomy may be required as well as debridement/removal of necrotic debris/tissue. Surgical arthrodesis of the involved articulation is indicated if comfortable, useful function cannot be attained. Any surgery should be deferred until the patient has received a 2–3-month course of chemotherapy. Chemotherapy includes isoniazid, ethambutol, and 2 months of streptomycin. However, if the bacterium is susceptible to both isoniazid and ethambutol, one may delete the streptomycin. Chemotherapy should be continued for at least 24 months. Rifampin is also an effective drug for skeletal tuberculosis.

ELECTIVE SURGERY—PROPHYLAXIS

Preventing infection must be foremost in the planning and implementation of all invasive diagnostic and therapeutic shoulder procedures. Fortunately, postoperative infection in the normal individual is uncommon—less than 5% in elective cases performed without prophylactic antibiotic coverage.

Basic Principles

Patients with active or recent infection should not be operated on electively. Careful and thorough preparation of the skin in the operative area prior to admission and just before the actual incision is essential. Strict attention to sterile technique during the draping and throughout the surgical procedure should be observed. Surgery should include limited dissection, gentle handling of the tissues, avoidance of prolonged traction, frequent irrigation to prevent desiccation, and meticulous hemostasis. Operative time should be minimized. Large and/or particularly bloody wounds should be drained but not for more than 24–36 hours. The postoperative dressing should be changed using sterile technique until the superficial tissues have healed and the wound is dry.

Prophylactic Antibiotics

Administration of prophylactic antibiotics in prosthetic and fracture implant surgery is accepted because of the extent of the tissue manipulation involved, the insertion of foreign material, the significant sequelae of postoperative sepsis, and the marked decrease in the occurrence of postoperative infection associated with their use. Controversy exists over the role of prophylactic antibiosis in clean, elective soft tissue surgery where the infection rate is low. However, the author and others advocate the use of cefazolin 30 minutes prior to the procedure and every 8 hours for 24 hours postoperatively in this setting (exceptions: arthroscopic and very minor open surgery).

Patients who have undergone shoulder prosthetic replacement surgery should also receive prophylactic antibiotic coverage whenever they develop a bacterial illness that can cause septicemia or whenever they are to undergo a surgical or dental procedure that can release large numbers of bacteria into their bloodstream. The particular antibiotic(s), its dosage, and the duration of therapy are dependent upon the particular clinical situation.

INFECTIONS FOLLOWING ELECTIVE SURGERY

These infections are uncommon and classified as either superficial or deep to the fascia layer.

Superficial Infection

Clinical signs include erythema, warmth, induration, direct tenderness, pain-free motion, mild fever, lymphangitis, and regional adenopathy. Laboratory studies and x-rays/scans are usually not helpful. Treatment includes immobilization, antibiotics, and local moist heat. The most common organisms are *Staphylococcus* and *Streptococcus*. Consequently, a first-generation cephalosporin or a penicillinase-resistant penicillin should be prescribed, and oral administration is usually sufficient. If marked improvement is not noted within 24–36 hours, however, intravenous antibiosis is begun. If still no improvement occurs, one must consider either the presence of an infected focus/abscess, in which case surgical exploration/evacuation is necessary, or a deep infection. Progressive range of motion and gradual increase in functional use of the shoulder is allowed as symptoms resolve.

Deep Infection

Most of these infections occur within the first 2 weeks postoperatively, especially after soft tissue procedures. Following internal fixation and prosthetic surgery, however, delayed infections may develop several months to 2 years postoperatively. Patients who have received a surgical implant are always at some risk for hematogenous seeding (12). *Staphylococcus* is the most common organism, but anaerobic Gram-negative and mixed infections are increasing in frequency. Regardless of the time of presentation, these infections are always serious, demand immediate attention, and may become chronic (Fig. 16.5).

Clinical signs and symptoms include spiking fevers, chills, painful motion, increasing shoulder pain, swelling, warmth, erythema, cellulitis, and serous drainage from the incision. Depending upon the virulence of the organisms, sepsis after fracture fixation and joint replacement surgery may follow an acute fulminant course, or the process may be insidious and indolent with mild signs and symptoms. Failure to diagnose and treat aggressively can lead to

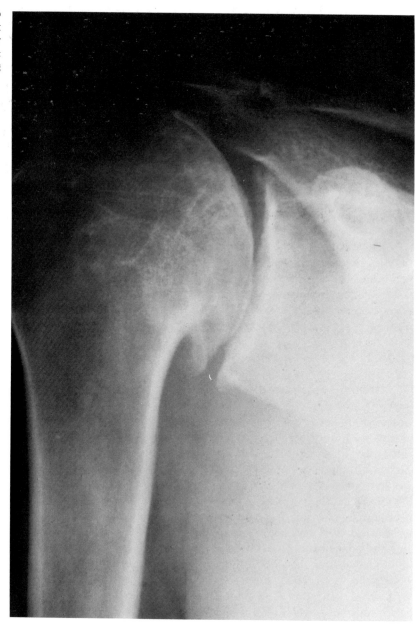

Figure 16.5. A 25-year-old male who developed an infection of the glenohumeral joint following surgery for a recurrent anteriorly disocating shoulder. Note the destruction of the articular surfaces and joint space narrowing 6 years following the infection.

chronicity with draining sinuses, an infected nonunion, prosthetic loosening, and severe bone stock destruction.

Diagnostic tests (hematologic and radiologic) all have limitations and may be incorrect. Definitive diagnosis depends upon a positive C/S of tissue or fluid, and this may be difficult with standard C/S techniques. One may need to infer the diagnosis from histologic examination of the involved tissues. Special laboratory techniques may be used to isolate pathogenic organisms.

TREATMENT FOLLOWING SOFT TISSUE PROCEDURES

One should perform a formal surgical exploration/debridement under anesthesia. The wound should be opened carefully until purulence is encountered. A specimen for Gram's stain and C/S is taken before irrigation is performed. All necrotic material should be debrided and the wound irrigated copiously. The joint capsule should be inspected, and a needle aspirate should be performed. If an infection is encountered, the joint should be irrigated and debrided. Whatever surgical repair is present should be protected as much as possible, but adequate exposure, debridement, and drainage are tantamount. Depending upon the nature of the infection, the appearance of the tissues, and one's own preference, the wound may be closed tightly over a CSI system, loosely over drains, or packed open and allowed to heal secondarily or closed at a later date. Initial antibiotic treatment is based upon the intraoperative Gram's stain and should be effective against *Staphylococcus*. The definitive agent, however, is based upon the final C/S result and should be given parenterally for 4–6 weeks, or at least 3 weeks after all indicators are normal. Shoulder rehabilitation is begun when clinical signs of infection have subsided.

TREATMENT FOLLOWING INTERNAL FIXATION OF FRACTURES

These demand immediate surgical attention. The wound should be reopened and specimens taken for Gram's stain and C/S. All necrotic tissue and devascularized bone should be meticulously removed. The wound should be irrigated copiously. The fracture reduction and stabilization should be examined. If secure and providing rigid fixation, the implant may be retained and covered with a layer of soft tissue. If the fixation is insecure or felt to predispose to continuing infection, the implant should be removed, the fragments repositioned, a new implant or external fixation/support (a safer alternative) ap-

plied for stability, and the fracture site covered with a layer of soft tissue. The wound may be closed tightly over a CSI system, closed loosely over drains, or packed open and allowed to heal secondarily or closed at a later date, depending upon the nature of the infection, the appearance of the tissues, and the surgeon's preference. Since the fracture itself may be infected, 6 weeks of appropriate intravenous antibiotic therapy is advisable. Once the infection has been eradicated, treatment is dictated by the nature of the fracture itself.

TREATMENT FOLLOWING PROSTHETIC IMPLANTATION (HEMIARTHROPLASTY OR TOTAL SHOULDER REPLACEMENT)

All infected tissue should be debrided and the wound thoroughly irrigated. If the infection is relatively acute and contained and the prosthesis is well fixed, it can be retained. However, this may be unsuccessful and may allow the development of a chronic infection with severe bone stock destruction, preventing future prosthetic reimplantation. If the prosthesis is loose or is felt to predispose to continuing infection, it (and the cement if present) should be removed. Several therapeutic options are then available, but there is very little in the shoulder literature to provide guidance. Choices include: (*a*) revision of the arthroplasty—one-stage, two-stage with a short interval between extraction and reimplantation, and two-stage with a long interval between extraction and reimplantation; (*b*) arthrodesis; and (*c*) acceptance of the resection arthroplasty (Fig. 16.6).

It is beyond the scope of this discussion to describe the complex decision-making process required to choose the best option and the details of the various procedures; however, a few general statements can be made. The therapeutic decision is based upon the type of infection and microorganisms present, the status of the glenohumeral bone stock and periarticular soft tissues, the overall medical status and age of the patient, and the experience of the attending surgeon. Prosthetic revision surgery offers the patient his best chance for as normal a shoulder as possible, but also poses the greatest risk of persistence or reactivation of the infection. Arthrodesis can be especially difficult to achieve in this setting, requires prolonged postoperative immobilization and rehabilitation, and eliminates glenohumeral range of motion. At the same time, however, it can help to eradicate the infection, provide significant pain relief, and improve overall shoulder function. Resection arthroplasty results in a relatively comfortable shoulder and usually either eradicates the

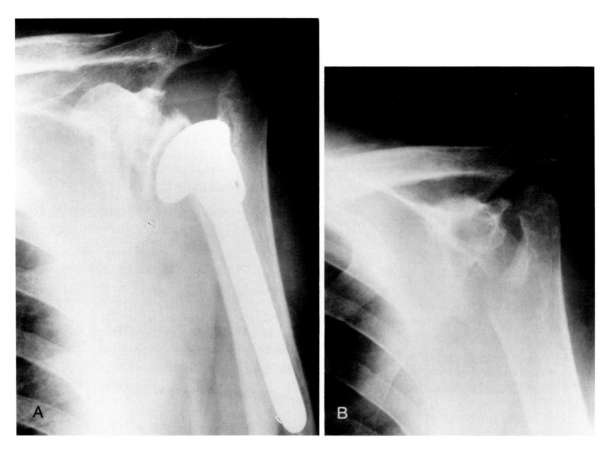

Figure 16.6. **A**, A 70-year-old male who developed an intra-articular *Staphylococcus epidermidis* infection following a total shoulder replacement. Note the displacement of the prosthetic components and bone stock destruction. **B**, X-ray appearance of the shoulder area following removal of the prosthetic components and debridement of the articulation.

infection or brings it under control, but leaves the individual with an essentially flail articulation.

If the prosthetic components are simply removed at the time of the original exploration/debridement, the wound may be closed tightly over a CSI system, loosely over drains, or packed open and allowed to heal secondarily or closed at a later date, depending upon the nature of the infection, the appearance of the tissues, and one's own preference. Six weeks of parenteral antibiotics based upon the intraoperative C/S are prescribed.

OPEN FRACTURES

These injuries are treated as an incipient infection. Further contamination should be prevented by covering the wound with a dry or saline-soaked sterile dressing, and the shoulder immobilized. Protruding bone ends should not be drawn back into the wound since this only introduces additional filth and bacteria into the soft tissues where it is much more difficult to locate and remove. As much as possible, the wound should be meticulously cleaned and debrided of all foreign material and devascularized tissue (bone and soft tissues) in the operating room and then copiously irrigated (preferably with a pulsatile lavage) in a systematic manner.

The fracture should be stabilized. This may require only immobilization of the extremity in a sling/splint arrangement. External fixation is an option in certain situations. Internal fixation is also a consideration but should be used with caution in an open wound. If it is used, foreign material should be kept to a minimum and used only to prevent unacceptable displacement of fracture fragments until definitive fixation in a clean area with intact soft tissues can be performed. "Clean wounds" may be closed loosely over drains. "Dirty wounds" should be packed open and reinspected/debrided/irrigated daily in the operating room until "clean" and ready for closure. Exposed bone, tendon, and neurovascular structures should be covered with viable soft tissue as soon as possible but not until the area is clean. Plastic surgery and sophisticated temporary/definitive coverage techniques may be required.

Patients should receive appropriate tetanus prophylaxis. Those with "clean" wounds should be started on an intravenous antibiotic effective against Gram-positive organisms, especially *Staphylococcus.* Those with "dirty" wounds should receive intravenous antibiotic coverage effective against Gram-positive organisms, including *Staphylococcus,* and as wide a spectrum of Gram-negative organisms as possible. An intraoperative C/S should be taken and antibiotic therapy adjusted accordingly. Intravenous antibiotic therapy should be continued for at least 48 hours after soft tissue coverage of the fracture has been provided. The extremity is immobilized until it is felt that the risk of infection has passed. Treatment is then dictated by the nature of the fracture itself.

References

1. Armbuster TG, Slivka J, Resnick D, Goergen TG, Weisman M, Master R. Extraarticular manifestations of septic arthritis of the glenohumeral joint. Am J Roentgenol 1977; 129:667–672.

2. Bateman JE. The shoulder and neck. Philadelphia: WB Saunders, 1972.

3. DePalma AF. Surgery of the shoulder. 3rd ed. Philadelphia: JB Lippincott, 1983.

4. Gelberman RH, Menon J, Austerlitz MS, Weisman MH. Pyogenic arthritis of the shoulder in adults. J Bone Joint Surg [Am] 1980;62A:550–553.

5. Kelly PJ, Coventry MB, Martin WJ. Bacterial arthritis of the shoulder. Mayo Clin Proc 1965;40:695–699.

6. Leslie BM, Harris JM, Driscoll D. Septic arthritis of the shoulder in adults. J Bone Joint Surg [Am] 1989; 71A:1516–1522.

7. Master R, Weisman MH, Armbuster TG, Slivka J, Resnick D, Goergen TG. Septic arthritis of the glenohumeral joint: unique clinical and radiographic features and a favorable outcome. Arthritis Rheum 1977;20:1500–1506.

8. Neer CS. Shoulder reconstruction. Philadelphia: WB Saunders, 1990.

9. Post M. The shoulder: surgical and nonsurgical management. 2nd ed. Philadelphia: Lea & Febiger, 1988.

10. Rockwood CA, Matsen FA, eds. The shoulder. Philadelphia: WB Saunders, 1990.

11. Rowe CR, ed. The shoulder. New York: Churchill Livingstone, 1988.

12. Stinchfield FE, Bigliani LU, Nev HC, Coss TP, Foster CR. Late hematogenous infection of total joint replacement. J Bone Joint Surg [Am] 1980;62A:1345–1350.

13. Toby EB, Webb LX, Voytek A, Grstina AG. Septic arthritis of the shoulder. Orthopaedic Transactions 1987;11:230.

17
Isolated Nerve Injuries about the Shoulder

Stephen J. McIlveen and Xavier A. Duralde

INTRODUCTION

Isolated nerve injuries about the shoulder can accompany a variety of types and degrees of trauma about the shoulder girdle. Injuries about the shoulder involving the acromioclavicular joint and rotator cuff as well as those that result in glenohumeral instability and subacromial impingement are more common and more widely recognized entities. But injuries involving the peripheral nerves about the shoulder are less common and may go undetected by the clinician. Injuries to the axillary, suprascapular, musculotendinous, long thoracic, and spinal accessory nerves will produce distinct clinical syndromes (44, 83, 86, 87, 91). The diagnosis of these nerve lesions can be difficult due to their often vague presentation. Repeat physical examination and electromyographic evaluation play an essential role in the assessment and follow-up of isolated nerve injuries about the shoulder (58). Greater awareness of these nerve lesions could lead to prompt recognition and treatment of these conditions. Controversy still exists regarding the management and prognosis of these injuries (8, 17, 24, 50, 88, 100). Some authors have recommended observation, citing an overall favorable prognosis (17, 88), whereas others advocate early surgery (16, 58, 74).

AXILLARY NERVE

Anatomy

The axillary nerve (circumflex nerve) is comprised of fibers from the 5th and 6th cervical nerve roots and takes its origin from the posterior cord of the brachial plexus near the level of the coracoid process and passes anterior to the subscapularis muscle and posterior to the axillary artery. The nerve courses posteriorly and inferiorly to the lower border of the subscapularis and enters the quadrilateral space. (Fig. 17.1)

It maintains a close anatomic relationship to the inferior capsule. This makes it potentially susceptible to direct traumatic injury during glenohumeral dislocations or surgical procedures involving the inferior joint capsule (Fig. 17.2). Also, compression injuries may occur such as with the use of crutches. As it passes through the quadrilateral space accompanied by the posterior humeral circumflex artery, it supplies branches to the inferior aspect of the capsule of the glenohumeral joint. The axillary nerve then divides into an anterior and posterior branch, which supplies the anterior and posterior portions of the deltoid muscle (Fig. 17.3). A small branch arises from the posterior branch, innervating the teres minor and posterior deltoid and supplies the skin overlying the deltoid. The posterior branch terminates as the lateral brachial cutaneous nerve of the arm. The anterior branch continues to wind around the surgical neck of the humerus, under the deltoid and extends to the anterior border of the deltoid, which it supplies. The anterior branch also provides a few small cutaneous branches to the skin overlying the deltoid.

Etiology and Incidence

Axillary nerve palsy is commonly caused by trauma about the shoulder. It is most often seen in association with surgical neck fractures, glenohumeral dislocation, or surgical procedures on the shoulder. Injuries to the axillary nerve may be isolated or occur in association with lesions of other peripheral nerves about the shoulder girdle (50).

Blunt trauma to the anterior aspect of the shoulder without fracture or dislocation occurs quite often in certain athletic activities such as football, wrestling, and gymnastics, resulting in axillary

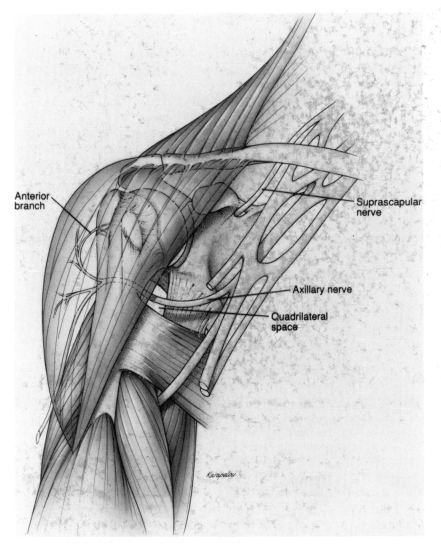

Anterior
branch

Suprascapular
nerve

Axillary nerve

Quadrilateral
space

Karpalov

Figure 17.1. The axillary nerve (circumflex nerve) takes its origin from the posterior cord of the brachial plexus near the level of the coracoid process and passes anteriorly to the subscapularis muscle, and then courses posteriorly and inferiorly to the lower border of the subscapularis and enters the quadrilateral space.

nerve injury (7). Berry and Brill (8) reported an axillary nerve palsy that occurred in a boxer after a match. In their series (8) of axillary nerve palsy following blunt trauma to the shoulder region, the mechanism of the palsy injury appeared to involve a stretch injury. The prognosis for recovery from this injury is worse than with axillary nerve palsy due to shoulder dislocation or humeral fracture (8, 17, 87). The formation of a hematoma and subsequent fibrous adhesions following blunt trauma to the axilla region may also impinge upon the nerve and cause neuropathy (61). The incidence of injury to the axillary nerve following acute anterior dislocation is significant, with a range reported in the literature from 9–18% (17, 20, 40, 54, 69, 72, 94). Pasila (72) reviewed 23 patients with shoulder dislocations and noted plexus lesions in 12% and a lesion of the axillary nerve in 9%. Blom and Dahlback (17) ex-

amined 73 patients using electromyographic studies and found a variety of nerve injuries in 35% of their cases overall, and a lesion of the axillary nerve in 18%. They also described spontaneous and satisfactory recovery over a 3–5-month period, and that surgical exploration was not indicated as recovery was satisfactory even in those patients who presented with complete initial paralysis and denervation (17). Leffer and Seddon (50) in their series found clinical evidence of axillary nerve injury in 13 patients associated with dislocation or fracture of the surgical neck of the humerus, in addition to a larger group of 31 patients with infraclavicular brachial plexus lesions. They reported that none of the patients with isolated axillary palsy achieved full recovery and that those with an associated posterior cord lesion had a better prognosis. Sunderland (88), however, stated that most cases of

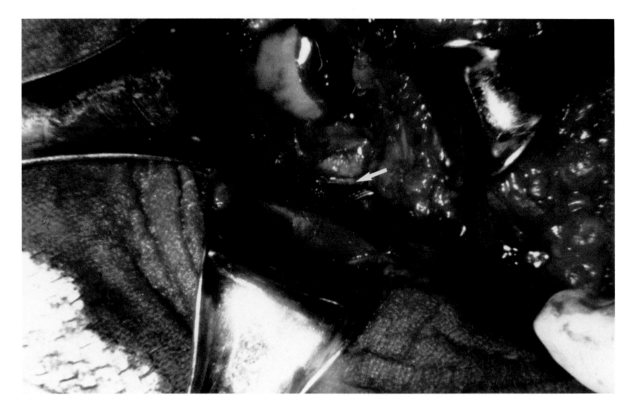

Figure 17.2. This intraoperative photo taken in a patient undergoing a total shoulder replacement demonstrates the close anatomic relationship of the axillary nerve (*white arrow*) to both the inferior capsule and the inferior aspect of the glenoid.

axillary nerve palsy recover spontaneously, although there may be a delay in recovery up to 12 months.

Inferior glenohumeral dislocation, or luxatio erecta, is a rare dislocation, usually caused by a hyperabduction injury to the arm. Mallon (55), et al., in their review of the literature found 80 cases of luxatio erecta, and in those cases in which the neurologic status was mentioned, 47 (59%) had some degree of nerve injury, and that the axillary nerve was most commonly injured. Follow-up of the nerve injuries was described in only 14 cases, and the recovery time varied from 2 weeks to 6 months. Neviaser (69), et al., in their series of patients with rupture of the rotator cuff following primary anterior dislocation of the shoulder, found the incidence of injury to the axillary nerve to be 7.8%.

In the series reported by Neer and McIlveen (66) of 61 four-part fractures-dislocations treated by prosthetic replacement, there were 14 patients with axillary nerve palsy, of which 12 recovered spontaneously. In this type of injury, the fractures are repaired if surgically indicated to obtain stability, and the rotator cuff is repaired if torn without waiting for recovery of axillary nerve function. Improvement of the rotator cuff and fulcrum action of the glenohu-

meral joint seems to aid the recovery of the axillary nerve (67). Spontaneous recovery of the axillary nerve following fracture or dislocation usually occurs within 6–9 months (67).

Axillary neuropathy may also occur as a result of chronic nerve entrapment. Cahill and Palmer (18) and others (60) have described the "quadrilateral space syndrome," which is an uncommon syndrome caused by entrapment of the axillary nerve and compression of the posterior humeral circumflex artery. There is usually no history of trauma, and the onset of symptoms is often insidious. Forward elevation and/or abduction and external rotation of the humerus aggravate the patient's symptoms, and discrete point tenderness is found posteriorly in the quadrilateral space. A subclavian arteriogram is needed to confirm the diagnosis. If positive, it will reveal occlusion of the posterior humeral circumflex artery with the arm in abduction and external rotation. Surgical decompression via the posterior approach may be considered for those patients with sufficient symptoms, localized tenderness over the quadrilateral space, and a positive subclavian arteriogram. Successful results with surgical decompression have been reported (18, 60).

Axillary nerve injury is a recognized and documented complication of the inferior capsular shift procedure (53, 64), and other procedures involving anterior shoulder repair (80). In 1980, Neer and Foster (64) discussed the concept of multidirectional instability of the shoulder and described the inferior capsular shift procedure. They reported three axillary neuropraxias in the first 40 patients despite care taken to protect the axillary nerve with blunt retractors. Bryan (14), et al., also reemphasized the proximity of the axillary nerve beneath the inferior capsule, which is the area of primary surgical attention in the inferior capsular shift procedure. There is an intimate relationship between the axillary nerve and the subscapularis, and because of its prominence within the operative field and its proximity to the inferior capsule, the axillary nerve is at risk for injury during the capsular shift procedure. The axillary nerve is in potential danger when the inferior flap is

being detached from the inferior humeral neck. By externally rotating the humerus, better capsular exposure is obtained and the nerve is relaxed. General retraction by a flat retractor such as a Darrach will further protect the nerve. Neer (67) has pointed out that with anterior approaches to the glenohumeral joint, the axillary nerve is placed in peril if the arm is held in abduction (19) and internal rotation, whereas having the arm at the side and in external rotation is a safer position. Superior translation of the inferior flap to eliminate the pouch compresses the axillary nerve slightly between the humerus and long head of the triceps insertion, but produces entrapment in cadaveric subjects (53).

Procedures utilizing the posterior exposure of the capsule for repair also poses danger to the axillary nerve. In the posterior approach it is important to find the interval between the infraspinatus muscle, which is supplied by the suprascapular nerve

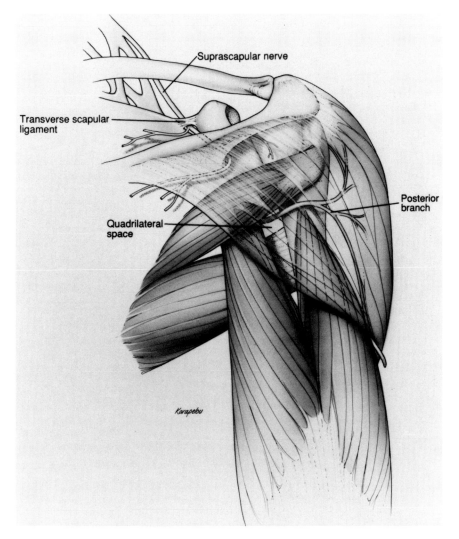

Figure 17.3. After the axillary nerve passes through the quadrilateral space, it divides into an anterior and posterior branch which supplies anterior and posterior portions of the deltoid muscle. A branch also arises from the posterior branch and innervates the teres minor and posterior deltoid, as well as supplying a skin overlying the deltoid.

from above, and the teres minor, which is supplied by the axillary nerve from below. It is a safe interval to enter the joint (67). Care must be taken during exposure of the posterior inferior capsule because the nerve is adjacent to the capsule on the inferior margin of the teres minor. The dissection of the capsule should be close to the humeral neck to avoid injury.

The anterior acromioplasty as described by Neer (63, 65) emphasizes preservation of the deltoid muscle origin, obtaining adequate exposure of the rotator cuff and decompression of impingement. Abbott (1) et al., in their 1949 review of surgical ex-

posures to the shoulder joint, warned that an extended anterior deltoid-splitting incision ran the risk of possible axillary nerve injury. In performing a deltoid-splitting approach, it is essential to know the exact location of the axillary nerve in the deltoid muscle. The length of the split of the deltoid must be limited to 5.0 cm from the acromion, and a stay suture is placed at the lower end of the split to prevent injury to the anterior branch of the axillary nerve by muscle retraction (67) (Fig. 17.4). Bryan (14) et al., in their study of cadaveric dissections of the axillary nerve, found that the nerve was endangered both in the anterolateral and anterior deltoid-splitting ap-

Figure 17.4. An intraoperative photo demonstrating the deltoid splitting approach to allow decompression of the impingement lesion, as well as adequate exposure of the rotator cuff. The length of the split of the deltoid must be limited to 5.0 cm from the acromion, and a stay suture is placed at the lower end of the split to prevent injury to the anterior branch of the axillary nerve by muscle retraction.

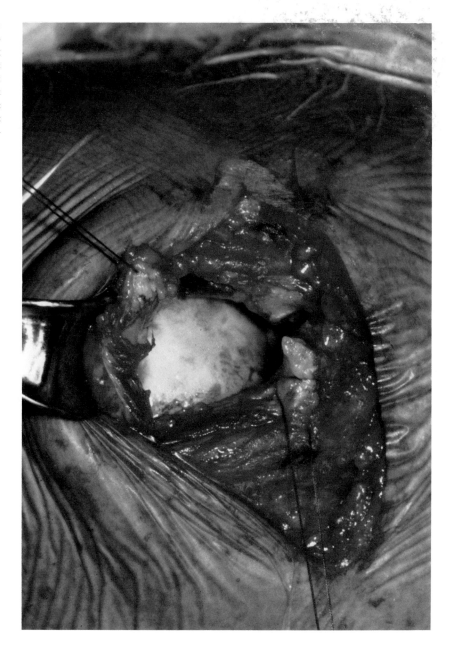

proaches. Furthermore, the more anterior incision had less inferior extensibility because the axillary nerve actually crosses superiorly as it nears its termination (14).

The relationship of the standard posterior shoulder arthroscopic stab wound 3–5 cm inferior to the acromial border and the main trunk of the axillary nerve has definite clinical importance. Bryan (14) et al. found that the arthroscopic trocar was often in close proximity to the axillary nerve, with an average perpendicular distance of 1.89 cm (range

0.5–4.0 cm) from the trocar to the main trunk of the nerve. They advised avoiding moving the posterior entry site and portal tract inferiorly to avoid injury.

Clinical Presentation

Axillary nerve compression will characteristically cause atrophy and weakness of the deltoid muscle. Clinical examination will reveal weakness of shoulder abduction and forward elevation (Fig. 17.5A and B). Altered sensation or sensory loss over-

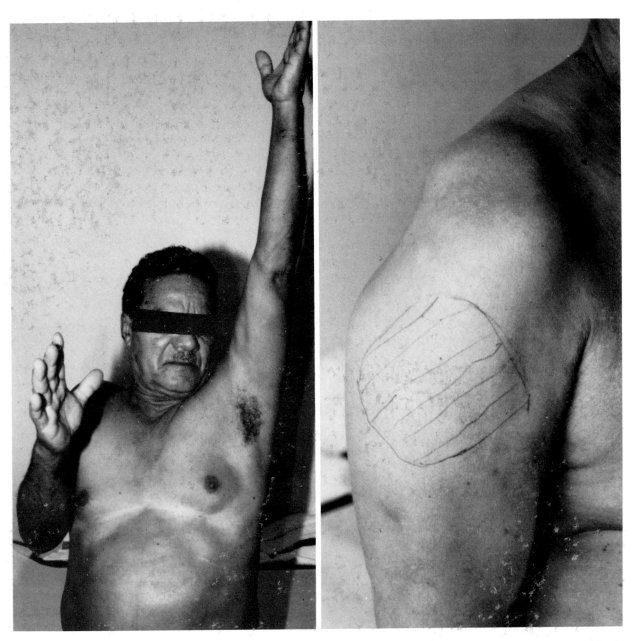

Figure 17.5. A, This patient with axillary neuropathy demonstrates weakness of active forward elevation. **B**, He also demonstrates atrophy of the deltoid muscle and altered sensation in the skin overlying the deltoid muscle, as indicated by the marked area.

lying the deltoid muscle may or may not be present (8, 59), as sensation is often intact and normal in the presence of complete deltoid paralysis (8). Weakness of the teres minor may be difficult to assess accurately due to the infraspinatus muscle, which is a more powerful external rotator (Fig. 17.6A and B).

Diagnosis

The differential diagnosis in a patient with a history of injury to the shoulder in whom axillary neuropathy is suspected includes lesions of the posterior cord of the brachial plexus or a more proximal root lesion. The thoracodorsal nerve arises proximal to the axillary nerve, and manual testing of the latismus dorsi muscle along with muscles innervated by the radial nerve helps to localize the lesion (61). Paralysis localized to the deltoid muscle without involvement of the adjacent muscles of C5 segmental origin tends to exclude a more proximal or root lesion (8). A spontaneous or sudden onset of a painful paralysis of the deltoid and adjacent muscles is a feature of neurologic amyotrophy or localized shoulder neuritis (8, 31). In this condition, the paralysis is isolated to the deltoid muscle in about 50% of patients, and in the remainder there is additional involvement of the serratus anterior, spinati, and other muscles. The onset of neurologic amyotrophy is spontaneous and is not a consideration in patients who have had trauma to the shoulder (8, 31).

Treatment

An EMG evaluation will confirm the diagnosis and indicate whether the injury to the axillary nerve is complete or incomplete. When the axillary nerve lesion has been demonstrated to be incomplete by both clinical examination and EMG testing, the prognosis is favorable, and gradual improvement is expected. Bateman (7) recommended splinting the shoulder in a position of partial abduction, and suggested that daily electrical stimulation and daily passive range of motion exercises be performed to prevent stiffness of the glenohumeral joint. When the axillary nerve lesion is complete by both clinical and electromyographic criteria, the patient should be reevaluated at monthly intervals. The pace of recovery of the axillary nerve is such that there should be some recovery noted between the 3rd and 4th month after this onset (8). If there is no evidence of clinical recovery at 2–4 months and no evidence of reinnervation on follow-up EMG studies by the 4th

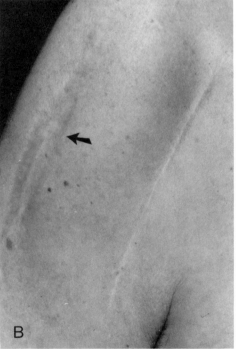

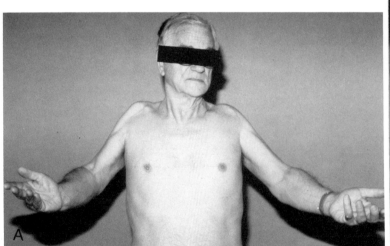

Figure 17.6. **A,** This patient demonstrates bilateral weakness of active forward elevation due to complete axillary nerve neuropathy present in both shoulders. The axillary nerve injuries were due to previous surgical incision and drainage of deltoid abscesses performed via a middle deltoid muscle-splitting approach performed as a child. **B,** A closer view (*arrow*).

month after onset, surgical exploration should be considered with neurolysis or possible nerve grafting (7, 8, 61) (Figs. 17.7, 17.8, and 17.9).

SUPRASCAPULAR NERVE INJURY

Anatomy

The suprascapular nerve originates from the upper trunk of the brachial plexus and is formed from the spinal roots of C5 and C6, with a variable contribution from the C4 nerve root. It branches from the upper trunk of the brachial plexus at Erb's point and runs laterally, crossing the posterior triangle of the neck, parallel and deep to the omohyoid muscle and deep to the trapezius muscle. The nerve then passes through the suprascapular notch of the scapula, which is bridged by a thick transverse scapular ligament. After entering the supraspinatus fossa, the nerve gives off two motor branches to the supraspinatus muscle, and then passes laterally within the fossa, providing sensory branches to the posterior capsule of the glenohumeral joint and the acromioclavicular joint. It then passes around the lateral border of the base of the spinous fossa to the infraspinatus fossa where the nerve terminates, supplying motor branches to the infraspinatus muscle (Fig. 17.10). Approximately 50% of individuals have a spinoglenoid ligament, which is an aponeurotic band that separates the supraspinatus and infraspinatus muscles (28, 62) (Fig. 17.11). The suprascapular nerve has no cutaneous distribution or innervation.

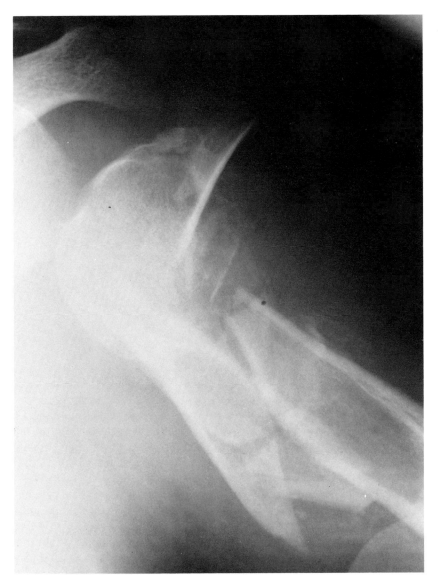

Figure 17.7. During the operative repair of this comminuted proximal left humerus fracture in a 34-year-old male who fell approximately 40 feet to the ground, a fragment of bone was found impaled into the anterior branch of the axillary nerve.

Figure 17.8. The fragment of bone held in the clamp was freed from its compression on the axillary nerve, which was identified by the two-vessel loops both above and below the sight of compression. The axillary nerve was found to be intact.

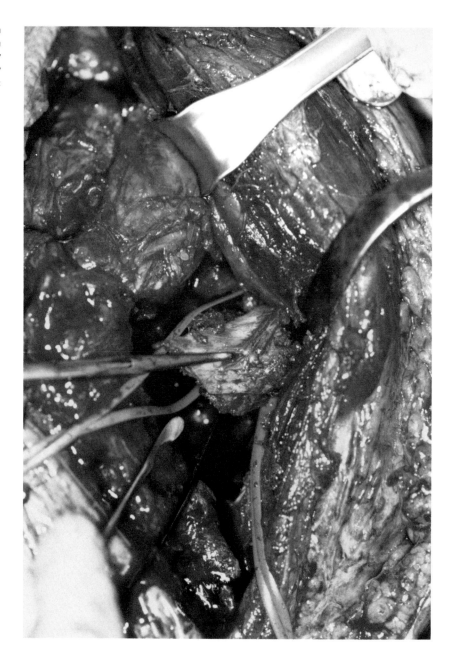

Etiology and Incidence

Suprascapular nerve injury is a well-described clinical entity, and numerous causes of injury to this nerve have been noted including blunt trauma to the shoulder (7, 100), anterior dislocation of the shoulder (102), and fractures of the suprascapular notch (27). In addition, sporting activities (7, 28) have been associated with suprascapular nerve injuries as well as upper extremity resistance exercises (2). Bryan and Wild (15) reported a suprascapular nerve injury in a professional baseball player who ex-

perienced sudden onset of pain after a long hard throw from centerfield.

A traction injury to the suprascapular nerve at its origin may result from a fall onto the point of the shoulder, resulting in a separating force that spreads the shoulder apart with elongation of the acromiomastoid dimension, as described by Bateman (7).

Suprascapular neuropathy may also be idiopathic (58, 62). Drez (24) reported four individuals with suprascapular nerve lesions, two of whom had no history of trauma. Although complications involving the suprascapular nerve following shoulder surgery may appear to be extremely rare, the potential for iatrogenic injury to the nerve certainly exists due to the proximity of the nerve to the operative field (10). Certain arthroscopic techniques may place the suprascapular nerve at risk for injury. These include placement of sutures for repair of detached anterior labrum and capsule that are directed posteriorly through drill holes in the glenoid neck, as well as tendon mobilization of the supraspinatus and infraspinatus needed for repair of massive rotator cuff tears, or glenoid osteotomies for treatment of posterior instability. Entrapment of the nerve secondary to a ganglionic cyst distal to the suprascapular notch, at the base of the scapular spine (32, 68, 90) as well as within the suprascapular fossa (49) have been reported.

Clinical Presentation

Suprascapular neuropathy may be difficult to diagnose. The patient with a suprascapular nerve injury may present with the same symptoms as that of a patient with a rotator cuff injury. There may be a history of trauma followed by a poorly localized pain. The sensation is usually intact, and weakness of external rotation and abduction as well as atrophy of the supraspinatus, infraspinatus or both can be observed, all of which resemble a rotator cuff injury (Fig. 17.12). Drez and Donovan (23, 24) have pointed out that in view of the similar features in both of these clinical entities, electromyography (EMG) and arthrography are important diagnostic tools to differentiate these conditions. Although the relief of

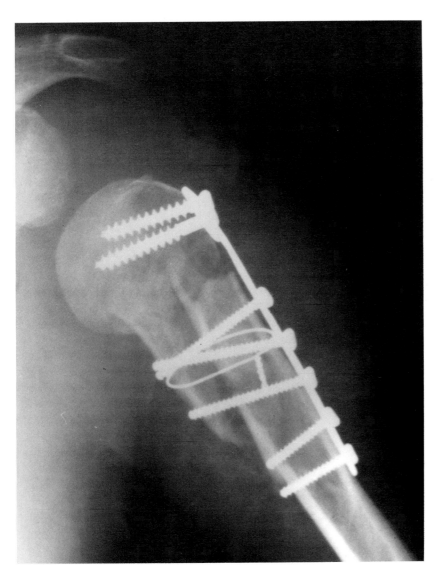

Figure 17.9. The immediate postoperative films following open reduction and internal fixation demonstrated subluxation due to marked deltoid atony.

Figure 17.10. The suprascapular nerve passes through the suprascapular notch of the scapular, which is bridged by a thick transverse scapular ligament. Upon entering the supraspinatus fossa, the nerve supplies motor branches to the supraspinatus muscle. It then passes around the lateral border of the base of the spinous fossa to the infraspinatus fossa, where the nerve terminates, supplying motor branches to the infraspinatus muscle.

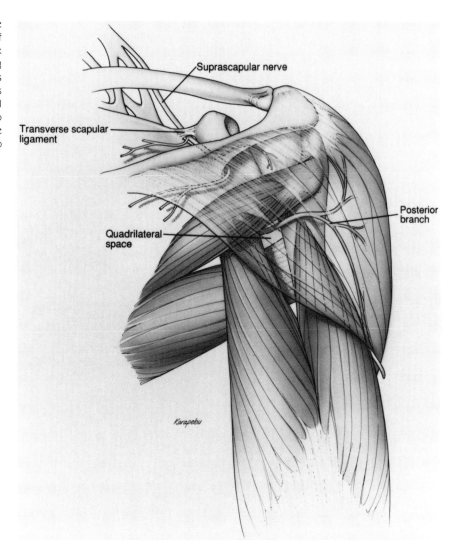

pain via infiltration of the scapular notch with local anesthetics may support the diagnosis of suprascapular nerve entrapment (33), only electromyography can confirm the diagnosis. The clinical presentation of the patient with a suprascapular neuropathy will vary, depending upon the anatomic site of neurologic compression. Three anatomic sites of compression or injury have been noted (62). The sites of possible injury include the origin of the nerve at Erb's point; the scapular notch beneath the scapular ligament and at the spinoglenoid notch, which is the site at which the nerve passes around the scapular spine to enter the infraspinatus fossa (Fig. 17.13).

Injuries to the nerve can also occur at the suprascapular notch. Injuries at this site are responsible for the so-called "suprascapular nerve entrapment syndrome" (SNES). Rengachary (77) et al. presented an anatomical study of the suprascapular notch, describing the "sling effect" of the suprascap-

ular nerve kinking against the transverse scapula ligament, resulting in the SNES. Fractures occurring in the scapular notch have also resulted in SNES (27). Alon (4) et al. reported on a 35-year-old patient with bilateral SNES due to an anomalous bifid transverse scapular ligament that was impinging on the nerve.

A nerve lesion may also occur at the spinoglenoid notch (3). This will result in denervation of the infraspinatus muscle, producing weakness of external rotation. Patients may be asymptomatic or have only mild pain because the injury may be distal to the sensory branches that innervate the glenohumeral joint capsule or acromioclavicular joint. Black and Lombardo (11) reported on four patients with suprascapular nerve injuries distal to the supraspinatus muscle branch who presented with shoulder pain and atrophy of the infraspinatus only. Ferretti (28) described isolated asymptomatic paralysis of the infraspinatus muscle in 12 volleyball players.

Diagnosis

The diagnosis of suprascapular nerve injury can be suspected by careful history and physical examination, but it can be confirmed and proven only by the appropriate EMG study. Plain radiographs in the AP projection with the beam directed 15–30° caudally are recommended views to recognize bony pathology in the notch, such as a fracture or a narrow notch where there has been nonfracture (61, 79). However, only by using EMG studies can a diagnosis of a suprascapular nerve injury and its actual anatomic site of injury or involvement be established with certainty. The study involves stimulating the nerve at Erb's point. The recording electrodes that have been placed in the supraspinatus and infraspinatus then measure the activity in the muscle. A prolonged latency time as compared with normal ranges of conduction of latency times (45) confirms the diagnosis of SNES and will also help to identify the anatomic site of compression of the nerve. Arthrog-

raphy or MRI studies can be used to rule out rotator cuff pathology.

Treatment

Once the diagnosis of suprascapular nerve injury has been confirmed, conservative measures of treatment are initiated. These include rest from stressful physical or athletic activities, analgesics, electrical stimulation, and possible injections of corticosteroids (7, 61, 78). Traction injuries to the suprascapular nerve due to blunt trauma to the shoulder itself or to the base of the neck usually have a favorable prognosis. When the site of the nerve injury is localized by EMG evaluation to be at the suprascapular or spinoglenoid notch, conservative measures may be less successful. If there is no clinical improvement or recovery and no electrical change in follow-up EMG seen noting improvement within the first several months (i.e., 6 months), then surgical exploration and decompression of the nerve

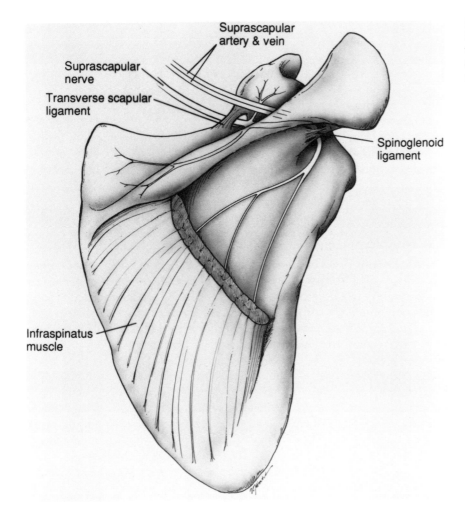

Figure 17.11. Approximately 50% of individuals have a spinoglenoid ligament, which is an aponeurotic band that separates the supraspinatus and infraspinatus muscles.

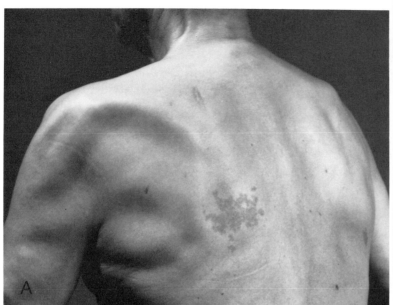

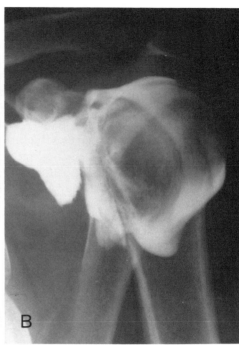

Figure 17.12. **A**, This 74-year-old male presented with weakness of active external rotation of his left shoulder. Physical examination revealed marked atrophy of the infraspinatus. **B**, His arthrogram was negative for a rotator cuff tear. EMG evaluation revealed a suprascapular neuropathy.

are indicated. Excision of the transverse scapular ligament does not have adverse structural consequences (76), and has been described as effective treatment for suprascapular nerve entrapment syndrome (SNES) (33, 76, 77). Ganglion cysts have been reported to compress the nerve as it winds around the scapular spine (32, 49, 90), and surgical exploration and decompression at the spinoglenoid notch by excision of a large ganglion cyst has been reported to achieve relief of symptoms (32).

The suprascapular nerve is at potential risk for injury due in part to its unique anatomy. Direct compression to the nerve, traction injuries, forceful upper extremity activities, and potential iatrogenic nerve injury are all possible mechanisms of injury to this nerve. Its presentation may resemble and mimic that of a full-thickness rotator cuff tear, and injury to the nerve should be considered in the differential diagnosis of shoulder pain. EMG evaluation is essential to make an accurate diagnosis. Often, improvement can be seen within the first few months. It should be noted that in many cases, the condition is a neuropraxia or axonotmesis that will usually recover if given sufficient time (11, 24). But if no improvement is seen or documented after several months, further follow-up diagnostic studies are necessary, and surgical decompression of the nerve in specific selected cases may be indicated.

MUSCULOCUTANEOUS NERVE INJURIES

Anatomy

The musculocutaneous nerve is derived from fibers from the C5 and C6 spinal roots with an occasional addition of C7. It originates from the lateral cord of the brachial plexus near the inferior border of the pectoralis minor and continues distally between the axillary artery and the median nerve. It then enters the upper arm by passing obliquely and distally through the coracobrachialis and between the biceps and brachialis muscles, which it innervates (Fig. 17.14). In approximately 50% of patients, the motor branch to the coracobrachialis muscle arises directly from the lateral cord of the brachial plexus proximal to the origin of the musculocutaneous nerve, or it branches from the musculocutaneous nerve just prior to where it penetrates the coracobrachialis muscle (61).

The musculocutaneous nerve becomes more superficial a short distance above the elbow as it exits the deep brachial fascia lateral to the biceps tendon at a point approximately 2–5 cm above the elbow crease. At this site, it terminates as the lateral antebrachial cutaneous nerve of the forearm, which then divides into the anterior and posterior terminal cutaneous branches. These branches innervate the skin of the radial aspect of the forearm.

The musculocutaneous nerve appears to be particularly vulnerable in its proximal course where it lies on the subscapular muscle (39). Bach (6) et al. found that the location of the muscular insertion of the musculocutaneous nerve into the coracobrachialis was a mean of 49 mm distal to the tip of the coracoid process. Of note was that of 61 specimens, three nerves had insertion sites at 20–25 mm distal to the coracoid tip. Bifurcation of the musculocutaneous nerve was seen in three specimens, and one smaller branch of the musculocutaneous nerve extended 10–15 mm proximal from the coracoid process. Flatow et al. (29), in their anatomic study of the musculocutaneous nerve and its relationship to the coracoid process, found that the distance from the coracoid to the point of entrance of the main nerve trunk into the coracoid brachialus muscle ranged from 31 to 82 mm with a mean of 66 mm. Small nerve twigs to the coracoid brachialus were found to enter the muscle as close as 17 mm below the coracoid. They concluded that the frequently cited range of 5–8 cm below the coracoid for the level of penetra-tion of the musculocutaneous nerve could not be relied upon as a safe zone, because 29% of the nerves in their study entered the muscle proximal 5 cm below the coracoid.

Etiology and Incidence

Isolated musculocutaneous nerve injuries about the shoulder are not common, but they have been reported in a variety of clinical situations. Musculocutaneous nerve injuries have been reported after heavy physical activity in young patients. Mastiglia (57) reported two cases of isolated nerve injuries, one in a 19-year-old student who was involved in competitive rowing, and the other in a 31-year-old participating in competitive model airplane flying. Isolated neuropathies have also been reported in weightlifters (12). Kim and Goodrich (42) have reported an isolated musculocutaneous nerve palsy that occurred in a 27-year-old man after throwing a football. Injury to the musculocutaneous nerve may also occur or complicate an anterior shoulder dislo-

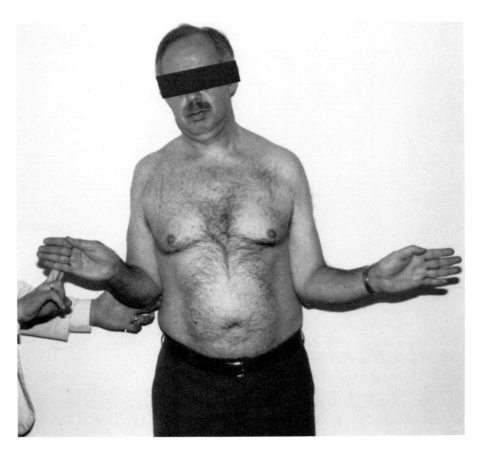

Figure 17.13.   This 52-year-old patient presented with the spontaneous onset of right shoulder pain, and on physical examination demonstrated weakness of active external rotation of his right shoulder. He was initially felt to have a rotator cuff tear, but the arthrogram was negative. EMG evaluation revealed axillary and suprascapular neuropathies.

Figure 17.14. The musculocutaneous nerve originates from the lateral cord of the brachial plexus near the inferior border of the pectoralis minor. It enters the upper arm by passing obliquely and distally through the coracobrachialis and between the biceps and brachialis muscles, which it innervates.

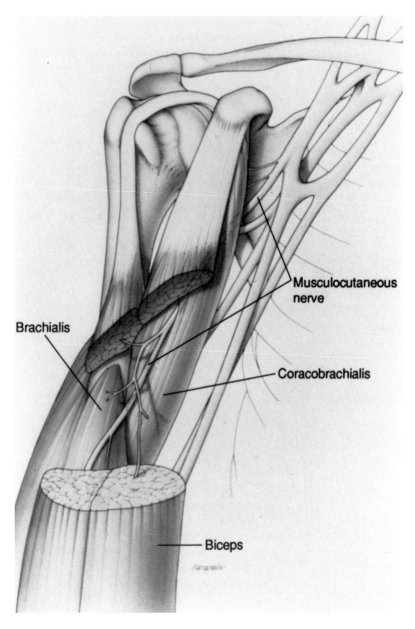

cation (17, 39), and often there are other nerve injuries associated with this (20, 54, 58, 72). Surgical procedures involving the anterior aspect of the shoulder have also been associated with complications related to musculocutaneous nerve injury (6, 80, 95). Bach et al. reported a musculocutaneous nerve injury in an 18-year-old competitive swimmer who had undergone a previous modified Bristow procedure for recurrent shoulder subluxations. Pitman (75) et al. pointed out the vulnerability of the musculocutaneous nerve to injury during shoulder arthroscopy, which was due to traction on the nerve. Factors responsible included joint distension, excessive traction and extravasation of fluid. Musculocutaneous

nerve injury has also been reported as a result of the position of the shoulder in abduction and external rotation during anesthesia when the surgical procedure did not involve the shoulder itself (25).

Clinical Presentation

The physical examination of a patient with musculocutaneous neuropathy usually demonstrates atrophy and weakness of the muscles it innervates, the biceps and brachial muscles (Fig. 17.15). There is also usually a sensory impairment located on the radial aspect of the forearm. Since isolated musculocutaneous nerve injuries are rare, other entities to be considered include brachial plexus injury, C5–C6 radiculopathy, or distal rupture of the biceps tendon at the elbow (61). Brachial plexus injuries usually produce widespread neurological abnormalities, and a C5–C6 radiculopathy will affect other muscles that are supplied by this root including the deltoid, supraspinatus, infraspinatus, and teres minor, whereas they are all normal with isolated injuries to the musculocutaneous nerve. Careful physical examination generally will reveal the proximal migration of the biceps muscle with a distal tend rupture, and there is no sensory loss (Fig. 17.16).

Treatment

Richards et al. (81) pointed out the importance of recognizing the potential for injury to the musculocutaneous nerve during either at Putti-Platt or Bristow procedure. He advocated isolating and protecting the nerve if the conjoint tendon required extensive mobilization or if the procedure was a revision of a previous shoulder repair. Mobilization

of the conjoint tendon places the musculocutaneous nerve at risk for injury. Incomplete lesions of the musculocutaneous nerve can be followed if they demonstrate progressive recovery, but lesions that do not demonstrate recovery or that fail to recover completely should be explored at 3 months (43). Complete lesions, however, should be explored at an earlier date and the appropriate repair performed (13).

LONG THORACIC NERVE INJURY

Anatomy

The long thoracic nerve (external respiratory nerve of Bell, posterior thoracic nerve) is formed from the spinal roots of C5, C6, and C7. The 5th and 6th cranial nerve root join after they pierce the scalenus medius muscle, and they are then united with the C7 contribution lateral to the muscle at the level of the 1st rib. The nerve then passes laterally beneath the brachial plexus and clavicle, dorsal to the axillary vessels and then continues down along the

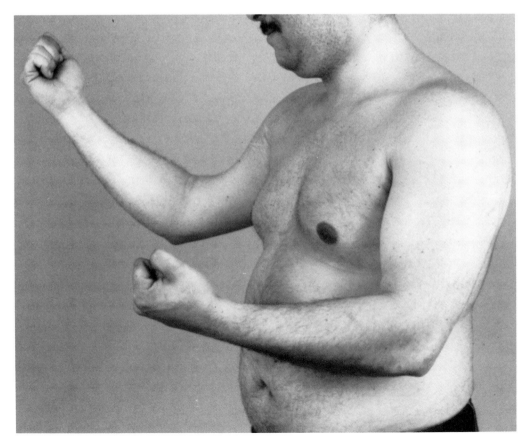

Figure 17.15. This patient demonstrates atrophy of the biceps and brachial muscles due to a complete musculocutaneous neuropathy that occurred during a surgical procedure intended to correct an anterior instability problem of the shoulder.

Figure 17.16. The long thoracic nerve passes laterally beneath the brachial plexus and the clavicle and continues down along the anterior lateral aspect of the chest wall, supplying branches to all the digitations of the serratus anterior muscle. A long thoracic nerve is a pure motor nerve, and its only function is innervation of the serratus anterior muscle.

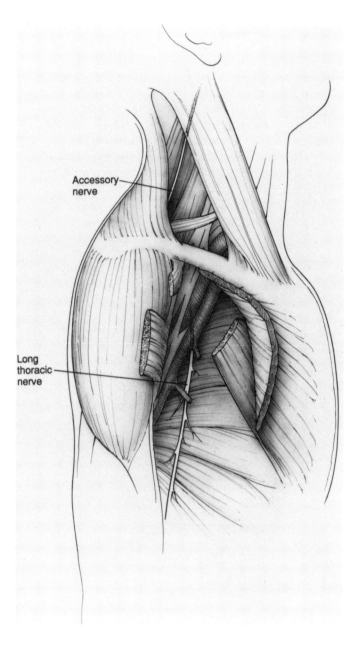

anterior lateral aspect of the chest wall supplying branches to all the digitations of the serratus anterior muscle (Fig. 17.17). The long thoracic nerve is a pure motor nerve, and its only function is innervation of the serratus anterior muscle. The fibers from C5 supply the upper part, C6 the middle part, and fibers from C7 supply the lower part of the muscle.

Etiology and Incidence

Isolated serratus anterior paralysis due to a long thoracic nerve lesion usually occurs as a result of an acute injury, or after carrying objects on the shoulder. Injuries include blunt and sharp trauma and traction on the neck or shoulder, which causes the shoulder to be depressed. Since the earliest report of an isolated serratus anterior muscle paralysis by Velpeau in 1937, similar injuries have been observed in numerous sports activities including archery, basketball, bowling, discus throwing, football, tennis, weightlifting, wrestling, as well as other sports (7, 30, 34, 35, 61, 85, 98). Viral infections of the nerve can also produce paralysis, or there may be no obvious cause of the paralysis (67).

Clinical Presentation

Patients with long thoracic nerve injury may present with an aching or burning sensation around the shoulder that may radiate down the arm or to the posterior scapular area (41). The patient usually has scapular pain and weakness in forward flexion, with inability to raise the arm above the horizontal level.

Physical examination reveals weakness and loss of normal forward elevation. Winging of the scapula is present, but the examination of the shoulder must include evaluation of this region from the back, or it may be missed (Fig. 17.18). Scapular winging can be best observed by having the patient flex the shoulder 90°, extend the elbows and internally rotate the shoulders, and push against a wall with both hands (Fig. 17.19). Several weeks may pass following an acute injury to the nerve before the trapezius muscle stretches sufficiently to allow marked scapular winging (35).

Diagnosis

Other conditions may also produce or cause winging of the scapula. These include trapezius muscle paralysis from a spinal accessory nerve injury, malunion or nonunion of scapula fractures, or diffuse shoulder girdle weakness in general (61).

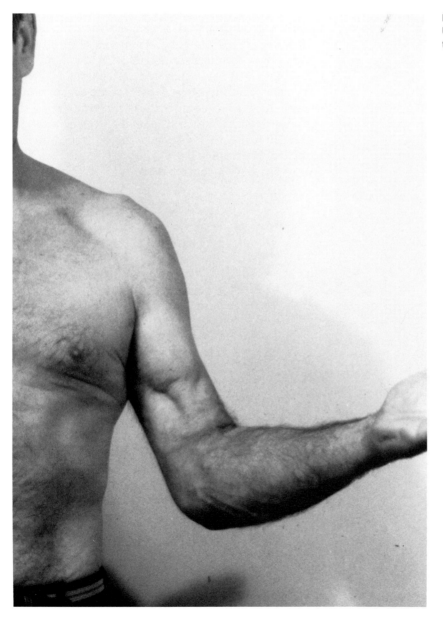

Figure 17.17. Proximal migration of the biceps muscle seen in a patient with a rupture of the biceps tendon at the elbow.

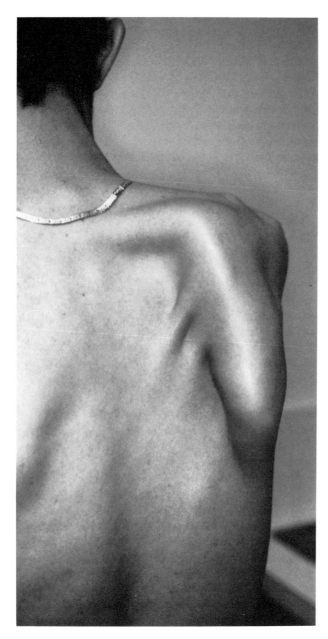

Figure 17.18. Paralysis of the serratus anterior muscle due to a long thoracic nerve injury, producing scapular winging.

Electromyographic evaluation will confirm the diagnosis of an isolated long thoracic nerve palsy. After the nerve is stimulated at Erb's point, the motor responses are reported over the serratus anterior muscle on the 5th rib lateral to the nipple. The findings of a prolonged latency and diminished amplitude of motor responses are consistent with a long thoracic neuropathy (52, 73).

Treatment

The treatment is conservative initially, and efforts must be made to eliminate excessive or repetitive use of the shoulder. Passive exercises are performed daily to prevent contracture and to stretch the rhomboid and pectoralis minor. Electrical stimulation of the nerve is also used to maintain muscle tone. Certain braces and orthotic devices have been developed to try to maintain the normal position of the scapula to relieve the serratus anterior muscle strain (92). The conservative approach should be considered for at least 9–24 months with the expectation that recovery of serratus anterior muscle function will occur (34, 101). Johnson and Kendall (41), in their review of 111 cases, reported an overall good response to conservative treatment. However, if the patients' symptoms and paralysis persist and become chronic, resulting in a significant disability, surgery may be considered. Muscle transfer procedures to substitute for the serratus anterior have been used, such as the transfer of the sternal head of the pectoralis major using a fascial extension into a hole made through the inferior angle of the scapula (56, 67), as well as other surgical procedures with varying degrees of success.

SPINAL ACCESSORY NERVE

Anatomy

The spinal accessory nerve (cranial nerve XI) is a motor nerve that innervates the trapezius muscle. It enters the neck by passing through the forearm and then pierces the sternocleidomastoid muscle, which it supplies, and then courses obliquely and superficially across the floor of the posterior triangle of the neck to the ventral border of the trapezius muscle. As it courses deep to the trapezius muscle, the accessory nerve communicates with C2, C3, and C4 and forms a plexus that continues to the deep surface of the trapezius muscle. The nerve continues distally and crosses the medial border of the scapula, and innervates the trapezius muscle on its deep surface (Fig. 17.20).

Etiology and Incidence

Injury to the spinal accessory (cranial nerve XI) nerve results in paralysis of the trapezius muscle, as it is the sole motor innervation of the trapezius (38, 71, 88). The injury may be blunt trauma, such as from a fall or a motor vehicle accident. The mechanism of injury with blunt trauma is usually either a direct blow to the area or a stretching of the nerve (51). Traction on the sternocleidomastoid muscle during carotid endarterectomy has also been observed to produce spinal accessory nerve injury (93). Bateman (7) reported falling on the point of the shoulder resulting in an elongation of the acromiomastoid dimension, causing a stretch injury to the spinal accessory nerve. He also described a crush injury to the nerve due to direct trauma, such as from a blow from a hockey or lacrosse stick in the posterior neck region where the nerve is superficial in its location (7). An injury to the spinal accessory nerve may also be penetrating, such as from a stab or a gunshot wound. Inadvertent injury may occur during a minor surgical procedure such as during a biopsy of a benign tumor or cervical lymph node (Fig. 17.21) (26, 71, 88, 97, 99). The spinal accessory nerve may be intentionally excised by necessity as part of a radical neck dissection for a malignant tumor, although in view of the deformity that may result, attempts are now made to spare the nerve (82, 84).

Clinical Presentation

As just described, the spinal accessory nerve has a superficial location on the floor of the posterior cervical triangle, where it lies in the subcutaneous tissue, allowing it to be susceptible to injury. A lesion of the spinal accessory nerve results in drooping of the shoulder, eventual asymmetry of the neck line, winging of the scapula, as well as weakness of forward elevation and abduction of the shoulder (Fig. 17.22). The balance of muscle forces about the scapula is altered, and the smoothness of the scapulohumeral rhythm is lost. Pain due to muscle spasm, radiculitis from traction on the brachial plexus, subacromial impingement, or frozen shoulder is often present and may be severe (9).

Initially, even though there is paralysis of the trapezius, the patient may only be aware of drooping of the shoulder and may not experience pain at the onset of the problem. However, a persistent ache and weakness about the shoulder girdle will often follow (61). Drooping of the shoulder with inability to shrug the shoulder, rotatory winging of the scapula with

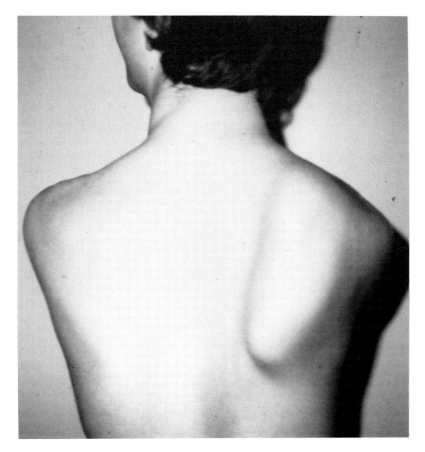

Figure 17.19. Scapular winging is best observed by having the patient flex the shoulder 90°, extend the elbows, and internally rotate the shoulders and push against a wall with both hands.

Figure 17.20. The spinal accessory nerve enters the neck and then pierces the sternocleidomastoid muscle, which it supplies, and then courses obliquely and superficially across the floor of the posterior triangle of the neck to the ventral border of the trapezius muscle. Distally, the nerve innervates the trapezius muscle on its deep surface.

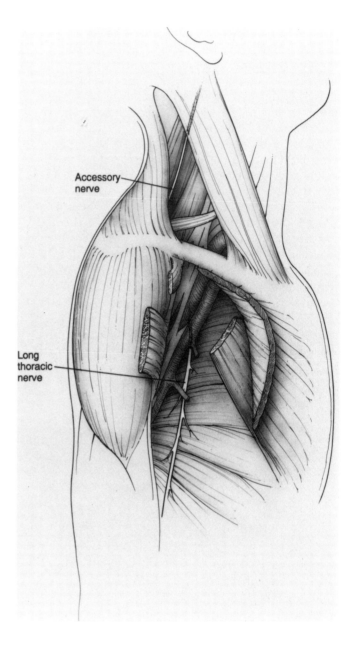

loss of stabilization of the medial scapula border, and weakness of forward elevation and abduction develops. Eventually, continued atrophy of the trapezius leads to an asymmetry about the neckline. Bigliani (9) et al. reported that the pain that develops can be quite severe due to muscle spasm, brachial plexus traction, frozen shoulder, or subacromial impingement.

Diagnosis

The diagnosis of paralysis of the trapezius may be difficult. A careful, thorough physical examination of the patient's neck, back, and chest is neces-

sary. Electromyographic studies are essential to confirm the diagnosis and will demonstrate denervation of the sternocleidomastoid and the three portions of the trapezius. EMG evaluation is necessary to assess which muscles are involved as well as the extent of their involvement, as this cannot be determined by physical examination alone.

Treatment

Conservative applications such as a sling, anti-inflammatory medications, muscle relaxants, and transcutaneous nerve stimulation may be beneficial in the immediate postinjury period, but are usually

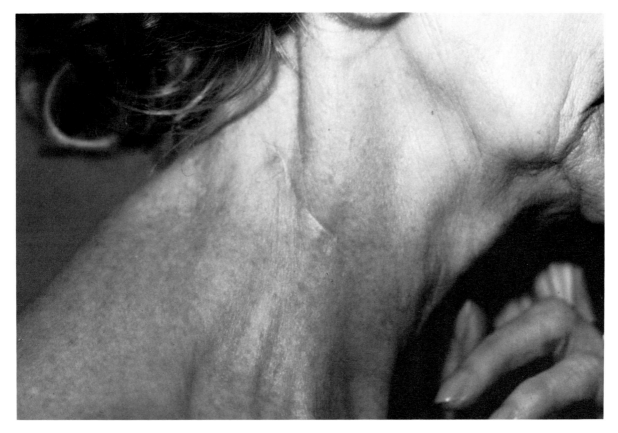

Figure 17.21. This patient had an injury to the spinal accessory nerve as a result of a biopsy of a cervical lymph node in the posterior triangle of the neck.

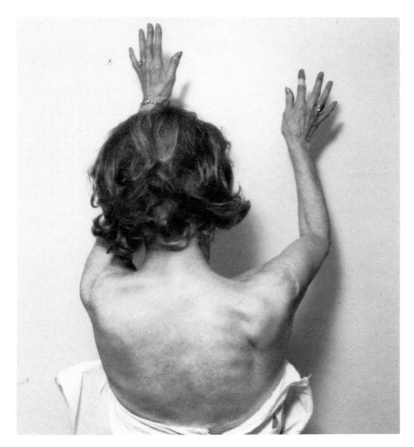

Figure 17.22. As a result of this inadvertent injury, she developed eventual lateral displacement and winging of the scapula, and weakness of forward elevation.

unsuccessful, especially in the active individual (9, 71, 88). Resistance exercises aimed at strengthening the adjacent scapular muscles are not sufficient to compensate or substitute for absent trapezius muscle function. Exploration and neurolysis of the closed nerve injury within 6 months after injury in the absence of any recovery seems to give the best results, whereas the results of neurolysis and grafting have been variable (5, 26, 36, 70, 97).

Scapula reconstruction stabilizing procedures have been used to substitute for the paralyzed trapezius. Fixation of the medial order of the scapular to the spinous process by the fascia lata as a static type of stabilization has been described (22, 37, 89, 96), but this does not compensate for the complex dy-

namic function of the trapezius muscle (51). Procedures involving transfer of the levator scapulae with fascia lata sling fixation have also been reported to be useful procedures (21, 99). Several series have reported successful results with a dynamic muscle transfer using the levator scapulae and rhomboid muscles (46, 47, 48). Bigliani (9) et al. have recently reported very favorable results using the transfer of the levator scapulae and rhomboid muscles, achieving a dynamic transfer to substitute for the paralyzed trapezius muscle (Fig. 17.23). They concluded that the transfer of the levator scapulae and rhomboid muscles was a valuable orthopaedic reconstructive procedure for the treatment of paralysis of the trapezius, when pain and diminished function of the

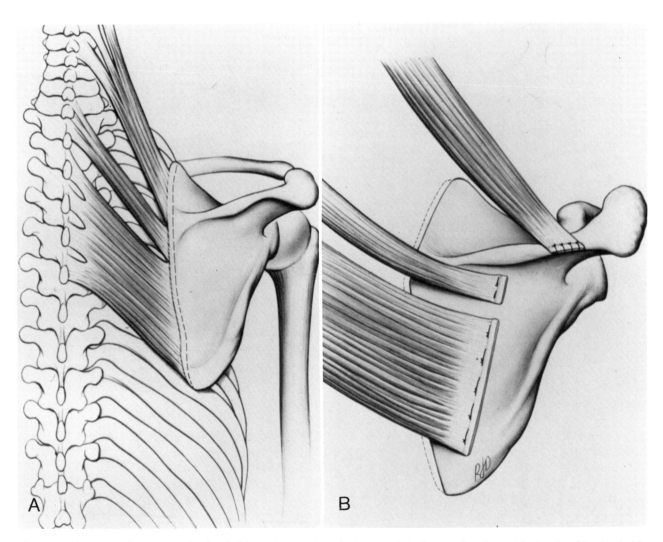

Figure 17.23. **A**, The levator scapula, rhomboideus minor, and rhomboideus major insert on the medial border of the scapula and assist the trapezius in the functions of the scapular rotation, elevation depression, and medial stabilization. **B**, The lateral transfer of the levator scapular to the scapular spine and the transfer of the rhomboid muscles to the scapular body improves the vectors through which the muscles must pull. (Reproduced with permission from Dr. Bigliani.)

extremity had been caused by irreparable nerve injury. They advocated that the procedure not be done as a primary procedure or when the spinal accessory nerve required exploration or repair, or both, but rather as a salvage procedure (9).

Acknowledgment.
Special thanks to Ms. Vaune J. Hatch, Medical Artist, Center for Bio-Medical Communications, College of Physicians & Surgeons of Columbia University, New York, New York for her illustrations.

References

1. Abbott LC, Saunders JBM, Hagey H, et al. Surgical approaches to the shoulder joint. J Bone Joint Surg 1949; 31A:235–244.

2. Agre JL, Ash N, Cameron MC, House J. Suprascapular neuropathy after intensive progressive resistive exercise: case report. Arch Phys Med Rehabil 1987;68:236–238.

3. AiIello I, Serra G, Traina GC, Tugnoli V. Entrapment neuropathy of the suprascapular nerve at the spinoglenoid notch. Ann Neurol 1982;12:314–316.

4. Alon M, Weiss S, Fishel B, et al. Bilateral suprascapular nerve entrapment syndrome due to an anomalous transverse scapular ligament. Clin Orthop 1988;234:31–33.

5. Anderson R, Flowers RS. Free grafts of the spinal accessory nerve during radical neck dissection. Am J Surg 1969; 118:769–799.

6. Bach BR, O'Brien SJ, Warren RF, et al. An unusual neurologic complication of the Bristow procedure. J Bone Joint Surg 1988;70A:458–460.

7. Bateman JE. Nerve injuries about the shoulder in sports. J Bone Joint Surg 1967;49A:785–792.

8. Berry H, Brill V. Axillary nerve palsy following blunt trauma to the shoulder region. A clinical and electromyographic review. J Neurol Neurosurg Psych., 45:1027–1032, 1982.

9. Bigliani LU, Perez-Snaz JR, Wolfe IN. Treatment of trapezius paralysis. J Bone Joint Surg 1985;67A:871–877.

10. Bigliani LU, Dalsey RM, McCann PD, April EW. An anatomic study of the suprascapular nerve. Arthroscopy 1990;6:301–305.

11. Black KP, Lombardo JA. Suprascapular nerve injuries with isolated paralysis of the infraspinatus. Am J Sports Med 1990;18:225–228.

12. Braddon RL, Wolfe C. Musculocutaneous nerve injury after heavy exercise. Arch Phys Med Rehabil 1978;59:290–293.

13. Bratton B, Kline DG, Coleman W, et al. Experimental interfascicular nerve grafting. J Neurosurg 1979;51:323–332.

14. Bryan WJ, Schander K, Tullos HS. The axillary nerve and its relationship to common sports medicine shoulder procedures. Am J Sports Med 1986;14:113–116.

15. Bryan WJ, Wild JJ. Isolated infraspinatus atrophy: a common cause of posterior shoulder pain and weakness in the throwing athlete. Am J Sports Med 1989;17:130–131.

16. Burge PD, Rushworth G, Watson NA. Patterns of injury to the terminal branches of the brachial plexus. J Bone Joint Surg 1985;67B:630–634.

17. Blom S, Dahlback LD. Nerve injuries in dislocations of the shoulder joint and fractures of the neck of the humerus. Acta Chir Scand 1970;136:461–466.

18. Cahill BR, Palmer RE. Quadrilateral space syndrome. J Hand Surg 1983;8:65–69.

19. Darrach W. Surgical approaches for surgery of the extremities. Am J Surg 1945;LXVII:237.

20. DePalma AF. Surgery of the shoulder. 3rd ed. Philadelphia: JB Lippincott, 1983:484–485.

21. Dewar FP, Harris RI. Restoration of function of the shoulder following paralysis of the trapezius by fascial sling fixation and transplantation of the levator scapulae. Ann Surg 1950;132:1111–1115.

22. Dickson FD. Fascial transplant in paralytic and other conditions. J Bone Joint Surg 1987;19:405–412.

23. Donovan WH. Rotator cuff tears versus suprascapular nerve injury: a problem in differential diagnosis. Arch Phys Med Rehabil 1974;55:424–428.

24. Drez D. Suprascapular neuropathy in the differential diagnosis of rotator cuff injuries. Am J Sports Med 1976; 4:43–45.

25. Dundore DE, DeLisa JA. Musculocutaneous nerve palsy: an isolated complication of surgery. Arch Phys Med Rehabil 1979;60:130–133.

26. Dunn AW. Trapezius paralysis after minor surgical procedures in the posterior clavicle triangle. South Med J 1974; 67:312–315.

27. Edeland HG, Zachrisson BE. Fracture of the scapular notch associated with lesion of the suprascapular nerve. Acta Orthop Scand 1975;46:758–763.

28. Ferretti A, Cerullo G, Russo G. Suprascapular neuropathy in volleyball players. J Bone Joint Surg 1987;69A:260–263.

29. Flatow EL, Bigliani LU, April EW. An anatomic study of the musculocutaneous nerve and its relationship to the coracoid process. Clin Orthop 1989;244:166–171.

30. Foo CL, Swann M. Isolated paralysis of the serratus anterior. J Bone Joint Surg 1983;65B:552–556.

31. Gaither JC, Bruyn GW. Neurologic amytrophy. In: Vinteen PJ, ed. Handbook of clinical neurology. Amsterdam: North Holland, 1970:8, 77–85.

32. Ganzhorn RW, Hocker JT, Horowitz M, Switzer H. Suprascapular nerve entrapment. J Bone Joint Surg 1981; 63A:492–494.

33. Garcia G, McQueen D. Bilateral suprascapular nerve entrapment. J Bone Joint Surg 1981;63A:491–492.

34. Goodman CE, Kenrick MM, Blum MV. Long thoracic nerve palsy: a follow-up study. Arch Phys Med Rehabil 1975; 56:352–355.

35. Gregg JR, Labosky D, Harty M, et al. Serratus anterior paralysis in the young athlete. J Bone Joint Surg 1979; 61A:825–832.

36. Harris HH, Dickey JR. Nerve grafting to restore function of trapezius muscle after radical neck dissection (a preliminary report). Ann Otol Rhinol Laryngol 1965;74:880–886.

37. Henry AK. An operation for slinging a dropped shoulder. Br J Surg 1927;15:95–98.

38. Hollinshead WH. Anatomy for surgeons, vol. 3, The back and limbs. 3rd ed. Philadelphia: Harper & Row, 1982.

39. Jerosch J, Castro WHM, Colemont J. A lesion of the musculocutaneous nerve. A rare complication of anterior shoulder dislocation. Acta Orthopaedica Belgica 1989;55:230–232.

40. Johnson JR, Bayley JIL. Early complications of acute anterior dislocation of the shoulder in middle-aged and elderly patients. Injury 1965;13:431–433.

41. Johnson JTH, Kendall HO. Isolated paralysis of the serratus anterior muscle. J Bone Joint Surg 1955;37A:567–574.

42. Kim SM, Goodrich JA. Isolated proximal musculocutaneous nerve palsy. Arch Phys Med Rehabil 1984;65:735–736.

43. Kline DG, Hudson AR. Complications of nerve injury and nerve repair. In: Lazar S, Greenfield J, eds. Complications in surgery and trauma. Philadelphia: JB Lippincott, 1983: 695-798.

44. Kopell HP, Thompson WAL. Peripheral entrapment neuropathies. Baltimore: Williams & Wilkins, 1963.

45. Kraft GN. Axillary musculocutaneous and suprascapular nerve latency studies. Arch Phys Med Rehabil 1972; 53:383-387.

46. Lange M. Die behandlung der irreparablem trapeziuslahmung. Langenbecks Arch Klin Chir 1951;270:437-439.

47. Lange Max. Die operative behandlung der irreparablem trapeziuslahmung. Tio Fakult Mecmuasim 1959;22:137-141.

48. Lagenslziold A, Rjoppy S. Treatment of paralysis of the trapesius muscle by the Eden-Lange operation. Acta Orthop Scand 1973;44:383-388.

49. Lauland T, Fedders O, Sgaard I, Kornum M. Suprascapular nerve compression syndrome. Surg Neurol 1984;22:308-312.

50. Leffer RD, Seddon H. Infraclavicular brachial plexus injuries. J Bone Joint Surg 1965;47B:9-22.

51. Logigan EF, McInnes JM, Berger AF, et al. Stretch-induced spinal accessory nerve palsy. Muscle Nerve 1988;II:146-150.

52. LoMonaco MD, Pasqua PG, Tonali P. Conduction studies along the accessory, long thoracic, dorsal scapular and thoracodorsal nerves. Acta Neurol Scand 1983;68:171-176.

53. Loomer R, Graham B. Anatomy of the axillary nerve and its relation to inferior capsular shift. Clin Orthop 1989; 243:100-105.

54. London PS. Treatment and after care for dislocation of the shoulder. Physiotherapy 1971;57:2-6.

55. Mallon WJ, Bassett FH III, Goldner RD. Lutatio Erecta: the inferior glenohumeral dislocation. J Orthop Trauma 1990;4:19-24.

56. Marmor L, Bechtol CO. Paralysis of the serratus anterior due to electric shock released by transplantation of the pectoralis major muscle. A case report. J Bone Joint Surg 1963;45A:156-160.

57. Mastiglia FL. Musculocutaneous neuropathy after strenuous physical activity. Med J Aust 1986;145:153-154.

58. McIlveen SJ, Bigliani LU, Duralde XA, D'Alessandro DF. Isolated nerve injuries about the shoulder. Orthop Trans Vol. II, 1987;2:247-248.

59. McIlveen SJ, Steinmann SJ, Bigliani LU. Rotator cuff tears and associated nerve injury. Presented at the 58th Annual Meeting of the AAOS, Anaheim, CA, March 11, 1991.

60. McKowen HC, Voorhies RM. Axillary nerve entrapment in the quadrilateral space. J Neurosurgery 1987;66:932-934.

61. Mendoza Francis X, Main K. Peripheral nerve injuries of the shoulder in the athlete. Clin Sports Med 1990;9:331-342.

62. Mestdagh M, Drizenko A, Ghestem P. Anatomical basis of suprascapular nerve syndrome. Anatomica Clinica 1981; 3:67-71.

63. Neer CS II. Anterior acromioplasty for the chronic impingement syndrome in the shoulder. J Bone Joint Surg 1972;54A:41.

64. Neer CS, Foster CR. Inferior capsular shift for involuntary and multidirectional instability of the shoulder. J Bone Joint Surg 1980;62A:897-907.

65. Neer CS. Impingement lesions. Clin Orthop 1983;173:70-77.

66. Neer CS II, McIlveen SJ. Replacement de la tete humerale avec reconstruction des tuberosities et de la coiffe elan les fractures deplaces. Results actuals et techniques. Rev Chir Orthop Supp V 1988;74:31.

67. Neer CS. Shoulder reconstruction. Philadelphia: WB Saunders, 1990:446.

68. Neviaser TJ, Ain BR, Neviaser RJ. Suprascapular nerve degeneration secondary to an attenuation by a ganglionic cyst. J Bone Joint Surg 1986;68A:622-628.

69. Neviaser RJ, Neviaser TJ, Neviaser JS. Concurrent ruptures of the rotator cuff and anterior dislocation of the shoulder in the older patient. J Bone Joint Surg 1988; 70A:1308-1311.

70. Norden A. Peripheral injuries to the spinal accessory nerve. Acta Chir Scand 1946;94:515,532.

71. Olarte M, Adams D. Accessory nerve palsy. J Neurol Neurosurg Psychiatry 1977;40:1113-1116.

72. Pasila M, Jaroma H, Kaviluoto O, Sundholm A. Early complications of primary shoulder dislocations. Acta Orthop Scand 1978;49:260-263.

73. Petrera JE, Trojaborg W. Conduction studies of the long thoracic nerve in serratus anterior palsy of different etiology. Neurology 1984;34:1033-1037.

74. Petrucci FS, Morelli A, Raimondi PL. Axillary nerve injuries. Twenty-one cases treated by nerve graft and neurolysis. J Hand Surg 1982;7:271-278.

75. Pitman MI, Nainzadeh N, Ergas E, Springer S. The use of somatosensory evoked potentials for detection of neuropratia during shoulder arthroscopy. Arthroscopy 1988; 4:250-255.

76. Post M, Mager J. Suprascapular nerve entrapment. Clin Orthop 1987;223:126-136.

77. Rengachary SS, Burr D, Luca S, et al. Suprascapular entrapment neuropathy; a clinical, anatomical and comparative study: II. Anatomical study. Neurosurgery 1979; 5:447-451.

78. Rengachary SS, Burr D, Lucas S, et al. Suprascapular entrapment neuropathy; a clinical, anatomical and comparative study. III. Comparative study. Neurosurgery 1979; 5:452-455.

79. Rengachary SS, Neff JP, Singer PA, et al. Suprascapular entrapment neuropathy: a clinical, anatomic and comparative study. I. Clinical study. Neurosurgery 1979;5:441-446.

80. Richards RR, Hudson AR, Waddell JP, Urbaniak JK. Injury to the brachial plexus during anterior shoulder repair. AAOS, 53rd annual meeting, New Orleans, 1986:55.

81. Richards RR, Hudson AR, Bertoid JT, Urbaniak JR, Waddell JP. Injury to the brachial plexus Kuring Putti-Platt and Bristow procedures. Am J Sports Medicine 1987; 15:374-380.

82. Roy PH, Bearhs OH. Spinal accessory nerve in radical neck dissections. Am J Surg 1969;118:800-804.

83. Seddon H. Surgical disorders of the peripheral nerves. Edingburgh: Churchill Livingstone, 1972.

84. Skolnick EM, Yee KF, Frieman MM, Golden TA. The posterior triangle in radical neck surgery. Arch Otolaryngol 1976;102:1-4.

85. Stanish WD, Lamb H. Isolated paralysis of the serratus anterior muscle: a weight training injury. Am J Sports Med 1978;6:385-386.

86. Stewart JD. Focal peripheral neuropathies. New York: Elsevier, 1987.

87. Sunderland S. Nerve and nerve injuries. Edinburgh and London: Churchill Livingstone, 1968.

88. Sunderland S. Nerves and nerve injuries. 2nd ed. New York: Churchill Livingstone, 1978.

89. Szubinski A. Ersatz des gelahmten trapezius durch fascien-zugel. Zentralbl Chir 1920;47:1172-1174.

90. Thompson RC, Schneider W, Kennedy T. Entrapment neu-ropathy of the inferior branch of the suprascapular nerve by ganglia. CORR 1982;166:185-187.

91. Thompson WAL, Koppell HP. Peripheral entrapment neu-ropathies of the upper extremity. N Engl J Med 1959; 260:1261-1265.

92. Truong XT, Rippel DV. Orthotic devices for serratus ante-rior palsy: some biomechanical considerations. Arch Phys Med Rehabil 1979;60:66-69.

93. Tucker JA, Gee W, Nichola GG, McDonald RM, Goodreau JJ. Accessory nerve injury during carotoid endarterectomy. J Vasc Surg 1987;3:440-444.

94. Watson-Jones R. Fractures and joint inquiries, vol 1. 4th ed. Edinburgh: Churchill Livingstone, 1952.

95. Weidmann E, Huggler AH. Die Lasion des nerves musculo-cutaneous bei der operativen Behandlung der habituellen Schulterluxation der Orthopade. 1978;7:192-195.

96. Whitman Armitage. Congenital elevation of scapula and pa-ralysis of serratus magnus muscle. JAMA 1932;99: 1332-1334.

97. Woodhall Barnes. Trapesius paralysis following minor surgical procedure in the posterior cervical triangle. Re-sults following cranial nerve suture. Am Surg 1952;136: 375-380.

98. Woodhead AB. Paralysis of the serratus anterior in a world class marksman. Am J Sports Med 1985;13: 359-362.

99. Wright PE, Simmons JCH. Peripheral nerve injuries. In: Edmonson AS, Crenshaw AH, eds. Campbell's operative or-thopaedics, vol 2. 6th ed. St. Louis: CV Mosby, 1980: 1642-1702.

99. Wright PG, Simmonsm JCH. Peripheral nerve injuires. In: Edmonson AS, Crenshaw AH, eds. Campbell's operative or-thopaedics, vol. 2. 6th ed. St. Louis: CV Mosby, 1980:1642-1702.

100. Yoon TN, Grabois M. Scapular nerve injury following trauma to the shoulder. J Trauma 1981;21:652-655.

101. Zeir FG. The treatment of winged scapula. Clin Orthop 1973;91:128-133.

102. Zoltan JD. Injury to the suprascapular nerve association with anterior dislocation of the shoulder. Case report and re-view of the literature. J Trauma 1979;19:203-206.

18
Complications of Shoulder Instability in the Competitive Athlete

Daniel E. Cooper, Jon J.P. Warner, Russell F. Warren

INTRODUCTION

Instability involving the athlete's shoulder accounts for a major portion of shoulder instability in general. In the younger age group, up to 80% of shoulder dislocations occur during sport (6, 10, 19, 39, 44, 74, 76, 80, 84, 86). In many ways, shoulder instability and its complications are no different for the athlete than for the nonathlete. The anatomy, pathology, and biomechanics are similar. However, the demands of his sport may render the athlete more disabled by instability or its complications than the nonathlete.

Therefore, with increasing career opportunities for the competitive athlete and his high demands for full function, it is imperative that the treating physician have a thorough understanding of the pathomechanics of shoulder instability, as well as the special needs of athletes for participation in their sports. It is no longer sufficient to accept as a good result simply the prevention of a subsequent dislocation. Rather, the competitive athlete must be assessed from a highly functional point of view. The ultimate goals for the athlete include stability, power, full range of motion, and return to sport.

CLASSIFICATION

It is important to organize the spectrum of shoulder instability by classification. In doing so, one should consider the etiology, frequency, direction, degree of instability, as well as any voluntary nature. A careful history and physical examination are critical in determining these factors and will greatly facilitate accurate diagnosis. Table 18.1 illustrates the classification system that we have developed.

Certain instability patterns are very common in the athlete, though they may differ dramatically. Rowe (76) has estimated that 95–98% of shoulder in-

stability is anterior in direction. Certainly, traumatic anterior instability is the most common form in the athlete. This may vary from frank, recurrent, dislocation due to "macrotrauma," to the less obvious recurrent anterior subluxation due to "microtrauma" of repetitive overuse, such as pitching (7, 32, 52, 80).

In contrast, many swimmers tend to have mild generalized ligamentous laxity, which has enabled them to excel in their sport (73, 82). They often present with evidence of multidirectional instability and secondary inflammation that may limit performance. Due to increased awareness since Neer's (62) description, multidirectional instability is more frequently diagnosed and recognized as an underlying component in the pathomechanics of many unstable shoulders.

Posterior instability is much less common, but may be disabling for the athlete who must lift weights (bench press) or block with the arm in the flexed and adducted position. These activities apply posteriorly directed translational force to the glenohumeral joint. Throwers may also have symptoms of posterior instability during the follow-through phase of throwing when there is a posterior translational force on the humeral head (29). It has been our experience that these patients mainly complain of pain or clicking with the aggravating activity and less commonly notice a sensation of instability. Apprehension to posterior translation in the flexed and adducted position is less frequently found on physical examination than is apprehension in those with anterior instability. In addition, the vast majority of these athletes are experiencing recurrent posterior subluxation, not dislocation. Frank posterior dislocation is uncommon in general and particularly in the athlete (26). It is more often seen in patients with seizure disorders or due to trauma in the older patient.

It is beyond the scope of this chapter to expound further on the classification and evaluation of shoulder instability in general. This is well covered elsewhere. Clearly, the physician caring for the athlete must have a good understanding of normal shoulder mechanics and the pathomechanics of the different types of shoulder instability. This, combined with a thorough history and physical examination, will ensure accurate diagnosis and appropriate management.

TREATMENT GOALS

Prior to determining treatment, the needs of the individual athlete must be assessed. The type of sport, age, position, level of ability, laxity, and arm dominance are all factors in decision making. For the football player with recurrent traumatic dislocation, the goal of treatment is to prevent recurrence and allow return to contact sport. Open procedures have been very successful in this setting. The pitcher with painful subluxation while throwing is a much more challenging problem. Inability to participate fully is this patient's main disability. If surgery restores stability but fails to allow return to throwing, then it has not been successful. This is where many open procedures have failed to live up to the patient's expectations.

Table 18.1.   Shoulder Instability Classification

1. Frequency
   * acute
   * recurrent
   * fixed (chronic)

2. Etiology
   * traumatic (macrotrauma)
   * atraumatic (voluntary, involuntary)
   * microtrauma
   * congenital
   * neuromuscular (Erb's palsy, C.P., seizures)

3. Direction
   * anterior
   * posterior
   * inferior
   * multidirectional

4. Degree
   * dislocation
   * subluxation
   * micro (transient)

REHABILITATION

Any discussion of shoulder instability in the athlete would be incomplete without emphasis on rehabilitation. Although less effective in the conservative management of recurrent traumatic (macrotrauma) instability, conservative rehabilitation is essential in the management of atraumatic instability and recurrent subluxation due to microtrauma.

For shoulder pain due to subluxation, rest is the important first phase of the rehabilitation. For the athlete with a first-time acute traumatic subluxation, we immobilize the shoulder for 5–6 weeks to allow healing and to decrease the recurrence rate. Then, mobilization and strengthening are begun. The throwing athlete with pain due to microsubluxation is initially rested with complete avoidance of throwing. Once the acute inflammation and pain have subsided, a strengthening and stretching program is instituted. We usually begin with Theraband and progress to free weights and finally isokinetic (Cybex) strengthening. Abduction in the scapular plane is used for supraspinatus strengthening. Internal rotation and external rotation strengthening is performed at the side and at 90° abduction to optimize cuff strengthening. Strengthening of the scapular stabilizers including the trapezius, serratus anterior, rhomboids, and latissimus dorsi is an integral part of the program. Gentle stretching exercises are used to restore full external and internal rotation.

COMPLICATIONS OF INSTABILITY

The complications of shoulder instability may be grouped into those arising from the instability itself and those arising from the treatment of that instability. Since shoulder instability is such a common problem in our athletic population, we are fortunate that resultant complications are infrequent. Many of these complications do not differ for the athlete compared with the nonathlete, although they may be more significant in adversely affecting the athlete's ability to participate competitively in his chosen sport.

Recurrent Anterior Dislocation

Recurrence is the most significant and most common sequelae of anterior shoulder instability in the athlete. It is well established that risk of redislocation is directly proportionate to youth and activity level (34, 37, 40, 41, 76, 79, 86). This, of course, places the young athlete at great risk for recurrence after initial shoulder dislocation.

Watson-Jones (97), in 1948, responded to the increasing popularity of surgical treatment of shoulder instability by urging orthopaedists to return to the basic principle of immobilization after acute dislocation. He advocated immobilization in full internal rotation for not less than 4 weeks. He also stated that he had never seen recurrence of anterior instability after treating several hundred patients in this manner. Subsequent reports, however, have not supported this claim.

McLaughlin (57), 2 years later, reported a 50% recurrence rate in 573 patients, but with only 18% follow-up. Recurrence was strongly related to age, being 90% in those less than 20 years. In 1956, Rowe (76) reported that overall recurrence of anterior dislocation was 58% in a series of 398 patients with 53% follow-up. Again recurrence was strongly related to age, being 94%, 79%, and 14% in those less than 20, 20–40, and over 40, respectively. This appreciation of the high ocurrence rate following initial dislocation stimulated closer analysis of the effect of immobilization.

Rowe and Sakellarides (79) did find decreased recurrence after immobilization and recommended 3 weeks in a sling. Then, in 1980, Kiviluoto (49) prospectively evaluated the effect of immobilization in 53 patients. In patients younger than 30, recurrence at 1-year follow-up was 50% in those treated in a sling for 1 week, and was 22% in those treated in a stockinette Valpeau bandage for 3 weeks. Henry and Genung (37), in reviewing 121 high-risk young athletic patients, found 85% recurrence after no immobilization and 90% after immobilization for a varied time period. Six of six patients who were immobilized for 6 weeks had recurrence within 18 months, but compliance was not documented.

In 1983, Hovelius (41) reported the 2-year follow-up results of a prospective multicenter study on the effect of immobilization after recurrence. Only those patients who were strictly compliant with the immobilization were included in the comparison. He found that 3–4 weeks immobilization had no effect on recurrence rate. Simonet and Cofield (86) reported an overall 33% recurrence after first-time anterior dislocation. Again, in patients younger than 20 years of age, the rate was much higher in athletes (82%) than in nonathletes (30%). In this group, immobilization of varying length was less of a factor in preventing recurrence than was avoidance of athletic participation for 6 weeks. This reduced the recurrence rate from 85% to 44% in patients under 30.

In support of immobilization, Yoneda (99) reported less frequent recurrence after 5 weeks' immobilization followed by 6 more weeks of muscle rehabilitation while continuing to limit abduction to less than 90°. Studies of ligament healing have demonstrated that it takes 6 weeks for substantial healing to occur and, therefore, support this practice (17).

The literature reflects that the vast majority (65–82%) of recurrences occur within the first 2 years after initial dislocation (19, 37, 40, 41, 76, 79, 86). Hovelius (40) in a 5-year follow-up of his initial series noted that recurrence was only 10% more frequent at 5-year vs. 2-year follow-up in patients under 30. There was no difference in those older than 30. Length of time left unreduced, reduction technique, and relaxation during reduction have not been shown to affect recurrence.

Although there are certainly conflicting reports in the literature, we believe that there is enough evidence to support the practice of immobilizing the shoulder for 5–6 weeks, followed by a strengthening program. We continue to use this regimen in most athletes who dislocate for the first time. A case can be made for allowing the high-risk athlete to return to play after regaining strength, and use of an orthosis that limits abduction and extension may be of use in this setting to help prevent recurrent dislocations and allow the athlete to complete the season. Surgical stabilization may then be performed in the off-season. If it is near the end of the season, and it is unlikely that the athlete will be able to return, then we believe that consideration of early stabilization is appropriate. This would apply only to the high-risk young athlete who participates in contact sport and who is unwilling to take the chance of suffering from recurrent instability the following season.

In addition, because of the frequency of functional disability in the throwing athlete after complete anterior dislocation, we use the same approach for throwers and prefer arthroscopic techniques, if possible. We must stress that we use this approach only for those with complete dislocation or macrosubluxation due to a specific traumatic episode, and that conservative treatment is more appropriate for those with repetitive microsubluxation. This is especially true for the elite pitcher whose performance is often limited after surgical stabilization.

Fracture

Fractures associated with shoulder instability have been reported in up to 50% of acute dislocations

(74). These include greater tuberosity, lesser tuberosity, glenoid rim, Hill-Sachs, humeral neck, scapular, and clavicular fractures. In general, older patients are more likely to sustain these fractures (34).

Greater tuberosity fractures occur in 10–15% of anterior dislocations (40, 41, 94). These are more common in the adolescent with open growth plates and in those older than 35 (Fig. 18.1) (41). Many authors have noted the decreased recurrence rate of anterior instability associated with these fractures (40, 41, 76, 94). This may be in part due to the age group in which they occur, but is also related to tuberosity fracture causing the dislocation, and there is minimal injury to the labrum and inferior glenohumeral ligament complex. Once the tuberosity fracture heals, this posterior mechanism for dislocation is eliminated, and recurrence is uncommon. Displaced greater tuberosity fractures usually spontaneously reduce with glenohumeral joint reduction, and although the rotator cuff may be torn, arthrography is usually negative in this setting (94).

Hill-Sachs impression fractures have been reported to occur in 11–50% of acute and 80–100% of chronic anterior dislocations (Fig. 18.2) (74, 94). Although the Bankart-Perthes lesion has been reported to be present in up to 85% of anterior dislocations, significant glenoid rim fractures occur in only 5–8% (Fig. 18.3) (74). Both the Hill-Sachs and glenoid rim fracture are rare in voluntary dislocations (78). Acute glenoid rim fractures should be fixed if they involve one-third or more of the width of the glenoid and create either subluxation of the humeral head or articular surface incongruity (Fig. 18.4). Excepting very large fractures, neither the Hill-Sachs nor the glenoid rim fracture has been shown to affect recurrence rates (41, 76, 79).

Rotator Cuff Tears

Tears of the rotator cuff associated with shoulder instability are frequent in older patients, but are rare in the young athlete (34). Although infrequent, tears may be associated with displaced

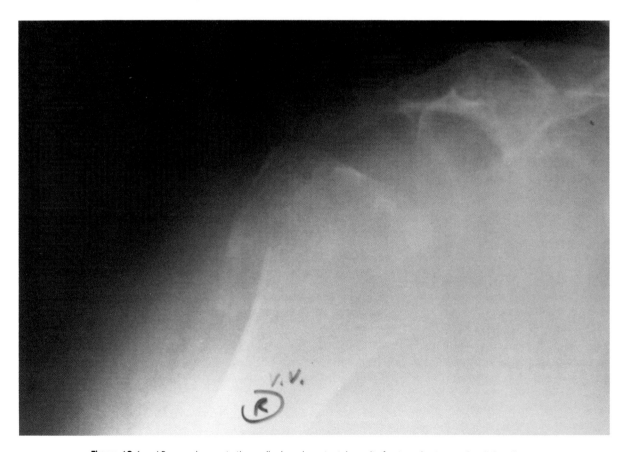

Figure 18.1.   AP x-ray demonstrating a displaced greater tuberosity fracture due to anterior dislocation. There is also an impacted humeral neck fracture.

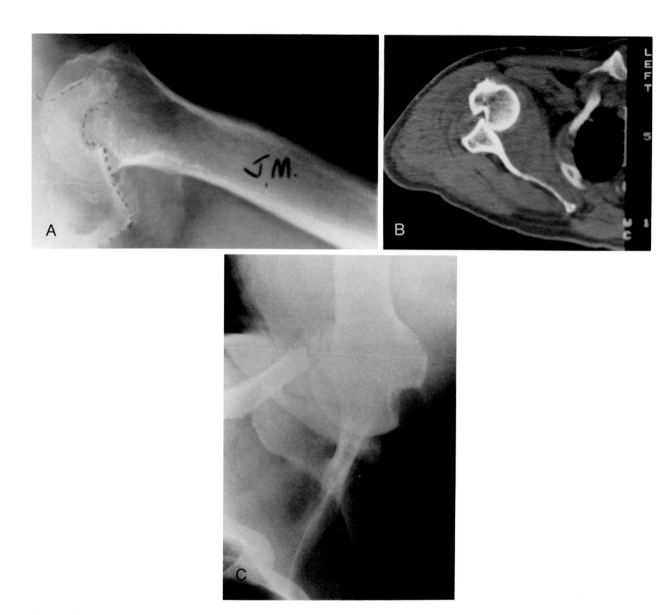

Figure 18.2. **A**, Axillary x-ray demonstrating the pathomechanics of the Hill-Sachs fracture. **B**, CT scan of the same shoulder (fixed anterior dislocation). **C**, Stryker notch view, which nicely reveals a large Hill-Sachs fracture.

greater tuberosity fractures. Partial-thickness rotator cuff tears may also occur in the throwing athlete with instability. It is believed that these tears may be a traction phenomenon (46, 68, 69, 95).

Rotator cuff tears are common over age 40 but rare in the high school or college athlete. Nevertheless, they should be considered if pain and weakness persist following reduction. In this setting, an arthrogram should be obtained by 3 weeks. If a tear is noted, early repair is recommended, as pain and weakness are likely to persist. In contrast, instability is less likely to persist because the pathogenesis of instability is a posterior mechanism (cuff failure)

that allows the humeral head to dislocate anteriorly, hinging on the intact anterior soft tissues.

Fortunately, the surgical repair is usually easy, as the injury is frequently an avulsion, and there is excellent tissue available. When performing a rotator cuff repair in this setting, the anterior labrum and capsule should be inspected and repaired if torn.

Neurovascular Injury

Nerve injury occurs in 5–15% of shoulder dislocations (19, 76). Although usually transient neurapraxia, injury may be more severe, causing permanent deficit. Since these are closed-traction injuries, there is no benefit of surgical exploration. Axillary nerve injury is most common, followed by the musculocutaneous nerve (19). Less often, radial, ulnar, median, or combined plexus injury may occur. It is imperative that neurologic examination, including motor and sensory testing, be performed prior to and after reduction. Following nerve injury, participation in contact sport should be delayed until strength returns.

Symptoms due to shoulder instability may be confused with a "burner" when paresthesias or the "dead arm" sensation prevails. A careful history and physical examination will usually distinguish the two.

Axillary artery injury due to shoulder dislocations has been sporadically reported. This injury is seen in the older population and has not been reported in the young athlete. Factors associated with risk of arterial injury include old age, attempted closed reduction of a fixed (chronically unreduced) dislocation, collagen vascular disease, and steroid use.

Impingement

Much attention has been given to impingement-type symptoms that occur in the throwing or swimming shoulder. Although inflammatory bursitis and cuff tendinitis may exist as separate entities due to overuse, it is also quite common for these to be a secondary sequela of recurrent subluxation (73). Because of only recent awareness of this association, it is difficult to determine their relative frequencies based on reports in the literature. Every young athlete with inflammatory conditions of the shoulder should be thoroughly evaluated for underlying instability. In a study by Altchek et al. (2) on multidirectional instability in athletes, 20% of patients requiring surgical stabilization had preoperative symptoms consistent with impingement or cuff tendonitis. It is probably best to discard the term "impingement" in association with shoulder instability, and instead refer directly to rotator cuff strain or tendinitis as a consequence of the instability.

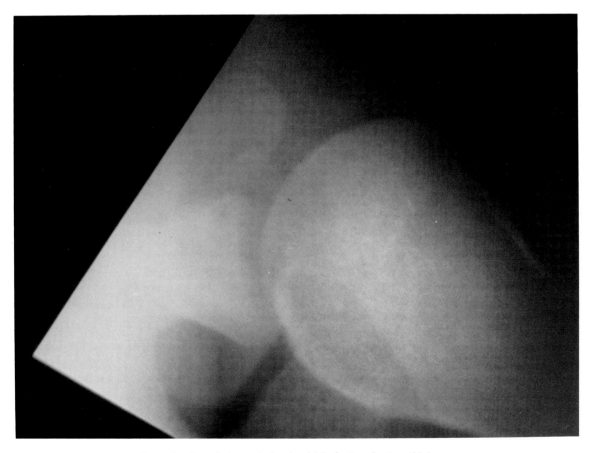

Figure 18.3. West point view of a large anterior glenoid rim fracture. Fractures this large are uncommon.

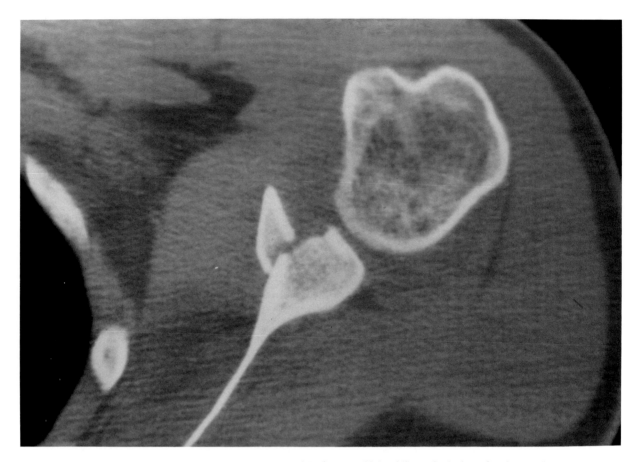

Figure 18.4. CT scan demonstrating a large glenoid rim fracture with instability and articular surface incongruity.

Arthritis

Samilson and Prieto (83) reviewed 70 patients with dislocation arthropathy and found it to be more common after posterior dislocations due to the frequency of missed diagnosis and delay in reduction. It is generally accepted that dislocation arthropathy is more common after certain surgical reconstructions than it is as a sequela of the instability itself. However, 10 of 15 shoulders with severe arthrosis and six of 14 with moderate arthrosis had had no operation for the dislocation (83). In addition, they found that young age at the time of initial dislocation was a favorable prognostic factor when considering the risk of subsequent degenerative changes (83).

COMPLICATIONS OF SURGERY FOR INSTABILITY

Cofield (19) has described the characteristics of the ideal surgical procedure for the unstable shoulder. They include:

- Low recurrence rate;
- Low complication rate;
- Low reoperation rate;
- Preserve motion;
- Do no harm (DJD);
- Applicable to most;
- Allow for joint inspection;
- Address pathology;
- Restore function; and
- Not too technically difficult.

The fact that there have been over 100 different procedures and modifications to treat shoulder instability is evidence that no one procedure has been able to meet all of these expectations. The following discussion reviews the complications and shortcomings of surgery for shoulder instability and special considerations of how they affect the competitive athlete.

Recurrence

ANTERIOR INSTABILITY

The numerous open procedures for anterior instability cannot be separated based on incidence of recurrence alone (Table 18.1). In reviewing the literature comprising over 2,300 cases, Rockwood (74) found that the average recurrence rate of reconstructions for anterior instability is 3%. Therefore, critical evaluation of the complications and functional results of each procedure are more important than selection based on rate of recurrence.

Recurrence is often caused by failure to correctly diagnose multidirectional laxity or inadequately addressing the primary pathology at the time of surgery. Capsular laxity, excessive tightness of repair, fixation failure, recurrent trauma, voluntary (intentional) instability, and posterior instability have all been associated with higher recurrence rates after surgery (19, 77). In contrast, regaining full motion has *not* been associated with increased recurrence (19, 77).

Recurrence in the form of anterior subluxation seems to be more frequent in procedures that fail to address the "essential lesion," whether that be capsular stripping from the glenoid neck (61), capsular laxity (62, 93), or capsular disruption (72, 90). While once proposed as a predominant factor in anterior instability, subscapularis deficiency as a primary cause is exceedingly rare (89).

A discussion of recurrence after shoulder reconstructions would not be complete without including arthroscopic capsulorrhaphy. Enthusiasm for this technique has escalated in hope of correcting instability but preserving motion, strength, and function. However, arthroscopic techinques must equal the low recurrence rates of open procedures. The recent reports of Johnson (47), Eckert and Richardson (21), and Gross (30) indicate that the recurrence after *staple* capsulorrhaphy is as high as 23%. However, both Morgan (58, 59) and Caspari (16) have reported less than 5% recurrence after arthroscopic *suture* capsulorrhaphy techniques used in properly selected patients. Our experience with the suture technique has also been favorable.

POSTERIOR INSTABILITY

Reconstructions for posterior instability have been reported to be less successful than anterior reconstructions (12, 35, 58, 64, 82, 91). Hawkins (35) reported poor results of treatment for posterior instability in 35 patients (50 shoulders). Forty-one shoulders had voluntary instability, and only 11 were attributed to trauma. In a study of 26 shoulders treated surgically (12), 17 glenoid osteotomies, six reverse Putti-Platts, and three biceps transfers were performed with recurrence of 41%, 83%, and 33%, respectively. This represents 50% recurrence. There was also a higher incidence of arthritis after glenoid osteotomy noted in this study. Kretzler (50) and Norwood (64) reported increased recurrence rates in voluntary or lax posterior dislocators after glenoid osteotomy. Results were somewhat better in those with definite traumatic etiology. Tibone (91) reported 30% recurrence after posterior staple capsulorrhaphy with 40% complications and none returning to throwing.

More recent authors have not expressed the same frustration in treating posterior instability. Bigliani (9) reported 25 posterior capsular shift procedures at 40-month follow-up with 88% good–excellent results and no recurrent instability. He emphasized accurate identification of those with willful dislocations and the importance of correcting capsular laxity with the procedure.

Our experience is more consistent with that of Bigliani. We distinguish between patients with microtrauma and those with macrotrauma. Fronek et al. (26) recently reported 27 patients with posterior subluxation treated in our institution. Sixteen had microtrauma without major disability, and 63% were successfully treated with rehabilitation alone. Eleven patients with either macrotrauma or major disability due to instability were treated surgically using a posterior modified capsular shift with 91% success. Bone-block procedures were rarely necessary, and the ability to voluntarily sublux the shoulder did not adversely affect the result. Many of these patients begin as purely involuntary subluxators, and with time are able to voluntarily reproduce the instability. This tends to be more positional than muscular in etiolgy. We would, however, caution against surgery in the patient with willful manipulative voluntary posterior instability. Surgery has been successful in returning several professional football players to their previous level of play.

Loss of Motion

During the first half of this century, most surgeons favored the use of procedures that did not address the primary pathology of anterior instability. Instead, limitation of external rotation was considered by many to be an essential component of reconstruction for anterior instability. Bankart (6) recognized that capsular stripping from the anterior inferior glenoid neck was present in most cases and encouraged repair of this "essential lesion." Using the Bankart procedure, Rowe (77) obtained good to excellent results in 97% with 3.5% recurrence. However, 24% of his patients regained only 75% of external rotation compared with the opposite shoulder. To prevent stiffness, he recommended complete external rotation to tighten the capsule while incising it, positioning in 20–30° external rotation for the repair and early postoperative motion, as this did not adversely affect results. Because of the technical difficulty of the Bankart procedure, many surgeons continued to use the Putti-Platt and Magnusson-Stack procedures for recurrent anterior instability. However, numerous reviews of these procedures have documented from 15–60° average loss of external rotation (1, 14, 32, 33, 48, 51, 52, 60, 66).

Thomas and Matsen (90) carefully documented motion in follow-up of 39 patients who had a modified Bankart procedure. External rotation averaged 68° at the side and 84° at 90° of abduction. Protzman (71) reviewed his experience with a modified Bankart procedure and found the average loss of external rotation to be 7° at the side and 12° at 90° of abduction.

The Bristow procedure was described in 1958 by Helfet (36). It rapidly gained popularity as a technically easy procedure that would allow full recovery of motion and function, even for the throwing athlete. Experience has now shown that, although the Bristow procedure is effective in preventing recurrence, it often results in a 10–20° average limitation in external rotation (8, 13, 23, 31, 38, 53, 55, 56, 63, 85). Hill (38), Halley (31), Lombardo (53), and Torg (92) all were unsuccessful in returning the throwing athlete to competition using the Bristow procedure. However, this was not simply related to loss of motion. For these reasons as well as more frequent complications and difficulty of revision, we have abandoned the use of the Bristow procedure.

In 1980, Neer (62) reported his experience with the capsular shift procedure for multidirectional instability. He emphasized the use of conservative treatment, but in cases requiring surgery, he considered 20° loss of external rotation ideal. All of his patients had multidirectional laxity, and 27% had had previous failed surgery. Six of seven swimmers were able to return to competitive swimming. In reviewing 42 cases of anterior/inferior instability treated at The Hospital for Special Surgery with a

"T" capsular shift modification of the Bankart procedure, Altchek et al. (2) found that the average loss of external rotation was 5° at the side and 4° at 90° of abduction. In addition, it was found that 85% of these patients with limited motion at follow-up had loss of motion preoperatively.

In evaluating the athlete for loss of motion, one should be aware that normal motion averages have been published (11). Average external rotation in males ranges from 90° (AAOS) to 104° (11). In addition, competitive throwers consistently have increased external rotation and decreased internal rotation in the dominant arm when compared with the nondominant arm. This side-to-side difference increases after the throwing "warm-up" (95).

At surgery, it is imperative not to use procedures that artificially capture the joint (i.e., Putti-Platt), but rather procedures that attempt to correct the primary pathology and restore motion. The lesion may be a torn labrum, a lax capsule/ligament, or a combination of both. If the labrum is torn without capsular stretching, then reattachment is sufficient. Conversely, if the capsule is lax, it must be tightened. In performing capsular procedures, we incise the capsule near the glenoid with the arm in full external rotation to avoid shortening. The capsule is advanced superiorly to create tension, not medially, to create a contracture (Fig. 18.5). While reattaching the capsule, we position the arm in about 40° abduction and 30° external rotation to avoid complete obliteration of the axillary pouch and to facilitate return of full motion postoperatively.

Return to Competition

It must be emphasized that when stability is restored, mild loss of external rotation is not a significant functional limitation for many athletes. Complete return of external rotation is not necessary for full participation in many sports, but it may severely limit participation in throwing, swimming, and racket sports. The throwing athlete, especially the pitcher, may have severe functional limitation due to loss of external rotation. Protzman (71) noted a direct correlation between functional result and recovery of motion.

Few studies have evaluated strength using isokinetic testing (38, 92). Post (70) has shown this to be much more sensitive in detecting loss of power and endurance than manual testing. Loss of strength and endurance most likely play a role in preventing return of the thrower to competition. Future studies

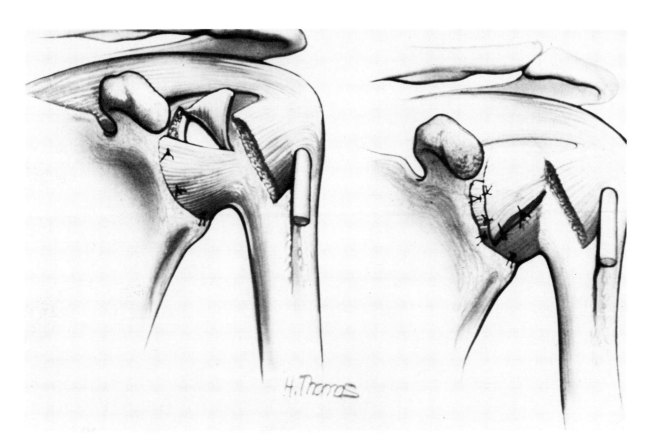

Figure 18.5.   Figure depicting our technique for "T"-type capsular shift to correct capsular laxity.

should more closely address this aspect of functional evaluation.

Jobe (45) recently has achieved improved return to competition after "capsulolabral" reconstruction in throwing athletes with anterior instability. Of 19 patients followed for 2 years, 79% returned to competitive throwing. Three of five professional pitchers returned. He emphasizes splitting the subscapularis longitudinally, reconstructing the inferior glenohumeral ligament-labral complex, and postoperative abduction splinting. The numbers in his review reveal that although shoulder instability in the competitive thrower is not rare, few of these athletes fail an adequate rehabilitation program and ultimately require surgery. The limited success of returning elite throwing athletes, especially pitchers, to preinjury function after surgery makes a strong case for adhering to the principles of conservative treatment until this has proven to have failed.

Metal Problems

Metal screws and staples have been used for capsulorrhaphy (20, 53), fixation of large glenoid rim fractures, bone-block procedures for deficient glenoids, and for the Bristow procedure (25, 27, 31–34, 38–40, 49, 63, 66, 72). In each of these settings, complications may arise due to incorrect placement, migration, loosening, breakage, and impingement or joint penetration, causing arthritis (Fig. 18.6). Samilson noted the frequent association of problems with metal implants with the presence of dislocation arthropathy (83).

Nonunion of the coracoid transfer after the Bristow procedure has been reported in 3–48% of cases (23, 38, 53, 75, 92). This incidence is very technique-dependent, but even large series reported by those experienced with the technique reveal that problems directly related to the screw occur in about 10% of cases (Fig. 18.7). Zuckerman and Matsen (100) reported 37 cases with complications due to metal implants, 21 of which were following the Bristow procedure. Hovelius (42) and, more recently, Young and Rockwood (75) have also emphasized the frequency of these complications after the Bristow procedure.

Small (88) found a 5.3% incidence of staple complications in 562 arthroscopic staple capsulor-

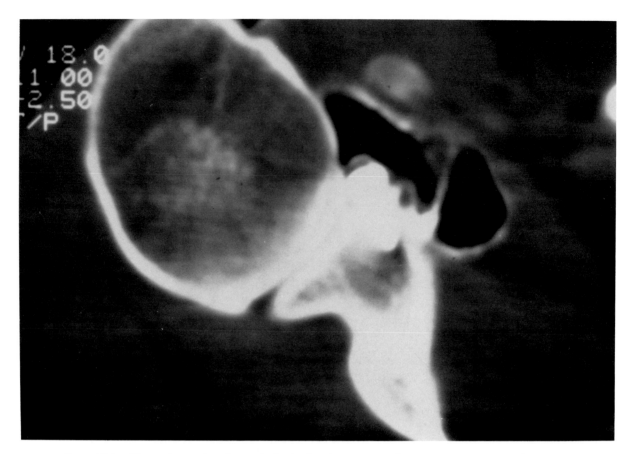

Figure 18.6. CT scan after metal staple capsulorrhaphy. The close proximity of the staple to the articular surface of the head may lead to wear and subsequent arthrosis.

rhaphies. This included 19 loose or migrated staples, six which impinged on the articular surface of the humeral head, two brachial plexus injuries, and two bent staples. Sisk and Boyd (87) reported similar problems in only five of 239 cases. Experience, caution, and proper technique can limit these complications. However, we prefer to avoid use of metal screws and staples in shoulder reconstructions.

Neurovascular Injury

Overall, the incidence of nerve injury during shoulder reconstructions is very low. Neer (62) reported three axillary neurapraxias in 40 inferior capsular shift procedures. Musculocutaneous nerve injury has occurred following excessive retraction on the conjoined tendon and more often is related to the Bristow procedure (5, 25).

To avoid nerve injury, the surgeon should exercise caution in retracting the conjoined tendon and subscapularis. Anterior dissection should be lateral to the conjoined tendon. It is important to know where the axillary nerve is, but it is not necessary to routinely visualize the nerve. In contrast, when operating for multidirectional instability, the nerve should be identified by palpation or observation and carefully avoided while dissecting the inferior capsule (62).

The average distance from the coracoid tip to muscular insertion of the musculocutaneous nerve has been reported to be 5.6 cm by Flatow (24), 4.7 cm by Burkhead (15), and 4.9 cm by Bach (5). This distance is less than 2.5 cm in 5% of specimens (5). In addition, transfer of the coracoid to the glenoid neck has been shown by Burkhead to move the nerve an average of 1.9 cm proximally. Therefore, great caution must be taken when dissecting in this region, especially for revision of the Bristow procedure.

Vascular injury is rare but has been reported due to screw migration after the Bristow procedure (4, 22, 43). Pseudoaneurysm formation may result and even cause compression of the brachial plexus.

Arthritis

Though infrequent, dislocation arthropathy is more often due to surgical intervention (83). Certain procedures such as the Eden-Hybbonette bone block and those employing internal fixation devices were more commonly associated with arthritis. Impingement or intra-articular placement of metal screws or staples may be associated. In addition, Hawkins (33) reported increased arthritic changes in patients with excessively tight Putti-Platt reconstructions (Fig. 18.8). An excessively tight anterior repair causes an internal rotation contracture and results in high compressive and shearing loads on the articular cartilage with subsequent arthrosis.

Wound Problems

Wound problems can occur in all patients. Widening of surgical scars about the shoulder is a common occurrence and may be of cosmetic concern, especially for women. This risk of scar widening is best minimized by keeping the incision within Langer's lines and performing a running subcutic-

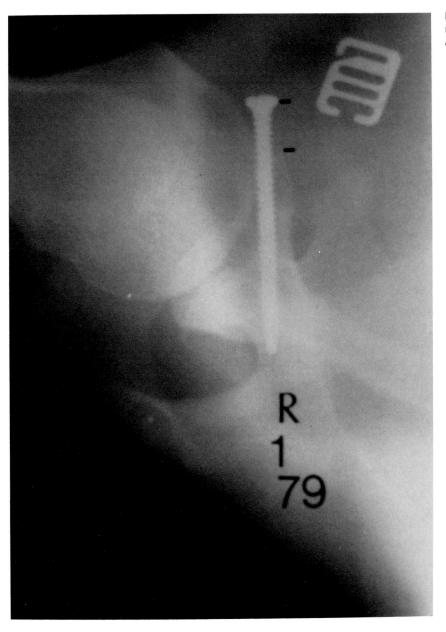

Figure 18.7. Axillary view demonstrating nonunion of a coracoid transfer to the anterior glenoid neck (Bristow procedure).

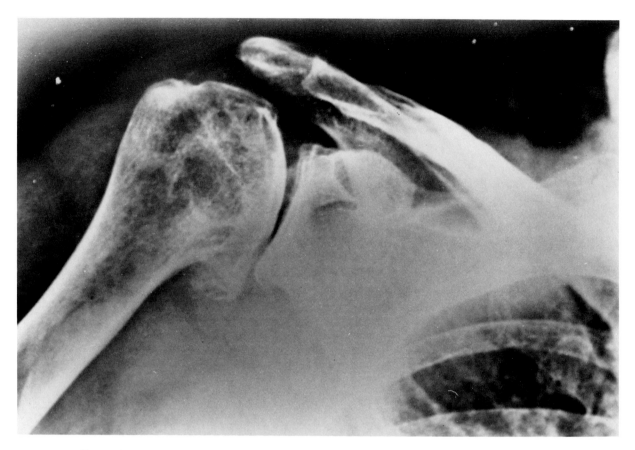

Figure 18.8. AP x-ray demonstrating severe arthritis in a shoulder after an excessively tight Putti-Platt procedure.

ular skin closure. Hematoma formation can be prevented by meticulous hemostasis and suction drainage. Prophylactic antibiotics will reduce infection rates. When these problems are encountered, early evacuation of hematoma or purulence is recommended to decrease morbidity.

POSTOPERATIVE MANAGEMENT

For the surgical patient, range of motion is tested on the table to determine the safe zone of motion, especially external rotation, for the postoperative rehabilitation program. This program is determined by the following factors: arm dominance, generalized laxity, direction of instability, type of repair, and the goals of the patient (i.e., thrower vs. football lineman).

For the football lineman, after anterior stabilization, the arm is protected in a sling for 5–6 weeks, allowing only pendulum exercises for the first 4 weeks. Thereafter, external rotation is slowly increased with elevation above 90° avoided for 6 weeks. At this time, gentle stretching exercises are used, followed by strengthening at 8–10 weeks. Although Rowe (77, 79, 81) has recommended early removal of the sling, we have seen patients fall after surgery and disrupt a repair that was not protected by sling immobilization. It is safer to protect the arm from sudden high loads for approximately 4 weeks.

The exception to this program is in the dominant arm of the throwing athlete, where we use a more aggressive approach to regain motion. Pendulum exercises are allowed immediately, and at 2 weeks, gentle exercises are initiated to regain flexion and external rotation. External rotation is allowed only to a degree that is predetermined at the time of surgery. The goal is to regain full forward flexion by the 6th postoperative week. Forced external rotation is avoided until the 6th week, when we begin gentle stretching in abduction/external rotation. The strengthening program previously described is started after adequate motion returns, usually from the 8th to 10th postoperative week. Participation in noncontact sports is allowed at 4 months, but contact sports and throwing are avoided until the 6th postoperative month.

ROLE OF ARTHROSCOPY

The arthroscope is an established tool for diagnostic purposes. In the majority of cases, a thorough history, physical examination, and radiologic workup will clarify the instability pattern. However, for cases where the diagnosis remains unclear, examination under anesthesia and diagnostic arthroscopy are of great value (18, 20). Recent success has been reported in the arthroscopic treatment of impingement syndrome and shoulder instability (16, 21, 27, 30, 47, 54, 59, 65, 98).

Pappas (67) described three types of shoulder instability: dislocation, subluxation, and "functional glenohumeral instability" due to labral tears that cause mechanical symptoms but do not represent true instability. He reported good results after simple arthroscopic excision of the labral tear. Andrews (3) has also reported limited success in excision of these lesions.

Our experience has been that if the labral tear is below the equator of the glenoid, there is usually associated instability. Simple labral debridement in this setting has not been very successful and may even worsen the instability. This is especially true if the attachment of the inferior glenohumeral ligament is compromised.

We currently use arthroscopic stabilization for selected patients with recurrent traumatic unidirectional anterior instability. The high incidence (85%) of Bankart lesions in this population lends itself to arthroscopic stabilization procedures. If there is evidence of multidirectional instability on examination under anesthesia (EUA) or generalized ligamentous laxity, then we prefer open reconstruction (96).

When performing arthroscopic stabilization, it is imperative to debride the soft tissue and prepare a bleeding bony bed at the anterior inferior glenoid site for reattachment. We use one of two arthroscopic techniques. The first involves passing absorbable sutures (0–PDS) through the avulsed capsule and inferior glenohumeral ligament. These sutures are then passed through drill holes in the glenoid using modified Beath needles (Biomet). The needles exit through the infraspinatus fossa, and the sutures are tied subcutaneously (Fig. 18.9). The second technique involves using a cannulated absorbable Maxon tack (Acufex) that secures the detached capsular complex to the glenoid rim. The tack is inserted over a guide wire into a predrilled hole (Fig. 18.10). Because of the frequency of complications due to metal staples, we do not advocate their use.

The recent reports of Caspari (16) and Morgan (59) confirm that these techniques are successful when used by experienced shoulder arthroscopists and with appropriate indications. Their results have equaled those of open procedures. However, when considering the role of arthroscopic stabilization techniques, several questions remain to be answered:

1. *Is the arthroscopic stabilization appropriate for the athlete who participates in contact sports?*

We have maintained that if arthroscopic stabilization techniques are effective, then once healing of the lesion has occurred, the athlete should be able to participate in contact sports. Therefore, it has been our approach to apply these techniques to these athletes as well when there is capsular stripping from the anterior glenoid neck. In this setting, we have found the technique to be successful. We do protect the repair by sling immobilization for 4 weeks, allowing only gentle pendulum exercises.

2. *What is the role of arthroscopic stabilization in the dominant arm of a throwing athlete?*

Because of the limited success of open procedures in throwers, we currently favor arthroscopic stabilization in an attempt to minimize scar formation. There is a balance between protection of the repair and the need for early rehabilitation to regain full motion and strength. We currently begin pendulum exercises within the first week and then allow gentle progression in range of motion. Forced external rotation is avoided for 6 weeks.

3. *What is the role of arthroscopic stabilization for acute anterior dislocations in the high-risk patient?*

Since Rowe (76) reported the extremely high rate of recurrence in young patients, surgeons have debated over the indications for surgery in the acute setting. We generally have favored waiting to operate on recurrent instability. However, we believe that there is a place for surgery after only one dislocation in the high-risk patient who wants to minimize his chances of recurrence. This may be preferred immediately or at the conclusion of the season. The role of arthroscopic stabilization in this setting is under investigation in several centers, including our own.

CONCLUSION

Complications of shoulder instability that are inherent to the injury itself will be best managed by awareness, early recognition, and appropriate treatment, as outlined. Those that are a result of surgical

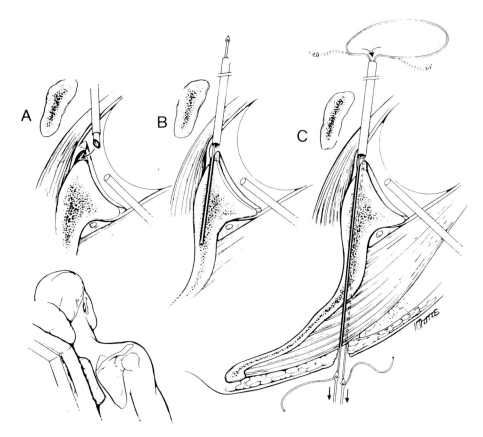

Figure 18.9. Technique of arthroscopic suture capsulorrhaphy. **A,** Abrasion of the anterior glenoid neck to create a well-vascularized bed and to optimize healing. **B,** Modified Beath needles are drilled across the scapula to exit in the infraspinatus fossa. **C,** The needles are passed posteriorly, delivering the sutures that are tied over fascia. The posterior exit point of the needles should err toward the inferior and medial aspect of the fossa in order to avoid damage to the suprascapular nerve as it courses around the base of the scapular spine.

treatment must be minimized by selection of a technique that is appropriate for the athlete's goals, skillful surgical employment of the technique, and appropriate rehabilitation based on intraoperative findings.

References

1. Aamoth GM, O'Phelan EH. Recurrent anterior dislocation of the shoulder: a review of forty athletes treated by sub-scapularis transfer (modified Magnuson-Stack procedure). Am J Sports Med 1977;5:188–190.
2. Altchek DW, Skyhar MJ, Warren RF, Ortiz G. T-plasty anterior repair for anterior-inferior multidirectional instability of the shoulder. Presented at the 4th International Conference on Surgery of the Shoulder, New York, NY, October 1989. Orthop Trans 1989;13:55.
3. Andrews JR, Carson WG. The arthroscopic treatment of glenoid labrum tears in the throwing athlete. Orthop Trans 1984;8:44.
4. Artz T, Huffer JM. A major complication of the modified Bristow procedure for recurrent dislocation of the shoulder. J Bone Joint Surg 1972;54A:1293–1296.
5. Bach BR, O'Brien SJ, Warren RF, Leighton M. An unusual neurological complication of the Bristow procedure. J Bone Joint Surg 1988;70A:458–460.
6. Bankart ASB. The pathology and treatment of recurrent dislocation of the shoulder joint. Br J Surg 1938;26:23–29.
7. Barnes DA, Tullos HS. An analysis of 100 symptomatic baseball players. Am J Sports Med 1978;6:62–67.
8. Barry TP, Lombardo SJ, Kerlan RK, et al. The coracoid transfer for recurrent anterior instability of the shoulder in adolescence. J Bone Joint Surg 1985;67A:383–387.
9. Bigliani LU, McIlveen SJ, Flatow EL, Dalsey RM. Operative management of posterior shoulder instability. Orthop Trans 1989;13:232.
10. Blazina ME. Shoulder injuries in athletes. J Am Coll Health Assoc 1966;15:143–145.
11. Boone DC, Azen SP. Normal range of motion of joints in male subjects. J Bone Joint Surg 1979;61A:756–759.
12. Boyd HB, Sisk TD. Recurrent posterior dislocation of the shoulder. J Bone Joint Surg 1972;54A:779–786.
13. Braly WG, Tullos HS. A modification of the Bristow procedure for recurrent anterior shoulder dislocation and subluxation. Am J Sports Med 1985;13:81–86.
14. Brav EA. An evaluation of the Putti-Platt reconstruction procedure for recurrent dislocation of the shoulder. J Bone Joint Surg 1955;37A:731–741.

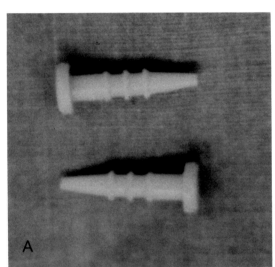

Figure 18.10. **A,** Absorbable Maxon tack (Acufex) used for arthroscopic capsulorrhaphy. The life of the standard tack is about 4 weeks, and there is now one with a life of 3 months. **B,** Arthroscopic photograph demonstrating placement of the tack through the inferior glenohumeral ligament and into the anterior glenoid neck.

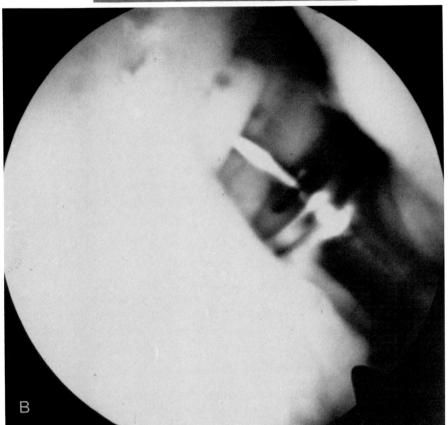

15. Burkhead WZ, Box G. Musculocutaneous and axillary nerve position after coracoid transfer. Presented at the 4th International Conference on Surgery of the Shoulder, New York, NY, October 1989. Orthop Trans 1989;13:232.

16. Caspari RB, Meyers JS, Savoie FH, Sutter J. Arthroscopic management of shoulder instability. Presented at the 4th International Conference on Surgery of the Shoulder, New York, NY, October 1989.

17. Clayton ML, Weir GJ, Jr. Experimental investigations of ligamentous healing. Am J Surg 1959;98:373–378.

18. Cofield RH, Irving JF. Evaluation and classification of shoulder instability: with special reference to examination under anesthesia. Clin Orthop 1987;223:32–42.

19. Cofield RH, Kavanagh BF, Frassica FJ. Anterior shoulder instability. In: American Academy of Orthopaedic Surgeons Instructional Course Lectures 1985;34:210.

20. DuToit G, Roux D. Recurrent dislocation of the shoulder. A twenty-four year study of the Johannesburg stapling operation. J Bone Joint Surg 1956;38A:1–12.

21. Eckert RR, Richardson AB, Derick GH. Arthroscopic

shoulder stapling for instability. Presented at the 4th International Conference on Surgery of the Shoulder, New York, NY, October 1989.

22. Fee HJ, McAvoy JM, Dainko EA. Pseudo aneurysm of the axillary artery following a modified Bristow operation. J Cardiovasc Surg 1978;19:65–68.

23. Ferlic DC, DiGiovine NM. A long-term retrospective study of the modified Bristow procedure. Am J Sports Med 1988;16:469–474.

24. Flatow EL, Bigliani LU, April EW. An anatomic study of the musculocutaneous nerve and its relationship to the coracoid process. Clin Orthop 1989;244:166–171.

25. Franken TH. Injury to the musculocutaneous nerve as a complication of operations for recurrent dislocation of the shoulder. J Bone Joint Surg 1984;66B:449.

26. Fronek J, Warren RF, Bowen M. Posterior subluxation of the glenohumeral joint. J Bone Joint Surg 1989;71A:205–216.

27. Fu FH, Klein AH. Shoulder arthroscopy: complications and pitfalls. Techniques in Orthopaedics 1988;3:27–32.

28. Gerber C, Ganz R. Clinical assessment of instability of the shoulder with special reference to anterior and posterior drawer tests. J Bone Joint Surg 1984;66B:551–556.

29. Glousman R, Jobe F, Tibone J, Moynes D, Antonelli D, Perry J. Dynamic electromyographic analysis of the throwing shoulder with glenohumeral instability. J Bone Joint Surg 1988;70A:220.

30. Gross RM. Arthroscopic shoulder capsulorrhaphy: does it work? Am J Sports Med 1989;17:495–500.

31. Halley DK, Olix ML. A review of the Bristow operation for recurrent anterior shoulder dislocation in athletes. Clin Orthop 1975;106:175–179.

32. Hastings DE, Coughlin LP. Recurrent subluxation of the glenohumeral joint. Am J Sports Med 1981;9:352–355.

33. Hawkins RJ. Paper #7, presented at the 4th Open Meeting of the American Shoulder and Elbow Surgeons, Atlanta, GA, February 1988.

34. Hawkins RJ, Koppert G. The natural history following anterior dislocation of the shoulder in the older patient. J Bone Joint Surg 1982;64B:255.

35. Hawkins RJ, Koppert G, Johnston G. Recurrent posterior instability (subluxation) of the shoulder. J Bone Joint Surg 1984;66A:169–174.

36. Helfet AJ. Coracoid transplantation for recurrent dislocation of the shoulder. J Bone Joint Surg 1958;40B:198–202.

37. Henry JH, Genung JA. Natural history of glenohumeral dislocation—revisited. Am J Sports Med 1982;10:135–140.

38. Hill JA, Lombardo SJ, Kerlan RK, et al. The modified Bristow-Helfet procedure for recurrent anterior shoulder subluxations and dislocations. Am J Sports Med 1981;9:283–287.

39. Hovelius L. Incidence of shoulder dislocation in Sweden. Clin Orthop 1982;166:127–131.

40. Hovelius L. Anterior dislocation of the shoulder in teenagers and young adults. J Bone Joint Surg 1987;69A:393–399.

41. Hovelius L, Eriksson GK, Fredin FH, et al. Recurrences after initial dislocation of the shoulder. J Bone Joint Surg 1983;65A:343–349.

42. Hovelius L, Korner GL, Lundberg GB, Akermark GC, Herberts SP, Wredmark GT, Berg E. The coracoid transfer for recurrent dislocation of the shoulder. J Bone Joint Surg 1983;65A:926–934.

43. Iftikhar TB, Kaminski RS, Silva I. Neurovascular complications of the modified Bristow procedure. J Bone Joint Surg 1984;66A:951–952.

44. Jobe FW. Unstable shoulders in the athlete. In: American Academy of Orthopaedic Surgeons Instructional Course Lectures 1985;34:228.

45. Jobe FW, Giangarra CE, Glousman RW. Anterior capsulolabral reconstruction in throwing athletes. Presented at the 4th International Conference on Surgery of the Shoulder, New York, NY, October 1989.

46. Jobe FW, Moynes DR, Tibone JE, Perry J. An EMG analysis of the shoulder in pitching. Am J Sports Med 1984;12:218–220.

47. Johnson LL. Arthroscopic stapling capsulorrhaphy. Presented at the 4th International Conference on Surgery of the Shoulder, New York, NY, October 1989.

48. Karadimas J, Rentis G, Varouchas G. Repair of recurrent anterior dislocation of the shoulder using transfer of the subscapularis tendon. J Bone Joint Surg 1980;62A:1147–1149.

49. Kiviluoto O. Immobilization after primary dislocation of the shoulder. Acta Orthop Scan 1980;51:915.

50. Kretzler HH. Scapular osteotomy for posterior dislocation of the shoulder. J Bone Joint Surg 1974;56A:197.

51. Leach RE, Corbett M, Schepsis A, Stockel J. Results of a modified Putti-Platt operation for recurrent shoulder dislocations and subluxations. Clin Orthop 1982;164:20–25.

52. Lipscomb AB. Treatment of recurrent anterior dislocation and subluxation of the glenohumeral joint in athletes. Clin Orthop 1975;109:122–125.

53. Lombardo SJ, Kerlan RK, Jobe FW, Carter VS, Blazina ME, Shields CL. The modified Bristow procedure for recurrent dislocation of the shoulder. J Bone Joint Surg 1976;58A:256–261.

54. Maki NJ. Arthroscopic stabilization for recurrent shoulder instability. Presented at the 4th International Conference on Surgery of the Shoulder, New York, NY, October 1989.

55. May VR. A modified Bristow operation for anterior recurrent dislocation of the shoulder. J Bone Joint Surg 1970;52A:1010–1016.

56. MacKenzie DB. The Bristow-Helfet operation for recurrent anterior dislocation of the shoulder. J Bone Joint Surg 1980;62B:273.

57. McLaughlin HL, Cavallaro WU. Primary anterior dislocation of the shoulder. Am J Surg 1950;80:615.

58. Morgan CD, Bodenstab AD. Arthroscopic Bankart suture repair: technique and early results. Arthroscopy 1987;3:111–122.

59. Morgan CD. Arthrosopic Bankart suture repair—two to five year results. Paper #7, 5th Annual Meeting, American Shoulder and Elbow Surgeons, Las Vegas, February 12, 1989. Orthop Trans 1989;13:231.

60. Morrey BF, Janes JM. Recurrent anterior dislocation of the shoulder. J Bone Joint Surg 1976;58A:252–256.

61. Moseley HF, Overgaard B. The anterior capsular mechanism in recurrent anterior dislocation of the shoulder. J Bone Joint Surg 1962;44B:913–927.

62. Neer CS, Foster CR. Inferior capsular shift for involuntary inferior and multidirectional instability of the shoulder. J Bone Joint Surg 1980;62A:897–907.

63. Nielsen AB, Nielsen K. The modified Bristow procedure for recurrent anterior dislocation of the shoulder. Acta Orthop Scand 1982;53:229–232.

64. Norwood AL, Terry GC. Shoulder posterior subluxation. Am J Sports Med 1984;12:25–30.

65. Ogilvie-Harris DJ, Wyley AM. Arthroscopic surgery of the shoulder. A general appraisal. J Bone Joint Surg 1986; 68B:201–207.

66. Osmond-Clarke H. Habitual dislocation of the shoulder. J Bone Joint Surg 1948;30B:19–25.

67. Pappas AM, Goss TP, Kleinman PK. Symptomatic shoulder instability due to lesions of the glenoid labrum. Am J Sports Med 1983;11:279–288.

68. Pappas AM, Zawacki RM, Sullivan TJ. Biomechanics of baseball pitching. Am J Sports Med 1985;13:216–222.

69. Perry J. Anatomy and biomechanics of the shoulder in throwing, swimming, gymnastics, and tennis. Clin Sports Med 1983;2:247–270.

70. Post M, Rabin S. A comparative study of clinical muscle testing and Cybex evaluation following surgery upon the shoulder. Presented at the 4th International Conference on Surgery of the Shoulder, New York, NY, October 1989.

71. Protzman RR. Anterior instability of the shoulder. J Bone Joint Surg 1980;62A:909–918.

72. Reeves B. Experiments on the tensile strength of the anterior capsular structures of the shoulder in man. J Bone Joint Surg 1968;50B:858–865.

73. Richardson AB, Jobe FW, Collins HR. The shoulder in competitive swimming. Am J Sports Med 1980;8:159–163.

74. Rockwood CA. Subluxations and dislocations about the shoulder. In: Rockwood CA, Green DP, eds. Fractures in adults. Philadelphia: JB Lippincott, 1984:722–860.

75. Rockwood CA, Young DC. Complications and management of the failed Bristow shoulder reconstruction. Presented at the 5th Open Meeting of the American Shoulder and Elbow Surgeons, Las Vegas, February 12, 1989. Orthop Trans 1989;13:232.

76. Rowe CR. Prognosis and dislocations of the shoulder. J Bone Joint Surg 1956;38A:957–977.

77. Rowe CR, Patel D, Southmayd WW. The Bankart procedure: a long-term end-result study. J Bone Joint Surg 1978;60A:1–16.

78. Rowe CR, Pierce DS, Clarke JG. Voluntary dislocation of the shoulder. J Bone Joint Surg 1973;55A:445–460.

79. Rowe CR, Sakellarides HT. Factors related to recurrences of anterior dislocation of the shoulder. Clin Orthop 1961; 20:40–47.

80. Rowe CR, Zarins B. Recurrent transient subluxation of the shoulder. J Bone Joint Surg 1981;63A:863–872.

81. Rowe CR, Zarins B, Ciullo JV. Recurrent anterior dislocation of the shoulder after surgical repair. J Bone Joint Surg 1984;66A:159–168.

82. Samilson RL, Prieto V. Posterior dislocation of the shoulder in athletes. Clin Sports Med 2:369–378.

83. Samilson RL, Prieto V. Dislocation arthropathy of the shoulder. J Bone Joint Surg 1983;65A:456–460.

84. Skyhar MJ, Warren RF, Altchek DW. Shoulder instability in athletes. In: Rockwood CA, Matsen F, eds. Surgery of the shoulder. Philadelphia: WB Saunders, 1989.

85. Shively J, Johnson J. Results of modified Bristow procedure. Clin Orthop 1984;187:150–153.

86. Simonet WT, Cofield RH. Prognosis in anterior shoulder dislocations. Am J Sports Med 1984;12:19–24.

87. Sisk TD, Boyd HB. Management of recurrent anterior dislocation of the shoulder. Clin Orthop 1974;103:150–156.

88. Small NC. Complications in arthroscopy: knee and other joints. Arthroscopy 1986;2:253–258.

89. Symeonides PP. The significance of the subscapularis muscle in the pathogenesis of recurrent anterior dislocation of the shoulder. J Bone Joint Surg 1972;54B:476–483.

90. Thomas SC, Matsen FA. An approach to the repair of avulsion of the glenohumeral ligaments in the management of traumatic anterior glenohumeral instability. J Bone Joint Surg 1989;71A:506–513.

91. Tibone JE, Prietto C, Jobe FW, et al. Staple capsulorrhaphy for recurrent posterior shoulder dislocation. Am J Sports Med 1981;9:135–139.

92. Torg JS, Balduini FC, Bonci C, Lehman RC, Gregg JR, Esterhai JL, Hensal FJ. A modified Bristow-Helfet-May procedure for recurrent dislocation and subluxation of the shoulder. J Bone Joint Surg 1987;69A:904–913.

93. Townley CO. The capsular mechanism in recurrent dislocation of the shoulder. J Bone Joint Surg 1950;32A:370–380.

94. Tullos HS, Bennett JB, Braly WG. Acute shoulder dislocations: factors influencing diagnosis and treatment. In: American Academy of Orthopaedic Surgeons Instructional Course Lectures 1985;34:364.

95. Tullos HS, King JW. Throwing mechanisms in sports. Orthop Clin NA 1973;4:709–720.

96. Warren RF. Subluxation of the shoulder in athletes. Clin Sports Med 1983;2:339–354.

97. Watson-Jones R. Recurrent dislocation of the shoulder. J Bone Joint Surg 1948;30B:6.

98. Wolf EM. Arthroscopic anterior shoulder capsulorrhaphy. Techniques in Orthopaedics 1988;3:67–73.

99. Yoneda B, Welsh RP, MacIntosh DL. Conservative treatment of shoulder dislocation. J Bone Joint Surg 1982; 54B:254–255.

100. Zuckerman J, Matsen F. Complications about the glenohumeral joint related to the use of screws and staples. J Bone Joint Surg 1984;66A:175.

19
Management of Resistant Subacromial Impingement Lesions in Competitive Athletes

James Tibone and James P. Bradley

INTRODUCTION

Athletes who participate in overhand sports commonly sustain injuries to the shoulder localized to the rotator cuff and ligamentous capsule. Chronic stress initiated by the repetitive high-velocity nature of these overhand throwing activities often predispose the shoulder to impingement syndrome and rotator cuff pathology. The sports most commonly implicated include: baseball, (especially pitching), tennis (serve, overhead smash), football, (quarterbacks), swimming, gymnastics, and javelin throwers.

Impingement syndrome associated with overhand athletes has been well documented in the literature. Sometimes the athlete will fail to improve after conservative or surgical management, and resistant impingement symptoms will persist. In athletes with resistant subacromial impingement symptoms, several entities must be carefully scrutinized to ensure proper treatment and recovery. They include: (*a*) correct diagnosis with special attention to underlying shoulder instability; (*b*) proper rehabilitation designed for rotator cuff and scapular rotator strengthening and stretching; and (*c*) proper surgical procedure and rehabilitation when indicated. Careful attention to the above problems should enable the orthopaedist to provide the athlete with the best chance for recovery and return to overhead athletics.

The purpose of this chapter is to highlight various common pitfalls associated with the conservative and operative management of resistant impingement syndrome in athletes and to discuss rarer maladies that occasionally mimic impingement syndrome. Knowledge of these problems will hopefully aid in the proper evaluation and treatment of impingement syndrome.

SUBACROMIAL IMPINGEMENT SYNDROME

The functional arc of motion of the shoulder in both athletes and the general population is forward, not lateral, and impingement of the rotator cuff and biceps tendon occurs against the anterior edge of the acromion, coracoacromial ligament, and undersurface of the acromioclavicular joint (22) (Fig. 19.1). Subacromial impingement usually is localized to the supraspinatus insertion on the humerus; however, it may also involve the adjacent long head of the biceps (9, 22, 23). Neer (23) emphasized that the subacromial bursa, supraspinatus tendon, long head of the biceps, and acromioclavicular joint should not be thought of as separate structures. Rather, recognize that they may all be involved together in the impingement process. The space available for the rotator cuff to pass beneath the coracoacromial arch is limited. Therefore, any processes that increase the volume of structures that pass beneath the coracoacromial arch or decrease the space available for the supraspinatus or biceps tendons will result in impingement. In athletes, the usual mechanism is an increase in volume by hypertrophy of the musculotendinous structures, or a local inflammatory response that causes edema and thickening of the cuff and subacromial bursa, secondary to microtrauma.

Throwing by virtue of its force, velocity, and repetition will predispose the shoulder to impingement by either of the aforementioned mechanisms. In older athletes, decreasing the size of the subacromial space by proximal migration of the humeral head with cuff degeneration or osteophyte formation will exacerbate the impingement.

Effective throwing requires the arm to be maximally extended, abducted, and externally rotated. During the throwing cycle, the arm moves from full external rotation into internal rotation, and the con-

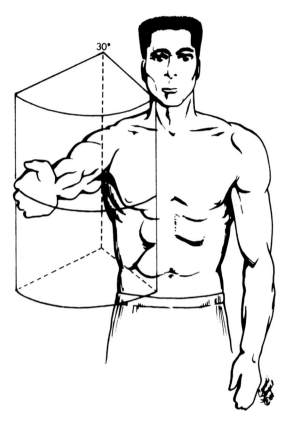

Figure 19.1. Demonstration of the functional arc of motion of the shoulder.

tracting rotator cuff muscles must pass directly under the coracoacromial arch (impingement area), potentially creating rotator cuff irritation and microtrauma. (Fig. 19.2)

Neer (23) described three progressive stages of impingement: stage I, edema and hemorrhage; stage II, fibrosis and tendinitis; stage III, bone spurs and tendon ruptures. Jobe (16) modified this classification into four stages with stage III divided into cuff tears of less than 1 cm and stage IV consisting of cuff tears greater than one centimeter.

Stage I Impingement

Overuse from overhead sports produces supraspinatus edema and hemorrhage. This lesion is predominant in young athletes, (less than 25 years of age), and responds well to activity modification and conservative treatment (reversible lesions).

Stage II Impingement

In athletes who incur several bouts of repeated mechanical irritation and inflammation (stage I impingement), the subacromial bursa will become fibrotic and thickened, which exacerbates the problem. Underlying supraspinatus tendinitis is also a

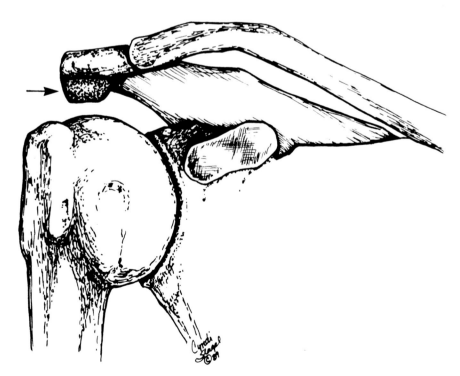

Figure 19.2. An acromial spur causing rotator cuff injury.

feature in stage II. This lesion is common in an older age group, (25–40 years of age), and is commonly responsive to conservative measures.

Stage III Impingement

Characteristically, this stage presents in persons over 40 years of age with a past history of multiple episodes of subacromial impingement (bursitis). The hallmark of this stage is the presence of a rotator cuff tear and associated bony osteophytes of the acromion and inferior distal clavicle. Conservative treatment of stage III lesions in athletes usually fails, and surgical management is generally indicated.

Stage IV Impingement

This stage corresponds to Neer's stage III impingement lesions, only the rotator cuff tear is greater than 1 cm. Surgical management is usually necessary.

In our experience, young overhand athletes with impingement syndrome usually respond to conservative treatment. Conservative treatment consists of rest from offending activity, anti-inflammatory medicine, occasional subacromial steroid injections in very painful cases, (not more than three in 1 year), and a supervised specific physical therapy protocol (10, 12, 13, 32). When these modalities fail, surgery is usually recommended; however, the literature is sparse on the results of surgery in an athletic population. Hawkins and Kennedy (10) reported that the results of anterior acromioplasty, done primarily for stage II disease, is unknown. They were surprised at the level of pain relief, yet the athletes were not always able to regain previous levels of competition. Neer (22) noted satisfactory results in 15 of 16 shoulders with incomplete rotator cuff tears (stage II) treated by open anterior acromioplasty. His subjects were all older than 40 years of age and had different functional demands than a younger overhand athletic population.

Tibone et al. (32) published a series on 35 shoulders in 33 athletes that had resistant stage I or II impingement treated by open anterior acromioplasty. Thirty-one of 35 shoulders (89%) were subjectively judged improved by the patients from their preoperative status. However, only 15 of 35 operated shoulders (43%) allowed return to the same preinjury level of competitive athletics, and only four of 18 athletes involved in pitching and throwing returned to their former preinjury status. He concluded that this operation was satisfactory for pain relief but does not allow an athlete to return to his former competitive status. Fly et al. (8) reported on 26 shoulders in 25 athletes younger than 40, who had arthroscopic subacromial decompression for stage I and II lesions. Twenty-two of the 26 shoulder patients (81%) showed a significant decrease in their pain. Overall, 77% of the patients returned to overhand athletics; however, only 46% were able to return to their previous level, and 31% returned to the same sport at a less intense level. The authors concluded that function is usually improved in the competitive athlete.

In the career high-demand athlete, however, the outcome with regard to pain, function, and return to previous sports is less predictable. Tibone and Elrod et al. (31) reported on 45 athletes with either a partial (30 patients) or a complete tear (15 patients) of the rotator cuff treated with anterior acromioplasty and repair of the tear. Thirty-nine (87%) of the patients stated that they were improved compared with their preoperative status, although only 34 patients (76%) felt that they had a significant reduction of pain. Objectively, 25 (56%) patients were rated as a good result, which allowed them to return to their former competitive status level without significant pain. Only 12 (41%) of the pitchers and throwers returned to their former competitive status. Seven (32%) of the 22 pitchers and throwers who had been active at a professional or collegiate level returned to the same competitive level. The authors concluded that acromioplasty combined with rotator cuff repair in a young athletic population provides satisfactory pain relief but does not guarantee that these patients will be able to return to their former competitive status.

Some investigators have recommended resection of the coracoacromial ligament for impingement syndromes in athletes (11, 26). This operation necessitates very little dissection and postoperative rehabilitation. Jackson (11) published a small series on nine patients in which at 1-year follow-up, five had been pain-free and returned to full function. Penny and Welsh (26) published a series on 20 athletes treated for biceps or supraspinatus impingements with a coracoacromial ligament resection. They report that 17 patients have returned to sporting activity without symptoms. This series, however, comprised only a small number of pitching injuries.

Athletes who participate in overhand sports activities including baseball, tennis, football, golf, javelin throwing, gymnastics, and swimming are predisposed to acquiring impingement syndrome. In most cases, the problem can be controlled with conservative treatment. Still, controversy surrounds the appropriate surgical management when conservative methods fail. In high-performance overhand athletes, the outcome as it affects return to their prior level, is unpredictable.

CAUSES OF RESISTANT SUBACROMIAL IMPINGEMENT

Improper Diagnosis

REFERRED PAIN

It is extremely important to remember that the shoulder is often the site of referred pain, most commonly from the cervical spine (C5–C6). Intradural, preforaminal, and postforaminal lesions of the neck can all precipitate shoulder pain (1). Ruptured intervertebral discs (preforaminal) remain the most common source of pain.

The character of the shoulder pain may often guide the orthopaedist to the site of pathology. Cervical spine pain is characterized by a deep burning pain in the posterior shoulder localized about the insertion of the levator scapulae and rhomboids. The pain will radiate down the arm to the fingers, associated with paresthesias in the fingers and less frequently in the forearm. The patient will sometimes be more comfortable with the shoulder abducted, allowing the forearm to rest on the top of his head. This maneuver presumably decreases some of the tension on the involved cervical roots. A good guideline is to ask the patient the site of maximal pain. If the patient points proximal to the lateral acromion, then the cervical spine or other proximal sites of pathology are likely. On physical examination, the Spurling test is helpful in uncovering cervical root irritation. The test entails lateral rotation of the cervical spine toward the painful shoulder and then application of cervical axial compression. Increasing pain or radiculopathy are positive findings (13).

Pleural referred pain should also be investigated. Especially noteworthy is Pancoast's tumor residing in the apex of the lung. Coincident Horner's syndrome (ptosis, miosis, anidrosis, and enophthalmos) may sometimes be the first clue to an apical tumor. Routine x-rays of the shoulder should always include the ipsilateral lung field to assess the pulmonary status.

Thoracic outlet syndrome may also produce pain, paresthesia, dysesthesia, numbness, weakness,

muscle atrophy, temperature changes, and trophic changes about the shoulder. This syndrome is caused by compression of the neurovascular bundle at or near the level of the thoracic outlet. Special tests such as Adson's, and costroclavicular maneuvers, as well as hyperabduction tests, will aid in its diagnosis (13).

Rarer sites of referred pain include gastric, pancreatic, cardiac, and diaphragmatic irritation (gallbladder, hepatic disorders) mediated through the phrenic nerve. A plethora of symptom complexes, some with subtle variations, may be evident when evaluating athletes with shoulder pain. Therefore, one should not assume that all shoulder pain in an athlete originates from the shoulder—a careful history and physical examination are essential.

Shoulder Pain Mimicking Impingement

Keep in mind that every athlete who presents with shoulder pain does not necessarily have impingement syndrome. The pain may be subcoracoid, glenohumeral, bony, neurologic, circulatory, or as discussed earlier, referred. A thorough understanding of the manifestations of impingement syndrome and a complete history and physical are very helpful.

AVASCULAR NECROSIS OF THE HUMERAL HEAD

Osteonecrosis of the humeral head can imitate impingement symptoms early in the course of the disease before obvious radiographic changes are apparent. The affected shoulder is painful, and wrist pain is a common feature. Lying on the shoulder is almost always painful; however, passive range of motion is maintained. Reduction of passive range of motion is noted as focal collapse of the humeral head, causing deformity, and a stiff shoulder occurs (24).

Radiographs are most helpful when they show a thin radiolucent line immediately below the subchondral cortex of the humeral head (Crescent sign) (Fig. 19.3). Bone scanning is usually abnormal before the typical radiographic changes of revascularization. Magnetic resonance scanning (MRI) is probably the most sensitive testing modality to show early avascular changes in the humeral head.

A complete past medical history commonly will alert the physician of the potential for osteonecrosis of the humeral head. A history of systemic adrenocorticoid drugs in moderate to high doses for several months may precede osteonecrosis. Spontaneous osteonecrosis has been noted in patients with systemic lupus erythematosus. Infrequent causes of osteonecrosis include primary or massive osteolysis (Gor-

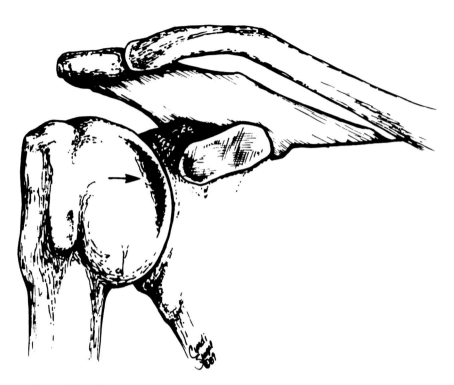

Figure 19.3.　Demonstration of a crescent sign seen in avascular necrosis of the shoulder.

ham's disease), sickle cell disease, Caisson disease, and pancreatitis (4, 24).

ACROMIOCLAVICULAR PATHOLOGY

One of the most prevalent causes of failed surgical treatment of impingement syndrome is neglecting to address acromioclavicular pathology (26). Acromioclavicular pathology can either be the primary cause of the pain or part of an associated degenerative process. Primary acromioclavicular pathology usually is preceded by a recent or remote acromioclavicular injury, and a thorough investigation to uncover this history should be sought. The subacromial bursa extends immediately below the acromioclavicular joint. This joint may very well degenerate because of extension of the inflammatory response of the impingement process (10, 26). Neer (22) noted the close anatomic proximity of the acromioclavicular joint to the supraspinatus tendon in abduction and reported that degenerative osteophytic lipping of this joint may continue to mechanically injure the supraspinatus muscle if not addressed. He further stated that one needs to understand the close anatomic relationships between the subacromial bursa, supraspinatus tendon, long head of the biceps, and acromioclavicular joint; thus, not thinking of these structures separately, but

rather recognizing that they may all be involved together (23).

Clinically, acromioclavicular symptoms usually localize to the acromioclavicular joint itself. However, the acromioclavicular joint may cause mechanical pain radiating toward the lateral border of the acromion or into the neck and trapezius (26). Acromioclavicular degeneration is best tested utilizing three maneuvers: (*a*) direct palpation; (*b*) adduction and internal rotation of the shoulder across the chest to compress the anterior joint together, causing pain; and (*c*) elevation of the arm to 90° of abduction, internal rotation, and extension to elicit pain by compressing the posterior aspect of the acromioclavicular joint (13, 26). Local injection of 1–2 cc xylocaine directly in the acromioclavicular joint may help verify the diagnosis by temporarily eliminating the pain during these maneuvers (26).

Routine radiographs of the acromioclavicular joint in any patient with suspected impingement syndrome are helpful. Acromioclavicular joint sclerosis, degeneration, or osteophytes (especially of the distal inferior clavicle) should be evaluated. A bone scan can confirm the inflammatory process in the acromioclavicular joint.

In the event that clinical and radiograph evidence of acromioclavicular degeneration is present, excision of the distal 1–2 cm of the clavicle in association with the primary procedure should be undertaken. If a history of acromioclavicular joint injury has been documented and clinical and radiographic evidence of acromioclavicular degeneration is present, then primary acromioclavicular pain mimicking impingement should be suspected.

FROZEN SHOULDER (ADHESIVE CAPSULITIS)

The etiology of frozen shoulder is not well understood; however, any stage of impingement syndrome may produce this process. Therefore, it is important to exclude the many other causes of frozen shoulder before implying that it is secondary to impingement. These other associations include: thyroid disorders, diabetes, autoimmune disease, immobilization, wrist fractures, and myocardial infarction (10, 28). Resistant subacromial impingement may, in fact, be caused by an underlying frozen shoulder, either as the primary cause of the shoulder pain or as a secondary manifestation of impingement syndrome. In either case, it must be addressed to ensure the proper conservative regimen or surgical procedure.

CALCIFIC BURSITIS

Although clinical findings of calcific bursitis are similar to impingement syndrome, it usually represents a distinct and separate pathologic process (10). Many authors feel that a metabolic rather than a local rotator cuff degenerative process may be the cause of calcific bursitis (19, 27). Clinically, calcification is rarely observed with degenerative rotator cuff disease (10). Many other conditions may produce periarticular calcifications. They include gout, hypervitaminous D, hyperparathyroidism, renal osteodystrophy, collagen vascular disease, pseudogout, and tumoral calcinosis (29).

LEVATOR SCAPULAE SYNDROME

This syndrome is a local tendinitis of the insertion of the levator scapulae to the superior medial scapula. The pain is deep, and the patients usually cannot localize the primary site of pain. Swimming, wrestling, boxing, gymnastics, karate, weightlifting, and golf have all been implicated (7). The mechanism is thought to be an acute or chronic overload of the levator scapulae at its insertion. During physical examination, however, the maximal tenderness is localized to the area of insertion of the levator scapulae in the posterior shoulder. Usually, the patient's symptoms resolve with a specific course of physical therapy and a steroid injection at the insertion of the levator scapulae (7).

SCAPULOTHORACIC BURSITIS

Located at the inferomedial angle of the scapula, the scapulothoracic bursa can become inflamed, especially in baseball pitchers. This condition is secondary to repetitive, high-velocity microtrauma applied to the anterior surface of the scapula, the underlying musculature, and the rib cage (30). Classically, the pain is localized to the inferior angle of the scapula during the cocking and acceleration stages of pitching and is alleviated at follow-through. A mass can often be palpated at the interomedial angle of the scapula. Usually, elevation to 60° and forward flexion to 30° enhances the examiner's ability to palpate the bursa sac. Shoulder range of motion is usually not affected. This condition may be associated with impingement and/or anterior instability seen in pitchers.

SUPRASCAPULAR NERVE ENTRAPMENT

Suprascapular nerve entrapment commonly occurs in the suprascapular notch; however, in the athlete, the nerve is often entrapped distally as it passes around the base of the acromion to innervate the infraspinatus. Athletes present with varied pain symptoms that are usually diagnosed as an impingement syndrome. On examination, there is obvious atrophy of the infraspinatus muscle with a normal-appearing supraspinatus. This has been seen in high-level pitchers. Because of the weakness of the rotator cuff, an impingement syndrome may coexist. This entrapment does not respond to surgical treatment. Good results have been attained with maximizing the residual infraspinatus muscle function and strengthening the remainder of the rotator cuff. The symptoms usually decrease with this exercise program, and the athletes are usually able to return to full competition.

LONG THORACIC NERVE INJURY

Injuries of the long thoracic nerve to the serratus anterior causes winging of the scapula. This can be diagnosed by having the patient perform a wall push-up and noticing the scapula being separated from the rib cage. Because of the weakness of the serratus anterior, the scapula cannot protract well with shoulder elevation. This can lead to a secondary impingement syndrome because of asyncrony of scapula thoracic motion with glenohumeral motion. With poor protraction of the scapula, the acromion does not elevate properly to allow proper clearance of the rotator cuff tendons. This can cause a very resistant impingement syndrome. Treatment consists of a therapy program to strengthen the serratus anterior and the trapezius muscle. The shoulder commonly responds to conservative care.

QUADRILATERAL SPACE SYNDROME

This is a very rare entity caused by compression of the posterior humeral circumflex artery and axillary nerve in the quadrilateral space (Fig. 19.4). Symptoms are insidious, with intermittent onset of pain and paresthesias in the upper extremity (8). Forward flexion and/or abduction and external rotation of the humerus aggravate the symptoms. As one would expect, throwing athletes seem to be the most susceptible, especially pitchers (25). The pain is poorly localized to the anterior shoulder, and sometimes paresthesias are noted in a nondermatomal distribution (3, 25). Palpation over the quadrilateral space causes pain, and hyperabduction and external rotation causes severe pain after several minutes. The diagnosis is made with a subclavian arteriogram.

It will demonstrate a patent posterior humeral circumflex artery with the arm at the side; however, occlusion of the artery occurs with the humerus hyperabducted and externally rotated (3, 5, 20, 25). Occlusion of the posterior circumflex artery indirectly indicates compression of the axillary nerve by fibrous bands that tether the quadrilateral space (3, 25). In patients with sufficient symptoms not improved by conservative treatment, a surgical decompression of the quadrilateral space is indicated (3, 5, 20, 25).

ROTATOR CUFF TENSION FAILURE WITHOUT IMPINGEMENT

Differentiating rotator cuff (supraspinatus) tension failure from incomplete rotator cuff tears secondary to progressive impingement is extremely difficult in throwing athletes. In either condition, the athletes present with impingement symptoms, one or more positive impingement signs (13), and commonly a positive impingement test (subacromial xylocaine injection). No definitive evidence by either history or physical exam has proven diagnostic. Arthroscopy is necessary to diagnose this condition.

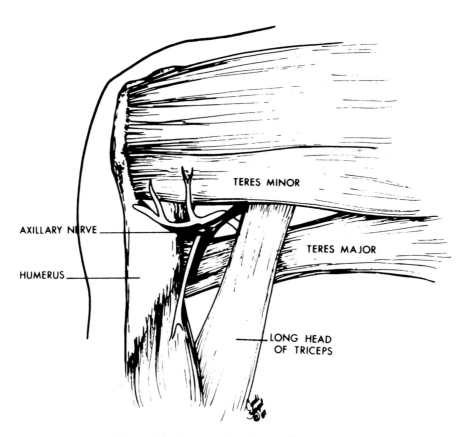

TERES MINOR

AXILLARY NERVE

TERES MAJOR

HUMERUS

LONG HEAD OF TRICEPS

Figure 19.4. Demonstration of the quadrilateral space.

Diagnostic arthroscopy has demonstrated a small incomplete undersurface tear of the supraspinatus at or near the greater tuberosity; however, the subacromial space has no signs of an inflammatory process typical of subacromial impingement. The appropriate treatment is not yet known. Currently, we advocate conservative treatment including rest from the offending activity, nonsteroidal anti-inflammatory drugs, and a rotator cuff and scapular rotator strengthening program.

ANTERIOR INSTABILITY WITH SECONDARY IMPINGEMENT

Anterior instability with secondary impingement is unique to groups of young (18–35-year-olds), throwing athletes, especially pitchers. Most throwing injuries commonly seen during training are related to overuse of the rotator cuff. Unrecognized anterior instability, or silent subluxation, is becoming more apparent as our diagnostic ability and awareness improve. There is a delicate balance between mobility and stability that makes the shoulder susceptible to injury when stressed by high athletic demands and poor throwing mechanics. A pathologic condition will occur when: (a) chronic overuse causes the physiologic healing response to lag behind the repetitive microtrauma; (b) when years of throwing cause increased external rotation with subsequent attenuation of the anterior capsule and associated subluxation; or (c) an imbalance in the shoulder's four-joint complex causes altered throwing mechanics (12).

The concept to appreciate in young overhand athletes is one of a progressive continuum of shoulder pathology: overuse leads to microtrauma leading to instability, leading to subluxation, leading to impingement, finally leading terminally to a rotator cuff tear. This cascade is termed the "instability complex" (2, 13, 14).

Overhand throwing athletes can usually be divided into one of four groups based on history, examination, and arthroscopic findings. Group I includes those with pure and isolated impingement and no instability, typically older athletes. Group II comprises patients with impingement findings with concurrent instability due to labral and capsular repetitive microtrauma: this is the most common group. Group III includes those patients who have impingement findings and associated instability due to hyperelasticity and a lax joint. Group IV consists of those people with isolated instability without impingement. It must be recognized that any of these groups can progress to a rotator cuff tear (12–15).

Treatment in all groups (I–IV) requires a specific supervised rehabilitation program, as described by Jobe (12, 13). Failure of this program will necessitate surgical intervention. Group I will require arthroscopic evaluation to confirm the diagnosis of pure impingement, followed by an arthroscopic resection of the coracoacromial ligament, subdeltoid bursa, and acromioplasty. Groups II–IV require a diagnostic arthroscopy to confirm the findings of anterior instability followed by an anterior (capsulolabral) reconstruction. In the event that a subacromial decompression is inadvertently done on Groups II–IV, it has been our experience that the impingement symptoms become worse due to the destabilizing effect on the already unstable shoulder (8, 12–15). The primary pathologic condition, namely the instability, must be treated.

Improper Rehabilitation

REHABILITATION OF IMPINGEMENT SYNDROME

The majority of patients with stage I impingement, and many of the patients with stage II impingement resolve with a supervised, specific rehabilitation program. Stages III and IV seem to have a more varied response and often fail conservative management.

Rehabilitation for impingement initially begins with rest from the offending activity. This does not mean placing the patient in a sling, for this would lead to further contracture of the rotator cuff. Anti-inflammatory medication has proven useful in decreasing the acute symptoms. The injection of steroids into the subacromial bursa and biceps tendon sheath is controversial. Kennedy and Willis (18) have demonstrated that collagen necrosis and diminished strength as well as failure were present in tendons injected with steroids for at least 2 weeks. The return to normal tendon strength and parallel arrangement of collagen fibrils after injection took many weeks. Realizing these shortcomings, injections should be over the tendons, not into them. We have had good responses to subacromial and biceps sheath injections. After an injection, we require three weeks of rest from competition or heavy weights, but continue light weights and stretching exercises. We permit no more than three steroid injections over a 1-year period.

The most important aspect of the rehabilitation protocol is a rotator cuff and scapular rotator strengthening program. The protocol entails rotator cuff strengthening by both internal and external rotation exercises with the arm at the side and, as symptoms permit, at 90° of abduction (Figs. 19.5 and 19.6). This can be accomplished isometrically, isotonically, or isokinetically. The supraspinatus can be isolated and strengthened with the upper extremity elevated to 90°, internally rotated and forward flexed to 30° (Fig. 19.7).

The scapular rotators are strengthened with three specific exercises: shoulder shrugs for the upper trapezius, push-ups for the serratus anterior, and chin-ups for the latissimus dorsi. While executing push-ups, hyperextension at the shoulder is avoided.

The coracobrachialis, long head of the biceps, and anterior deltoid are strengthened with forward flexion terminating at 90° to avoid the impingement arc. The pectoralis major and anterior deltoid are strengthened using horizontal adduction exercises with the arm abducted to 90°.

Periodically, athletes may not be relieved of incapacitating pain with conservative management. In such cases, a complete review of the work-up is undertaken to delineate any other possible pathology or concomitant condition. In the event of pure recalcitrant subacromial impingement, we advocate an arthroscopic subacromial decompression including: resection of the coracoacromial ligament; resection of the subdeltoid bursa; anterior acromioplasty; and resection of inferior distal clavicular osteophytes.

Improper Surgical Procedures

BICEPS TENODESIS

Bicipital tendinitis in athletes is usually secondary to impingement, and rarely, if ever, is the biceps involved primarily. Some authors treating middle-aged people have reported that biceps tenodesis for bicipital tendinitis has produced favorable results in more than 90% of patients (17). We do not, however, advocate biceps tenodesis in athletes for two basic reasons. First, sacrificing the long head of the biceps humeral head depressor function in throwing athletes is detrimental to throwing mechanics. Second, biceps tendinitis is usually secondary to impingement, which will require a subacromial decompression.

ISOLATED RESECTION OF THE CORACOACROMIAL LIGAMENT

Jackson (11) first indicated that in chronic impingement syndrome in athletes, isolated resection of the coracoacromial ligament allowed five of nine patients to return to competition, but follow-up was short. Later, Penny and Welsh (26) reported similar results when comparing formal acromioplasty with isolated coracoacromial ligament resection. They felt that acromioplasty was only effective because the coracoacromial ligament was resected and that acromioplasty was not required in most patients. Their series had few athletes involved in overhead sports. In our clinic, however, isolated coracoacromial ligament resection in throwing athletes has been disappointing with regard to allowing athletes to return to competition. This procedure seems to be inadequate, and in our experience, subacromial decompression, either open or arthroscopic, has provided better overall results.

IMPROPER ACROMIOPLASTY

Successful subacromial decompression requires the surgeon to: (a) perform a subacromial bur-

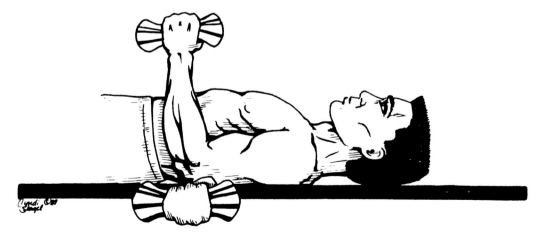

Figure 19.5.   Demonstration of internal rotation exercises with the patient supine.

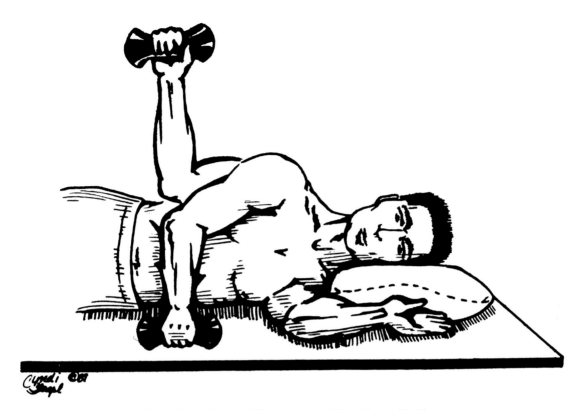

Figure 19.6. External rotation exercises with the patient on his side.

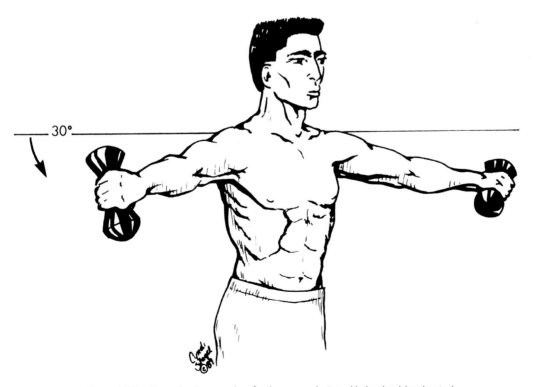

Figure 19.7. Strengthening exercises for the supraspinatus with the shoulder elevated in the plane of the scapula in full internal rotation.

sectomy to evaluate the rotator cuff and permit adequate visualization of the coracoacromial ligament and anterior acromion; (b) release and partially resect the coracoacromial ligament; and (c) perform an adequate acromioplasty to allow an impingement free range of motion. These goals can be attained by either arthroscopic or open techniques. Failure to achieve these objectives may add to persistent subacromial impingement symptoms.

In our experience, failure to perform an adequate acromioplasty is the leading cause of resistant subacromial impingement after subacromial decompression. The completed acromioplasty should eradicate the hooklike process of the anterior acromion including any spurs arising from the acromion. Osteophytes of the inferior distal clavicle should be actively sought out and removed (6). Morrison and Jackson (21) recommended that the excised bone should consist of a wedge 2 cm wide × 2 cm deep with a thickness tapering from .7 cm anteriorly to .2 cm posteriorly. Ellman advised that the entire undersurface of the anterior acromion should be burred and continued posteriorly for 2.5 cm, including any distal clavicular spurs (Fig. 19.8). In addition, 6–8 mm of the anterior edge of the acromion should be resected (6).

Technical errors can be avoided by adhering to these principles, especially remembering to remove adequate bone during the acromioplasty.

IMPROPER CARE OF THE DELTOID

In open subacromial decompression, the appropriate care of the deltoid is extremely important. Two common problems are: removing too much of the deltoid from the acromion, and failure to reattach the deltoid properly.

We prefer to detach the deltoid muscle from the anterolateral acromion with electrocautery in a "Y" type incision (Fig. 19.9). The total distance of the superior limbs of the "Y" rarely exceeds 2.5 cm (a little over 1 cm for each superior limb). Excessive takedown of the deltoid is not needed for adequate exposure and increases the risk of suture line disassociation during early rehabilitation.

The anterior deltoid is always reattached to the acromion utilizing no. 1 nonabsorbable suture through several small drill holes in the acromion (at

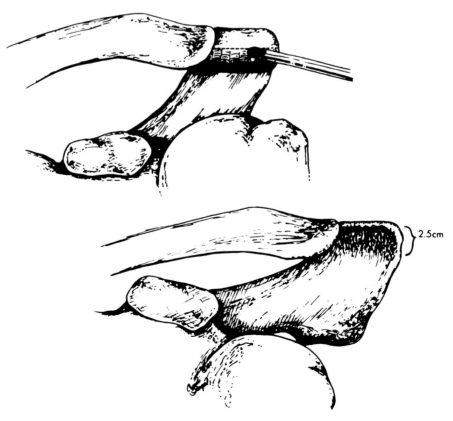

Figure 19.8. Part of the undersurface of the acromion that should be resected in an acromioplasty.

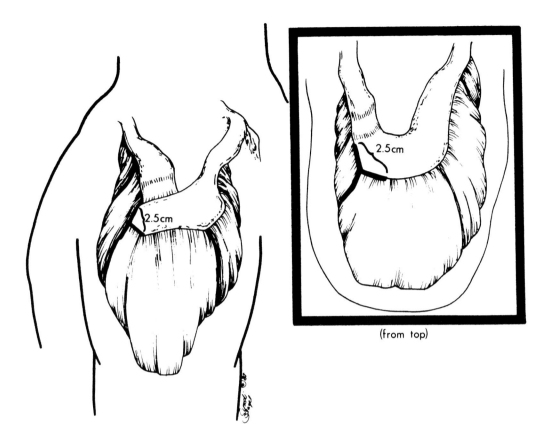

Figure 19.9. The detachment and split of the deltoid during an open acromioplasty.

least four). The repair is then augmented with simple (no. 1) absorbable suture at the deltoid acromial suture line (Fig. 19.10). Meticulous surgical technique and a secure acromial deltoid repair is helpful in avoiding postoperative detachment of the anterior deltoid. If detachment and muscle retraction occur, subsequent deltoid repair is very difficult.

ACROMIONECTOMY

In the past, acromionectomy had been used to treat impingement syndrome and rotator cuff pathology, with poor results. Patients referred to this clinic after acromionectomy have presented with recalcitrant anterior shoulder pain and deltoid weakness. We feel total acromionectomy should be avoided when contemplating surgical treatment of impingement syndrome secondary to the aforementioned problems. There is no salvage procedure after acromionectomy.

UNRECOGNIZED DISTAL CLAVICULAR SPURS

Many authors have stressed that distal clavicular undersurface spurs are a component of the im-

pingement process (9, 10, 22). It should be emphasized that if present, these spurs should be excised to help abate the impingement process. Failure to address this problem may lead to resistant impingement symptoms (Fig. 19.11).

SUMMARY

The specific emphasis in this chapter has been on entities that may cause resistant subacromial impingement in an athletic population. Knowledge of these problems will hopefully aid in the proper evaluation and treatment of impingement syndrome. A summary of basic problems associated with resistant impingement include: (a) attaining the correct diagnosis with emphasis on potential underlying shoulder instability, or possible referred pain; (b) proper initial, as well as postoperative rehabilitation with special attention given to the scapular rotators and rotator cuff; (c) selection of the appropriate surgical procedure; and (d) potential surgical problems. We have tried to give some insight into the possible causes of resistant subacromial impingement and

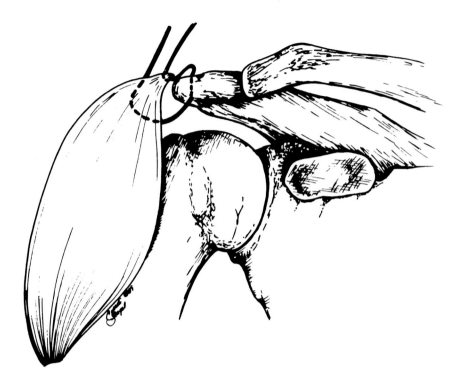

Figure 19.10.   The reattachment of the deltoid to the acromion with suture through bone.

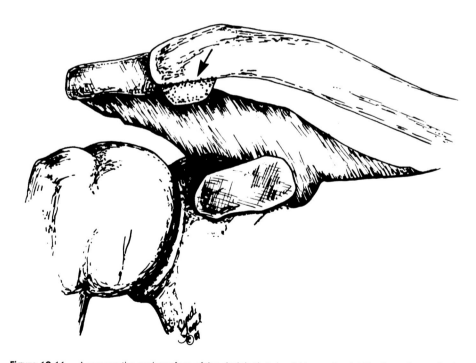

Figure 19.11.   A spur on the undersurface of the clavicle that should be excised at the time of acromioplasty.

hope this chapter is helpful in promoting accurate diagnosis, appropriate conservative or surgical treatment, and subsequent rehabilitation and recovery.

References

1. Bateman JE. Neurologic painful conditions affecting the shoulder. Clin Orthop 1983;173:55.
2. Bradley JP, Perry J, Jobe FW. The biomechanics of the throwing shoulder. Perspectives in Orthopedics 1990;1:49–59.
3. Cahill BR, Palmer RE. Quadrilateral space syndrome. J Hand Surg 1983;8:65–69.
4. Cannon SR. Massive osteolysis. J Bone Joint Surg 1986;68B:24.
5. Cormier PJ, Matalon TAS, Wolin PM. Quadrilateral space syndrome: a rare cause of shoulder pain. Radiology 1988;167:797–798.
6. Ellman H. Arthroscopic subacromial decompression: Analysis of one to three year results. Arthroscopy 1987;3:173–181.
7. Estwanik JJ. Levator scapulae syndrome. Physician Sports Med 1989;17:57–68.
8. Fly WR, Tibone JE, Jobe FW, et al. Arthroscopic subacromial decompression in athletes less than 40 years old. Submitted for publication.
9. Hawkins RJ, Hobeika PE. Impingement syndrome in the athletic shoulder. Clin Sports Med 1983;2:391–405.
10. Hawkins RJ, Kennedy JC. Impingement syndrome in athletes. Am J Sports Med 1980;8:151–158.
11. Jackson DW. Chronic rotator cuff impingement in the throwing athlete. Orthop Trans 1977;1:24.
12. Jobe FW, Bradley JP. Rotator cuff in baseball: Prevention and rehabilitation. Sports Med 1988;6:377–386.
13. Jobe FW, Bradley JP. The diagnosis and nonoperative treatment of shoulder injuries in athletes. Clin Sports Med 1989;8:419–437.
14. Jobe FW, Bradley JP. The treatment of impingement syndrome in overhand athletes: a philosophical basis, Part I. Surgical Rounds in Orthopedics 1990;19–24.
15. Jobe FW, Bradley JP. The treatment of impingement syndrome in overhand athletes: surgical technique, part II. Surgical Rounds in Orthopedics 1990;39–41.
16. Jobe FW, Jobe CM. Painful athletic injuries of the shoulder. Clin Orthop 1983;173:117–124.
17. Justis EJ. Nontraumatic disorders. In: Crenshaw, ed. Campbell's Operative Orthopedics. St. Louis: CV Mosby, 1987;2247–2261.
18. Kennedy JC, Willis RB. The effects of local steroid injections on tendons: a biomechanical and microscopic correlative study. Am J Sports Med 1976;4:210–213.
19. McCarty DJ, Gatter RA. Recurrent anterior inflammation associated with focal apatite crystal deposition. Arthritis Rheum 1966;9:804.
20. McKowen JC, Voorhies RM. Axillary nerve entrapment in the quadrilateral space: case report. J Neurosurg 1987;66:932–934.
21. Morrison DS, Jackson DW. Correlation of acromial morphology and the results of arthroscopic subacromial decompression. The American Shoulder and Elbow Surgeons Fourth Open Meeting, Atlanta, Georgia, February 7, 1988.
22. Neer CS, II. Anterior acromioplasty for the chronic impingement syndrome in the shoulder. J Bone Joint Surg 1972;54A:41–50.
23. Neer CS, II, Welsh RP. The shoulder in sports. Orthop Clin North Amer 1977;8:583–591.
24. Nills JA. Arthritis of the shoulder. In the Shoulder. Rowe, New York: Churchill Livingstone, 1988.
25. Pedler MR, Ruland LJ, III, McCue FC, III. Quadrilateral space syndrome in a throwing athlete. Am J Sports Med 1986;14:511–513.
26. Penny JW, Welsh RP. Shoulder impingement syndromes in athletes and their surgical management. Am J Sports Med 1981;9:11–15.
27. Resnick CS, Resnick D. Crystal deposition disease. Semin Arthritis Rheum 1983;2:39B.
28. Rowe CR, Leffert RD. Idiopathic chronic adhesive capsulitis ("frozen shoulder"). In: Rowe CR, ed. The Shoulder. New York: Churchill Livingstone, 1988:155–163.
29. Rowe CR. Tendinitis, bursitis, impingement "snapping scapula and calcific bursitis." In: Rowe CR, ed. The Shoulder. Rowe, New York: Churchill Livingstone, 1988:105–130.
30. Sisto DJ, Jobe FW. The operative treatment of scapulothoracic bursitis in professional pitchers. Am J Sports Med 1986;14:192–194.
31. Tibone JE, Elrod B, Jobe FW, et al. Surgical treatment of the rotator cuff in athletes. J Bone Joint Surg 1986;68A:887–891.
32. Tibone JE, Job FW, Kerlan RK, et al. Shoulder impingement syndrome in athletes treated by an anterior acromioplasty. Clin Orthop 1988;198:134–140.

Index

Page numbers followed by an *f* denote figures; page numbers followed by a *t* denote tables.